T0145398

Tongue Image Analysis

David Zhang · Hongzhi Zhang
Bob Zhang

Tongue Image Analysis

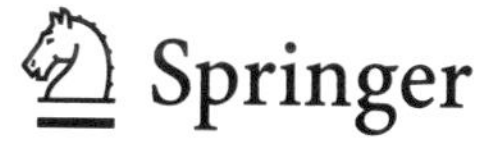

David Zhang
The Hong Kong Polytechnic University
Hong Kong
China

Hongzhi Zhang
School of Computer Science
and Technology
Harbin Institute of Technology
Harbin
China

Bob Zhang
Department of Computer and Information
Science
The University of Macau
Taipa
Macao

ISBN 978-981-10-9547-4 ISBN 978-981-10-2167-1 (eBook)
DOI 10.1007/978-981-10-2167-1

Softcover reprint of the hardcover 1st edition 2017

Printed on acid-free paper

This Springer imprint is published by Springer Nature
The registered company is Springer Nature Singapore Pte Ltd.
The registered company address is: 152 Beach Road, #22-06/08 Gateway East, Singapore 189721, Singapore

Preface

The tongue, as the primary organ of gustation, conveys abundant valuable information about the health status of the human body, i.e., disorders or even pathological changes of internal organs can be reflected by the human tongue and observed by medical practitioners. Tongue diagnosis (TD), a noninvasive diagnostic method using inspection of the appearance of human tongue, has played an indispensable role in Traditional Chinese Medicine (TCM) for over 2,000 years. In recent years, for the purpose of academic research, significant information technologies, including digitalized data acquisition, image processing, and pattern recognition have been widely used in tongue diagnosis to improve its diagnostic validity and accuracy. Computerized tongue diagnosis (CTD), as a result, has become a fundamental part of the revolution that has taken place at an ever-increasing pace over the past decade in TCM. The growing importance and rapid progress in CTD has brought about an independent and burgeoning branch in the TCM research field, and also resulted in urgent and extensive requirements for tongue image analytical techniques.

By its very nature, tongue image analysis is cross-disciplinary in several aspects. First, before a tongue image can be analyzed, it is imperative that the basic principles of TD should be mastered. For instance, we should know what kinds of visible information are crucial for the visual inspection process of TD. This mainly includes several aspects in the TCM and computer vision (CV) research fields. Next, in order to get useful data, a special acquisition system should be carefully designed to guarantee that all the information is included in the signal acquired by the imaging sensor. This incorporates the interaction of optics of matter to the geometry and radiometry of imaging and industrial design. Finally, after being captured and converted into digital form, the tongue image should be processed, analyzed, and classified by the computer. In this chain of processes, many areas from computer science and mathematics are involved, e.g., computer architecture, algebra, analysis, statistics, algorithm theory, graph theory, system theory, and numerical mathematics, all of which have a partial or strong association with tongue image analysis.

Today, the field of modern tongue diagnosis is becoming more technical. Although practitioners need to understand the basic theory and practice of computer science such as image processing and pattern recognition, they also need guidance on how to actually address thorny problems such as automatic segmentation, color distortion, and robust classification of tongue images which are very helpful to the practicing CTD scientist.

It is the purpose of this book, as briefly and concisely as possible, to give the reader a straightforward and intuitive introduction to basic and advanced techniques in tongue image processing and analysis and their typical applications in CTD systems. It features the most current research findings in all aspects of tongue image acquisition, preprocessing, classification, and diagnostic support methodologies, from theoretical and algorithmic problems to prototype design and development of CTD systems.

In the first two chapters, the book begins with a very high-level description of CTD on a need-to-know basis which includes an overview of CTD systems and Traditional Chinese Medicine (TCM) as the context and background knowledge of tongue image analysis. From Chaps. 3 to 13, the principal part of the book then provides useful algorithms as well as their implementation methods of tongue image analysis. The most notable extensions, at a know-how level, include detailed discussions on segmentation, chromatic correction, and classification which are arranged in systematic order as follows.

The first preprocessing step of tongue image processing and CTD, automated tongue image segmentation is difficult due to two special factors. First, there are many pathological details on the surface of the tongue, which have a large influence on edge extraction. Second, the shapes of tongue bodies captured from various persons are quite different. So far, there is no single solution that can address all the problems in automated tongue image segmentation. From Chaps. 3 to 7, the book presents five different segmentation approaches to solve domain problems based on different kinds of tongue images. These methods are robust to noise caused by a variety of shapes and irrelevant information from non-tongue parts such as lips, beard, and facial skin. After segmenting the tongue area from its surroundings, a study on tongue shape analysis by using the tongue contour and its geometric features is then introduced in Chap. 8 as the end of Part II.

Part III makes a sound exposition of the quantitative classification of tongue images beginning with the correction of the color feature in tongue image. Color inconsistency is the second problem CTD scientists have to face before analyzing the tongue image. Since the colors of the tongue image produced by digital cameras are usually device-dependent, this is a serious problem in computer-aided tongue image analysis which relies on the accurate rendering of color information. In Chaps. 9 and 10, the book introduces an optimized tongue image colorchecker and correction scheme which enhances the color consistency between different acquisition devices. It has long been a controversial topic that the TCM physician mainly explores the nonquantitative features in the traditional diagnosis process. To diagnose a wide range of health conditions, CTD should examine quantitative features of the tongue. From Chaps. 11 to 13, the book describes three tongue classification methods with excellent comprehensive performances.

In this book, some clinical applications based on the tongue image analyzing methods are also presented, for the show-how purpose, in the CTD research field. Case studies highlight different techniques that have been adopted to assist the diagnosis of diseases and health. From Chaps. 14 to 17, the book discusses relationships between diseases and the appearance of the human tongue in terms of quantitative features. In Part IV, we present case studies in the field of visual inspection for appendicitis, diabetes, and some other common diseases. Experimental results of the performance under different challenging clinical circumstances have shown the superiority of the techniques in this book.

The principles of tongue image analysis in this book are illustrated with plentiful graphs, tables, and practical experiments to simplify problems. In this way, readers can easily find a quick and systematic way through the complicated theories and they can later even extend their studies to special topics of interest. All the techniques presented in the book are well supported by experimental results using a large tongue image database, which was collected from 5,222 subjects (Over 9,000 images) by our dedicated developed image acquisition device. All these subjects were diagnosed (patient-subjects) or labeled (healthcare-subjects) into different health status (healthy, sub-healthy, and various diseases) in the hospital. To the best of our knowledge, this is the largest and most comprehensive database in the research community. This book will be of benefit to researchers, professionals, and graduate students working in the field of computer vision, pattern recognition, clinical practice, and TCM, and will also be useful for interdisciplinary research. We anticipate that physicians, biomedical scientists, engineers, programmers, and students of computers will find this book and the associated algorithms useful, and hope that anyone with an interest in computerized diagnostic research will find the book enjoyable and informative.

The book is the result of years of research on computational TCM diagnosis. Since 1998, under grant support from the National Natural Science Foundation of China (NSFC), Hong Kong Polytechnic University, and Harbin Institute of Technology, we have studied this topic. The authors would like to thank Dr. Zhaotian Zhang, Dr. Xiaoyun Xiong, and Dr. Ke Liu from NSFC for their consistent support to our research work.

Some of the material in the book, e.g., the tongue images and acquisition devices, has been under development for almost a decade. Portions of the book appeared in earlier forms as conference papers, journal papers, or experiments by my research group at The Hong Kong Polytechnic University and Harbin Institute of Technology. Therefore, these parts of the text are the newest updates based on our research.

I would like to gratefully acknowledge the Institute of Electrical and Electronic Engineers (IEEE) and Elsevier Publishers, for giving me permission to reuse texts and figures that have appeared in some earlier publications.

We would like to thank our colleagues and Ph.D. students, i.e., Prof. Kuanquan Wang, Prof. Naimin Li, Prof. Edward C. Mignot, Dr. Bo Pang, Dr. Xingzheng

Wang, Dr. Zhi Liu, and Dr. Zhenchao Cui, for their contributions to the research achievements on computational TCM diagnosis. It is also our honor to collaborate with them in this fascinating and ever-growing research field. I would also like to express my sincere thanks to all individuals and organizations who have contributed visual material for this book.

Finally, the work in this book was mainly sponsored by the NSFC Program under Grant No. 61332011, 61020106004, 61271093, 61272292, 61471146, and 61271344, Shenzhen Fundamental Science and Technology Development Fund (FDCT) of Macao SAR (FDCT/128/2013/A and FDCT/124/2014/A3), the University of Macau (MRG026/ZYB/2015/FST), Research Fund (JCYJ20130401152508661), and the Key Laboratory of Network Oriented Intelligent Computation, Shenzhen, China.

Kowloon, Hong Kong
June 2016

David Zhang

Contents

Part I
Background

Chapter 1
Introduction to Tongue Image Analysis

Abstract Tongue diagnosis is one of the most important and widely used diagnostic methods in Chinese medicine. Visual inspection of the human tongue offers a simple, immediate, inexpensive, and noninvasive solution for various clinical applications and self-diagnosis. Increasingly, powerful information technologies have made it possible to develop a computerized tongue diagnosis (CTD) system that is based on digital image processing and analysis. In this chapter, we first introduced the current state of knowledge on tongue diagnosis and CTD. Then, for the computational perspective, we provided brief surveys on the progress of tongue image analysis technologies including tongue image acquisition, preprocessing, and diagnosis classification.

1.1 Tongue Inspection for Medical Applications

Visual inspection of the human tongue, as a notable diagnostic approach, has been applied in various medical applications. In Western medicine, from the nineteenth century, the tongue has been found to be able to provide crucial signs for early diagnosis, and symptomatology of the tongue has been employed as an important index in human health and disease (Haller, 1982; Reamy, Richard, & Bunt, 2010). For instance, the color of the tongue can indicate Parkinson's disease (Matison, Mayeux, Rosen, & Fahn, 1982), nutritional deficiency (Jeghers, 1942), or even AIDS (Faria et al., 2005; Peng & Xie, 2006), and tongue fissure, as a typical kind of texture anomaly, has been found to be closely associated with Melkersson–Rosenthal syndrome (Ozgursoy et al., 2009), Down's syndrome (Avraham, Schickler, Sapoznikov, Yarom, & Groner, 1988), diabetes (Farman, 1976), and some other kinds of diseases (Grushka, Ching, & Polak, 2007; Zargari, 2006; Scheper, Nikitakis, Sarlani, Sauk, & Meiller, 2006; Han et al., 2016).

Moreover, in Traditional Chinese Medicine (TCM), as one of the most valuable and widely used diagnostic tools, the tongue has played an indispensable role for over 2000 years (Maciocia, 1995, 2004; Giovanni, 2015; Tang, Liu, & Ma, 2008; Fei, & Gu, 2007). Various kinds of tongue image features, including the tongue's

D. Zhang et al., *Tongue Image Analysis*, DOI 10.1007/978-981-10-2167-1_1

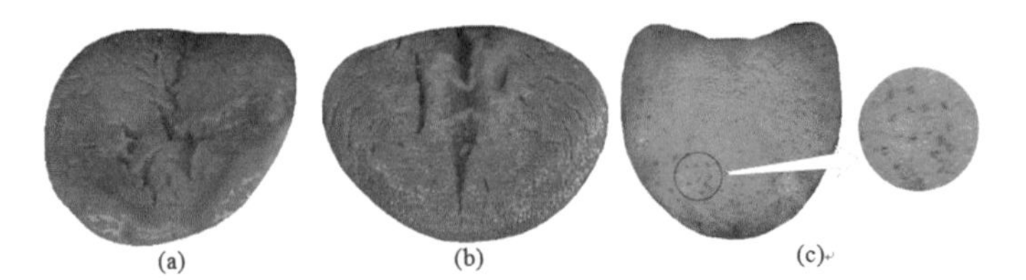

Fig. 1.1 Typical tongue image samples with different texture styles. **a** Is tongue fissure, **b** is tongue crack, **c** an image with a local substance (*red point*). Different texture styles convey various pathological information of internal organs, for example, *red point* is usually found on the tongue of subjects with appendicitis

color, texture, and geometrical shape, have been inspected and analyzed by TCM doctors in order to retrieve significant pathological information of the human body. For example, Fig. 1.1 shows three typical tongue texture styles: tongue fissure, tongue crack, and red point. These different texture styles have been discovered to be highly related with the health status of the human body. Yang, Zhang, and Nai-Min (2009) observed that people with irregular tongue crack features may be in an unhealthy state, and a red point is usually found on the tongue of subjects with appendicitis (Pang, Zhang, & Wang, 2005). In addition, the tongue shape is also used to indicate particular pathologies. Figure 1.2 presents some typical samples of various tongue shapes which are believed to convey pathological information of different internal organs (Huang, Wu, Zhang, & Li, 2010).

Among all features which can be extracted, the tongue's chromatic feature plays the most important role in evaluating a person's health condition (Nai-Min, Zhang, & Kuan-Quan, 2011). Tongue color is an essential attribute of the tongue body which

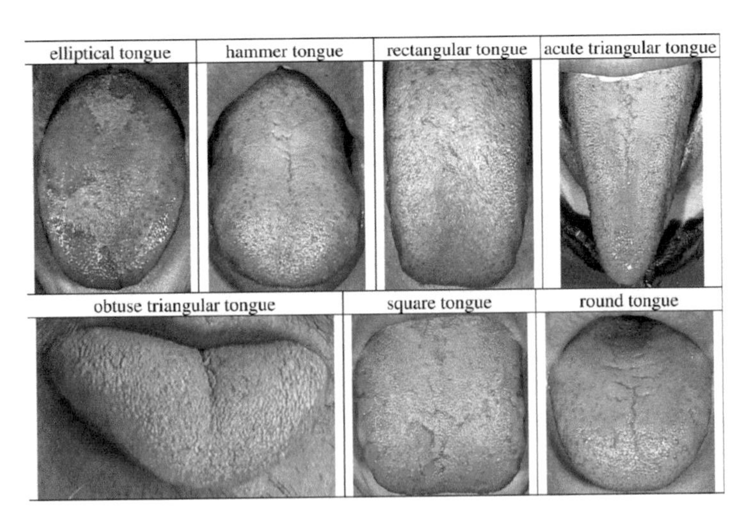

Fig. 1.2 Typical samples of various tongue shapes. Reprinted from Huang et al. (2010), with permission from Elsevier

possesses abundant medical information. According to the principle of tongue diagnosis in Traditional Chinese Medicine, TCM practitioners believe that pathological changes of internal organs can affect the color of the tongue body, and thus they can make a diagnostic decision based on this kind of color clue. Usually, tongue color is analyzed in two parts: substance color and coating color. Substance and coating are two essential parts of the surface of a tongue: tongue substance is usually the main body or the basis of a tongue while the coating is made up of materials floating above the tongue substance (Nai-Min, Zhang, & Kuan-Quan, 2011). The tongue colors of these two parts are different from each other, the tongue substance color is usually reddish colors including red, deep red, light red, and purple, and the tongue coating color is normally white, gray, black, or yellow. Figure 1.3 presents several typical images with various types of color features. Color patterns inspected from tongue images may lead to distinct diagnostic results. For example, a tongue body with a light red substance and white coating (as Fig. 1.3f shows) may indicate the healthy status of the person. Visual inspection of the human tongue offers a simple and immediate solution for medical diagnosis. If there is a severe disorder of the internal organs, tongue inspection instantly distinguishes the main pathological process. Hence, it is of great importance both in medical application and self-diagnosis to monitor one's state of health on a daily basis. In addition, tongue diagnosis is a kind of noninvasive diagnostic technique which accords with the most promising direction in the twenty-first century: no pain and no injury. Also, the tongue inspection process is inexpensive, and thus, this technique can be easily popularized.

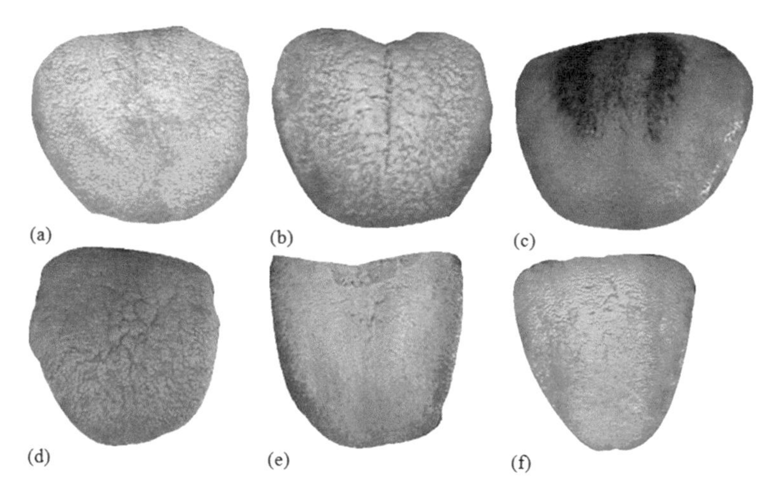

Fig. 1.3 Typical tongue images with various color patterns are critical for medical analysis in TCM. Colors of substance and coating in these images are **a** white and red, **b** gray and deep red, **c** black and deep red, **d** yellow and deep red, **e** gray and red, and **f** light red and white

1.2 Computerized Tongue Diagnosis System

As tongue inspection has a prominent role in both early warning signal provision and disease diagnosis, it has become more and more popular both in clinical medicine and in biomedicine. However, traditional tongue diagnosis has inevitable and intrinsic limitations which hinder its medical applications. First, since the tongue is visually observed by the human eye rather than recorded by a quantitative digital instrument, it is difficult or even impossible to quantitatively process tongue images, such as digital data storage, computer-aided image analysis and data transmission via the Internet for use in telemedicine applications. Second, the judging process of tongue diagnosis is subjective, which mostly depends on the medical experience and knowledge of the doctor. In other words, different doctors may achieve different results from the same visual expression on the human face. In view of this, attempts (Lukman, He, & Hui, 2008; Feng, Wu, Zhou, Zhou, & Fan, 2006; Chiu, 1996; Pang, Zhang, Li, & Wang, 2004; Chiu, 2000; Zhang, Pang, Li, Wang, & Zhang, 2005; Zhang, Wang, Zhang, Pang, & Huang, 2005) have been made to build an objective and quantitative tongue diagnosis system, i.e., a computerized tongue diagnosis system, which has been found to be an effective way to overcome the above problems.

By applying the technique of digital image processing (Sonka, Hlavac, & Boyle, 2014; Gonzalez & Wintz, 2007) and pattern recognition (Anzai, 2012; Duda, Hart, & Stork, 2012), the computerized tongue diagnosis system is proposed to make the inspection objective and repeatable so that it prevents human bias and errors. The schematic diagram of one typical computerized tongue diagnosis system is shown in Fig. 1.4. Similar to a typical pattern classification system, this system mainly consists of four modules: image acquisition, preprocessing, feature extraction, and decision-making. A lot of work has already been done concerning the development of these modules.

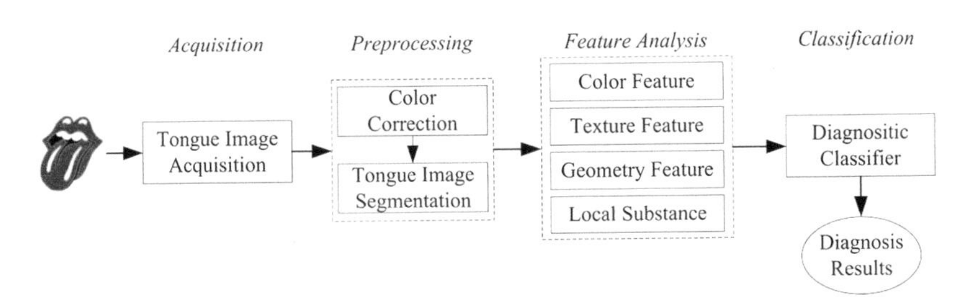

Fig. 1.4 Schematic diagram of a typical computerized tongue diagnosis system. This system mainly consists of four modules: image acquisition, preprocessing, feature extraction, and decision-making

1.3 Research Review on Tongue Image Analysis

The development of a computerized tongue image analysis and diagnosis system is believed to be an essential and effective way to solve the intrinsic problems in TCM which are unreliability and inconsistency. A lot of research work has been done on this topic to promote the standardization and modernization of tongue diagnosis in TCM.

1.3.1 Tongue Image Acquisition

Digital tongue image acquisition is the first step to realize computerized tongue diagnosis. With the development of digital imaging technology, the use of digital cameras in tongue inspection has been investigated for several years. According to the use of the illumination and imaging principle, there are generally two types of tongue image acquisition systems: the hyperspectral imaging system and the color imaging system.

The development of the hyperspectral tongue imaging system is generated by the growing interest in hyperspectral imaging in the research community (Chang, 2003; Kim, Chen, & Mehl, 2001; Mooradian, Weiderhold, Dabiri, & Coyle, 1998; Vo-Dinh, 2004; Zavattini et al., 2006). Researchers believe that by capturing images under illumination with a series of consecutive wavelengths (usually ranges of 400–800 nm with very narrow bandwidths), more valuable information could be retrieved for classification or recognition purposes. Liu and Li et al. developed a series of tongue imaging systems based on hyperspectral imaging technology (Du, Liu, Li, Yan, & Tang, 2007; Li, Wang, Liu, Sun, & Liu, 2010; Li, Wang, Liu, & Sun, 2010; Li, Liu, Xiao, & Xue, 2008). Also, related processing and matching algorithms were implemented (Liu, Yan, Zhang, & Li, 2007; Li & Liu, 2009; Zhi, Zhang, Yan, Li, & Tang, 2007). In their system, a series of tongue images was captured in 120 spectral over the waveband (400–1000 nm) at an interval of 5 nm. Hence a full 120-band hyperspectral image cube was acquired. Figure 1.5 shows two groups of hyperspectral images acquired from two persons. The left one was captured from a healthy person, and the other one was obtained from a patient with chronic cholecystitis.

Another type of tongue imaging system was implemented following the framework of a typical digital color imaging system. Tongue images were acquired under white illumination by various types of color imaging cameras. As these types of imaging devices are simple and easy to be implemented, researchers have paid more attention to this direction, and nearly ten imaging systems have been developed which possess various imaging characteristics (Pang et al., 2004; Chiu, 2000; Zhang et al., 2005; Yu, Jin, Tan, et al., 1994; Wong & Huang, 2001; Cai, 2002; Jang et al., 2002; Wei et al., 2002; Wang, Zhou, Yang, & Xu, 2004; Kim, Jung, Park, & Park, 2009; He, Liu, & Shen, 2007). These developed acquisition devices

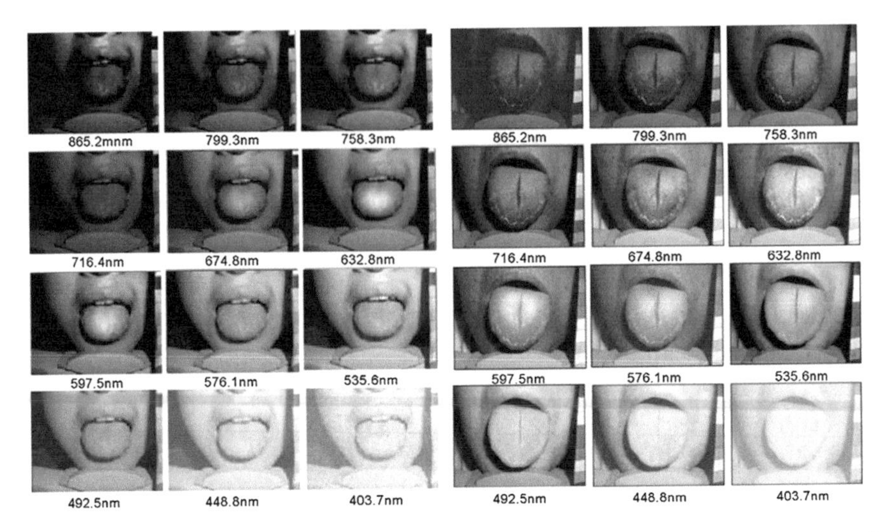

Fig. 1.5 Typical hyperspectral image samples of two individuals. These images were extracted between 403.7 and 865.2 nm wavelength. Reprinted from Zhi, Zhang, Yan, Li, and Tang (2007), with permission from Elsevier

mainly differ in the selection of lighting source and imaging camera. For instance, Wong and Huang (2001), Jang et al. (2002), and Zhang et al. (2005) utilized a halogen tungsten lamp as the lighting source, while Chiu (2000), Pang et al. (2004), and Wei et al. (2002), employed a fluorescent lamp. Due to the inconsistency among these devices, the quality of the captured tongue images varied.

1.3.2 *Tongue Image Preprocessing*

Tongue image preprocessing is essential for accurate and effective feature extraction. In computerized tongue diagnosis systems, two steps are commonly involved: one is color correction which aims to correct color variations caused by system components and to render the acquired tongue image into a device-independent color space. The other is image segmentation which extracts the tongue region from the original image which almost always includes lips, parts of the face, and the teeth.

1.3.2.1 Color Correction

Color images produced by digital cameras suffer from device-dependent color space rendering, i.e., the generated color information is dependent on the imaging characteristics of the specific camera. Furthermore, there are usually noises over the color images due to slight variations of the illumination. Therefore, in order to render the color image in high quality, color correction is necessary for accurate image acquisition and is often regarded as a prerequisite before further image analysis.

Research on color correction algorithms has been extensively conducted in the color science area. Several correction algorithms have been proposed for different tasks (Wang et al., 2004; Kim et al., 2009; He et al., 2007; Chang & Reid, 1996; Wandell, 1987; Finlayson, 1996; Barnard & Funt, 2002; Yamamoto et al., 2007; Vrhel & Trussell, 1999; Yamamoto & James, 2006; Vrhel, Saber, & Trussell, 2005). The polynomial-based correction method (LuoHong & Rhodes, 2001; Cheung, Westland, Connah, & Ripamonti, 2004) and neural network mapping (Cheung et al., 2004) are most commonly used. However, according to related literatures, there have been few published works that focused on the color correction of tongue images. In Zhang, Wang, Jin, and Zhang (2005), the authors proposed a novel color correction approach based on the Support Vector Regression (SVR) algorithm, and their experimental results confirmed the effectiveness of the proposed technique. Hu, Cheng, and Lan (2016) used the support vector machine (SVM) to predict the lighting condition and the corresponding color correction matrix according to the color difference of images taken with and without flash. In Zhuo et al. (2015), a kernel partial least squares regression based method was also proposed to obtain consistent correction by reducing the average color difference of their color patches.

1.3.2.2 Image Segmentation

Usually, in addition to the main tongue body, captured tongue images contain much other irrelevant information, such as lips, part of the face, and other non-tongue parts. Therefore, in order to improve the accuracy of tongue image analysis, we need to first extract the tongue region from the noisy background.

Image segmentation has been a classical problem for a long time, and a lot of segmentation algorithms have been proposed for distinct tasks (Sonka et al., 2014; Shi & Malik, 2000; Pal & Pal, 1993; Zhu & Yuille, 1996; Felzenszwalb & Huttenlocher, 2004; Shi, Li, Li, & Xu, 2014; Cui, Zhang, Zhang, Li, & Zuo, 2013; Wu & Zhang, 2015). In order to make these existing methods suitable for tongue image segmentation, researchers have made modification or revision of them. For example, based on the active contour model (Kass, Witkin, & Terzopoulos, 1988), Wu, Zhang, and Bai (2006) proposed a segmentation algorithm using the watershed transform to get the initial contour and converging with the active contour model to extract the tongue edge. Zhang et al. achieved this goal by employing the polar edge detector as the initial contour generator (Zhang, Zuo, Wang, & Zhang, 2006). Pang et al. proposed an algorithm named the bi-elliptical deformable contour (Pang et al. 2005a; Pang, Wang, Zhang, & Zhang, 2002) which combines a novel bi-elliptical deformable template (BEDT) with the traditional active contour model to improve the segmentation accuracy. Additionally, other segmentation algorithms have also been proposed. Wang, Zhou, Yang, and Wang 2004 applied the JSEG algorithm, which is a well-proposed method for unsupervised segmentation, for tongue segmentation. Yu, Yang, Wang, and Zhang 2007 and Ning, Zhang, Wu, and Yue 2012 developed their algorithms based on the gradient vector flow. All the above-proposed algorithms are reported to achieve acceptable performance.

1.3.3 Qualitative Feature Extraction

Based on the principle of tongue diagnosis in TCM, there are four main types of tongue features which can be extracted for medical analysis, i.e., color, texture, geometric shape, and local substance. Much work has been done to accurately and effectively extract these features (Cui, Liao, & Wang, 2015; Cui et al., 2014; Kim et al., 2014).

Tongue color is considered to be the most prominent feature which conveys plenty of valuable pathological information for medical diagnosis. Li and Yuen (2002) proposed several statistical metrics, including the color coordinate metric, color histogram metric, and sorted metric, to match the color content of different tongue images. Pang et al. extracted the mean and standard deviation of color values across entire tongue images to compare healthy samples with samples of appendicitis and pancreatitis (Pang et al., 2005a; Zhang et al., 2005). Following the diagnostic procedure in TCM, Huang and Li developed several tongue color centers which could be employed as class centers for disease classification (Li & Yuen, 2000; Huang & Li, 2008; Huang, Zhang, Zhang, Li, & Li, 2011; Huang, Zhang, Li, Zhang, & Li, 2011). Additionally, Wang, Yang, Zhou, and Wang (2007) considered the Earth Mover's Distance (EMD) (Rubner, Tomasi, & Guibas, 2000) as a classification metric for disease diagnosis.

Most traditional algorithms were directly applied to the task of tongue texture feature extraction. For instance, the Gabor wavelet was applied to extract Gabor Wavelet Opponent Color Features (GWOCF) for tongue image diagnosis (Yuen, Kuang, Wu, & Wu, 2000, 1999). The Grey Level Co-occurrence Matrix (Haralick, Shanmugam, & Dinstein, 1973) has also been utilized (Pang et al., 2005a; Zhang et al., 2005) to diagnose appendicitis and pancreatitis.

There has not been much research on the tongue geometrical shape and local substance features. Huang et al. extracted various geometric features, including tongue length, width, and diameter of the inscribed circle, in order to automatically classify tongue shapes (Huang, Wu, Zhang, & Li, 2010). The red point feature, which is a typical local substance feature, was extracted (Miao, 2007) using the Gabor wavelet. It is believed to be highly correlated to appendicitis. Also, Fungiform Papillae, as one kind of tiny substance in the surface of the human tongue, have been extracted by Gabor filter banks to predict various pathological conditions (Huang & Li, 2010).

1.3.4 *Diagnostic Classification*

After extraction of all kinds of features from tongue images, these features are supposed to be related to various pathological decisions including human health status or disease type. This is a classical pattern classification problem and many algorithms can be used for this task. As a powerful tool to effectively process fuzziness and uncertainty in the procedure of tongue diagnosis, the Bayesian network (Heckerman, 1997) was utilized for computerized tongue diagnosis in several studies (Pang et al., 2004; Wang & Zong, 2006; Ikeda & Uozumi, 2005). The reported experimental results show that this algorithm is suitable for tongue diagnosis and promising results were obtained. Moreover, in order to handle the fuzziness issue in tongue diagnosis, a diagnostic system for tongue analysis using fuzzy theory was developed (Watsuji, Arita, Shinohara, & Kitade, 1999). Five algorithms, i.e., ID3, J48, Naive Bayes, Bayes Net, and SVM, which are all implemented in WEKA, were compared to classify 457 tongue instances. The result shows that the Support Vector Machine performs the best among all these approaches (Hui, He, & Thach, 2007).

1.4 Issues and Challenges

Benefitting from the great improvement of image processing (especially gray image processing) and pattern classification technology in the past several years, several modules in the computerized tongue diagnosis system (as Fig. 1.4 shows) such as tongue image segmentation, texture feature extraction, and design of a diagnostic classifier have been greatly developed. Researchers started to pay more attention to these topics. Many related works could be found in imaging processing and the pattern recognition domain. However, several elementary but important issues have still not been well settled, which have impeded the development of this kind of system in recent years. First, although feature extraction and classification technology of tongue images have been well developed, tongue image acquisition technology, which is regarded as the basis of the computerized tongue diagnosis system, has not been greatly improved. Thereby, developed algorithms and obtained analytical results may not be reliable and convincing, and may suffer from limited applicability. Second, as the most important medical indicator, tongue color has not been well studied. For example, several important questions, including how to ensure that color information is captured in high fidelity, how to compensate for the noise and variations caused by the imaging system, what are the characteristics of tongue colors, and how to extract the most effective tongue color features for diagnostic purpose, have not been well answered. Figure 1.6 shows these most essential research topics which have not been well studied with green rectangular blocks.

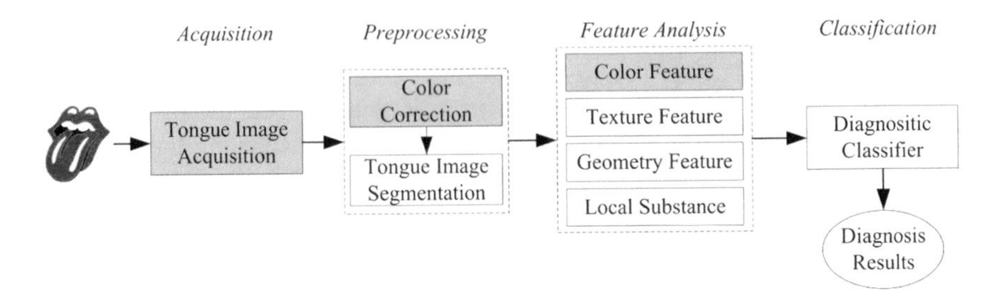

Fig. 1.6 Three modules which need to be further developed in the computerized tongue diagnosis system

1.4.1 Inconsistent Image Acquisition

Image acquisition is the most fundamental and vital part in the tongue diagnosis system. To date, nearly ten imaging systems have been implemented. However, due to the lack of fundamental research on guidance for designing tongue imaging systems, these systems were developed with inconsistent system components. Various types of imaging cameras and lighting sources which have different imaging characteristics have been utilized. Therefore, the quality of acquired tongue images varies considerably in these systems. Figure 1.7 shows three images acquired by the same camera for the same tongue body under three different kinds of lighting conditions. The color properties of these three images vary, and hence derived diagnostic results may be inconsistent even for the same tongue body. Also, images captured by the same camera at different times may be different due to inappropriate operation problems. Figure 1.8 shows images with different types of deficiencies of this type, i.e., inappropriate exposure and motion blur. This kind of imperfection would also greatly affect the analysis results. For instance, this kind of inconsistent image representation makes images captured by different devices noninterchangeable and nonsharable. Thereby, developed algorithms and obtained

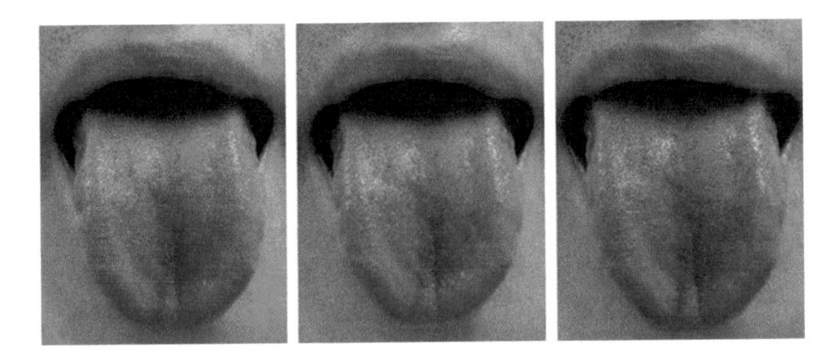

Fig. 1.7 Three tongue images captured by the same digital camera under different illumination conditions from the same tongue body. Color inconsistency can be easily observed among these three images

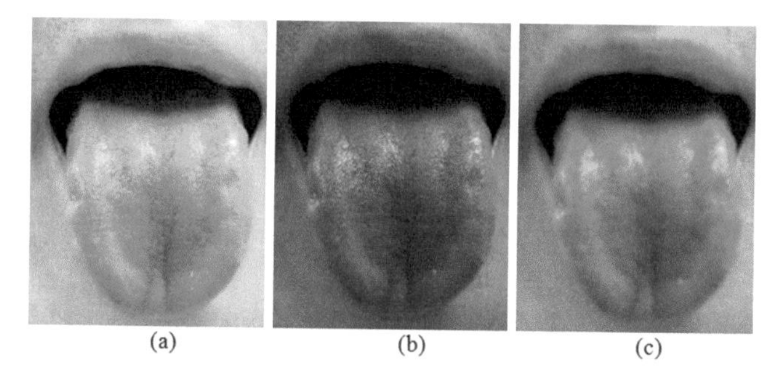

Fig. 1.8 Problem images acquired by a camera with inappropriate operation. **a** Over exposed image, **b** under exposed image, and **c** motion blur image

results on these captured images would be unstable and inconvincible. In view of this situation, it is crucial and urgent to conduct an in-depth requirement analysis in order to develop a high-quality and consistent tongue imaging system.

1.4.2 Inaccurate Color Correction

Tongue color correction is of great importance for high fidelity and accurate tongue image rendering. However, this issue has not yet been well addressed because of two main problems.

First, correction algorithms dedicated for tongue color correction have not been well developed. Although research on color correction methods in the color science area has been extensively conducted, these existing methods cannot be directly applied to tongue color correction because they are designed to process general imaging devices, such as digital cameras and cathode ray tube/liquid crystal display (CRT/LCD) monitors and printers, whose color gamut covers the whole visible color gamut and is much larger than the tongue color gamut. Therefore, in order to develop suitable tongue correction methods and thus to improve the correction accuracy, further optimization and improvement of the current correction methods need to be implemented and tested.

Second, besides the color correction algorithm, another problem which hinders the improvement of the accuracy of tongue color correction is the development of a tongue colorchecker. The colorchecker, which is usually utilized as a reference target for correction model training, plays a crucial role in the correction process. Currently, the Munsell colorchecker (MSCC) chart, which was designed in 1976 and regarded as the de facto standard is most commonly used in tongue color correction. However, this MSCC chart is designed to process natural images and is not specific for tongue colors, and thus it is too general to be applied for tongue color correction. Most colors in the MSCC chart are unlikely to appear in tongue images (e.g., green and yellowish green), and more theoretically, the color gamut (i.e., the range of colors) spanned by the MSCC chart colors is much larger than the limited color gamut of human tongue colors. In order to improve the accuracy of tongue color correction, developing a new colorchecker focused on tongue colors, i.e., a tongue colorchecker, is urgently needed to promote the correction performance so as to improve the tongue image quality.

1.4.3 Subjective Tongue Color Extraction and Classification

There are still many ambiguous and subjective factors involved in tongue image feature extraction. For example, because of the lack of knowledge about the tongue color distribution, and because the range of tongue colors and centers for typical color types cannot be objectively defined, the identification of different color types of tongue images is normally subjectively decided by TCM professionals based on their personal medical knowledge or experience (Wang et al., 2004, 2007; Kim et al., 2009; Kim, Do, Ryu, & Kim, 2008; Park, Lee, Yoo, & Park, 2016), which makes their obtained results unstable and imprecise. There are still no objective and precise definitions for each color category, such as what is the color center value of this "red" type and how to decide what kind of color belongs to the "red" type. Therefore, in-depth investigation of objective tongue color feature extraction is urgently needed in order to promote the development of computerized tongue image analysis.

References

Haller, J. S. (1982). The foul tongue: A 19th century index of disease. *Western Journal of Medicine, 137*(3), 258–264.

Reamy, B. V., Richard, D., & Bunt, C. W. (2010). Common tongue conditions in primary care. *American Family Physician, 81*(5), 627–634.

Matison, R., Mayeux, R., Rosen, J., & Fahn, S. (1982). "Tip-of-the-tongue" phenomenon in Parkinson disease. *Neurology, 32*(5), 567–570.

Jeghers, H. (1942). Nutrition: The appearance of the tongue as an index of nutritional deficiency. *New England Journal of Medicine, 227,* 221–228.

Faria, P. D., Vargas, P. A., Saldiva, P., Böhm, G. M., Mauad, T., & Almeida, O. D. (2005). Tongue disease in advanced AIDS. *Oral Diseases, 11*(2), 72–80.

Peng, B., & Xie, S. (2006). *Atlas of tongue diagnosis for AIDS patients*. Shelton: People's Medical Publishing House.

Ozgursoy, O. B., Ozgursoy, S. K., Tulunay, O., Kemal, O., Akyol, A., & Dursun, G. (2009). Melkersson-Rosenthal syndrome revisited as a misdiagnosed disease. *American Journal of Otolaryngology, 30*(1), 33–37.

Avraham, K. B., Schickler, M., Sapoznikov, D., Yarom, R., & Groner, Y. (1988). Down's syndrome: Abnormal neuromuscular junction in tongue of transgenic mice with elevated levels of human Cu/Zn-superoxide dismutase. *Cell, 54*(6), 823–829.

Farman, A. G. (1976). Atrophic lesions of the tongue: A prevalence study among 175 diabetic patients. *Journal of Oral Pathology, 5*(5), 255–264.

Grushka, M. W., Ching, V., & Polak, S. (2007). Retrospective study: Prevalence of geographic and fissured tongue in patients with burning mouth syndrome. *Oral Surgery, Oral Medicine, Oral Pathology, Oral Radiology & Endodontology, 103*(6), 789.

Zargari, O. (2006). The prevalence and significance of fissured tongue and geographical tongue in psoriatic patients. *Clinical and Experimental Dermatology, 31*(2), 192–195.

Scheper, M. A., Nikitakis, N. G., Sarlani, E., Sauk, J. J., & Meiller, T. F. (2006). Cowden syndrome: Report of a case with immunohistochemical analysis and review of the literature. *Oral Surgery, Oral Medicine, Oral Pathology, Oral Radiology & Endodontology, 101*(101), 625–631.

Han, S., Yang, X. I., Quan, Q. I., Pan, Y., Chen, Y., Shen, J., et al. (2016). Potential screening and early diagnosis method for cancer: Tongue diagnosis. *International Journal of Oncology, 48*(6), 2257–2264.

Maciocia, G. (1995). *Tongue diagnosis in Chinese medicine*. Seattle: Eastland Press.

Maciocia, G. (2004). *Diagnosis in Chinese medicine: A comprehensive guide*. London: Churchill Livingstone.

Giovanni, M. (2015). *The foundations of Chinese medicine*. Elsevier Science Health Science Div.

Tang, J.-L., Liu, B.-Y., & Ma, K.-W. (2008). Traditional Chinese medicine. *Lancet, 372*(8), 1938–1940.

Fei, Z., & Gu, Y. (2007). *Mirror of health: Tongue diagnosis in Chinese medicine*. Beijing, China: People's Medical Publishing House.

Yang, Z. H., Zhang, D. P., & Nai-Min, L. I. (2009). Physiological and pathological tongueprint images of human body. *Journal of Harbin Institute of Technology, 41*(12), 73–77.

Pang, B., Zhang, D., & Wang, K. (2005). Tongue image analysis for appendicitis diagnosis. *Information Sciences, 175*(3), 160–176.

Huang, B., Wu, J., Zhang, D., & Li, N. (2010). Tongue shape classification by geometric features. *Information Sciences an International Journal, 180*(2), 312–324.

Nai-Min, L. I., Zhang, D., & Kuan-Quan, W. (2011). *Tongue diagnostics*. Academy Press (Xue Yuan).

Lukman, S., He, Y., & Hui, S. C. (2008). Computational methods for traditional Chinese medicine: A survey. *Computer Methods and Programs in Biomedicine, 88*(3), 283–294.

Feng, Y., Wu, Z., Zhou, X., Zhou, Z., & Fan, W. (2006). Knowledge discovery in traditional Chinese medicine: State of the art and perspectives. *Artificial Intelligence in Medicine, 38*(3), 219–236.

Chiu, C. (1996). The development of a computerized tongue diagnosis system. *Biomedical Engineering Applications Basis Communications, 8*, 342–350.

Pang, B., et al. (2004). Computerized tongue diagnosis based on Bayesian networks. *IEEE Transactions on Biomedical Engineering, 51*(10), 1803–1810.

Chiu, C. (2000). A novel approach based on computerized image analysis for traditional Chinese medical diagnosis of the tongue. *Computer Methods and Programs in Biomedicine, 61*(2), 77–89.

Zhang, D., Pang, B., Li, N., Wang, K., & Zhang, H. (2005). Computerized diagnosis from tongue appearance using quantitative feature classification. *The American Journal of Chinese Medicine, 33*(06), 859–866.

Zhang, H. Z., Wang, K. Q., Zhang, D., Pang, B., & Huang, B. (2005). Computer aided tongue diagnosis system (pp. 6754–6757). IEEE.

Sonka, M., Hlavac, V., & Boyle, R. (2014). *Image processing, analysis, and machine vision*. Australia: Cengage Learning.

Gonzalez, R. C., & Woods, R. E. (2007). *Digital image processing* (3rd ed): Upper Saddle River, NJ: Prentice Hall.

Anzai, Y. (2012). *Pattern recognition and machine learning*. Amsterdam: Elsevier.

Duda, R. O., Hart, P. E., & Stork, D. G. (2012). *Pattern classification*. New York: Wiley.

Chang, C. (2003). *Hyperspectral imaging: Techniques for spectral detection and classification* (Vol. 1). Springer Science & Business Media.

Kim, M. S., Chen, Y. R., & Mehl, P. M. (2001). Hyperspectral reflectance and fluorescence imaging system for food quality and safety. *Transactions of the ASAE, 44*(3), 721.
Mooradian, G., Weiderhold, M., Dabiri, A. E., & Coyle, C. (1998). Hyperspectral imaging methods and apparatus for non-invasive diagnosis of tissue for cancer. Google Patents.
Vo-Dinh, T. (2004). A hyperspectral imaging system for in vivo optical diagnostics. *Engineering in Medicine and Biology Magazine, IEEE, 23*(5), 40–49.
Zavattini, G., Vecchi, S., Mitchell, G., Weisser, U., Leahy, R. M., Pichler, B. J., et al. (2006). A hyperspectral fluorescence system for 3D in vivo optical imaging. *Physics in Medicine & Biology, 51*(8), 2029.
Du, H., et al. (2007). A novel hyperspectral medical sensor for tongue diagnosis. *Sensor Review, 27*(1), 57–60.
Li, Q., Wang, Y., Liu, H., Sun, Z., & Liu, Z. (2010a). Tongue fissure extraction and classification using hyperspectral imaging technology. *Applied Optics, 49*(11), 2006–2013.
Li, Q., Wang, Y., Liu, H., & Sun, Z. (2010). AOTF based hyperspectral tongue imaging system and its applications in computer-aided tongue disease diagnosis (pp. 1424–1427).
Li, Q., Liu, J., Xiao, G., & Xue, Y. (2008). Hyperspectral tongue imaging system used in tongue diagnosis (pp. 2579–2581). IEEE.
Liu, Z., Yan, J. Q., Zhang, D., & Li, Q. L. (2007). Automated tongue segmentation in hyperspectral images for medicine. *Applied Optics, 46*(34), 8328–8334.
Li, Q., & Liu, Z. (2009). Tongue color analysis and discrimination based on hyperspectral images. *Computerized Medical Imaging and Graphics, 33*(3), 217–221.
Zhi, L., Zhang, D., Yan, J. Q., Li, Q. L., & Tang, Q. L. (2007). Classification of hyperspectral medical tongue images for tongue diagnosis. *Computerized Medical Imaging and Graphics, 31*(8), 672–678.
Yu, X., Jin, Z., Tan, G., et al. (1994). System of Automatic Diagnosis by Tongue Feature in Traditional Chinese Medicine. *Chinese Journal of Scientific Instrument, 1*, 13.
Wong, W., & Huang, S. (2001). Studies on externalization of application of tongue inspection of TCM. *Engineering Science, 3*(1), 78–82.
Cai, Y. (2002). A novel imaging system for tongue inspection (pp. 159–164): IEEE; 1999.
Jang, J. H., Kim, J. E., Park, K. M., Park, S. O., Chang, Y. S., & Kim, B. Y. (2002). Development of the digital tongue inspection system with image analysis (pp. 1033–1034). IEEE.
Wei, B. G., Shen, L. S., Wang, Y. Q., Wang, Y. G., Wang, A. M., & Zhao, Z. X. (2002). A digital tongue image analysis instrument for Traditional Chinese Medicine. *Chinese Journal of Medical Instrumentation* [*Zhongguo yi liao qi xie za zhi*], *26*(3), 164–166.
Wang, Y., Zhou, Y., Yang, J., & Xu, Q. (2004). An image analysis system for tongue diagnosis in traditional Chinese medicine. In *Computational and Information Science* (pp. 1181–1186): Springer.
Kim, J., Jung, Y., Park, K., & Park, J. (2009). A digital tongue imaging system for tongue coating evaluation in patients with oral malodour. *Oral Diseases, 15*(8), 565–569.
He, Y., Liu, C., & Shen, L. (2007). Digital camera based tongue manifestation acquisition platform. *World Science and Technology-Modernization of Traditional Chinese Medicine and Materia Medica, 5*.
Chang, Y., & Reid, J. F. (1996). RGB calibration for color image analysis in machine vision. *Image Processing, IEEE Transactions on, 5*(10), 1414–1422.
Wandell, B. A. (1987). The synthesis and analysis of color images. *IEEE Transactions on Pattern Analysis and Machine Intelligence,* (1), 2–13.
Finlayson, G. D. (1996). Color in perspective. *IEEE Transactions on Pattern Analysis and Machine Intelligence, 18*(10), 1034–1038.
Barnard, K., & Funt, B. (2002). Camera characterization for color research. *Color Research & Application, 27*(3), 152–163.
Yamamoto, K., Kitahara, M., Kimata, H., Yendo, T., Fujii, T., Tanimoto, M., et al. (2007). Multiview video coding using view interpolation and color correction. *IEEE Transactions on Circuits and Systems for Video Technology, 17*(11), 1436–1449.

Vrhel, M. J., & Trussell, H. J. (1999). Color device calibration: a mathematical formulation. *IEEE Transactions on Image Processing, 8*(12), 1796–1806.

Yamamoto, K., Kitahara, M., Kimata, H., Yendo, T., Fujii, T., Tanimoto, M., et al. (2006). Color calibration for multicamera system without color pattern board. *Monash University DECSE Technical Report MECSE-4-2006.*

Vrhel, M., Saber, E., & Trussell, H. J. (2005). Color image generation and display technologies.

Luo, M. R., Hong, G., & Rhodes, P. A. (2001). A study of digital camera colorimetric characterization based on polynomial modeling. *Color: Research and applications, 26*(1), 76–84.

Cheung, V., Westland, S., Connah, D., & Ripamonti, C. (2004). A comparative study of the characterisation of colour cameras by means of neural networks and polynomial transforms. *Coloration Technology, 120*(1), 19–25.

Zhang, H., Wang, K., Jin, X., & Zhang, D. (2005). SVR based color calibration for tongue image (pp. 5065–5070). IEEE.

Hu, M. C., Cheng, M. H., & Lan, K. C. (2016). Color correction parameter estimation on the smartphone and its application to automatic tongue diagnosis. *Journal of Medical Systems, 40*(1), 1–8.

Zhuo, L., Zhang, P., Qu, P., Peng, Y., Zhang, J., & Li, X. (2015). A K-PLSR-based color correction method for TCM tongue images under different illumination conditions. *Neurocomputing, 174*(9), 815–821.

Shi, J., et al. (2000). Normalized cuts and image segmentation. *IEEE Transactions on Pattern Analysis and Machine Intelligence, 22*(8), 888–905.

Pal, N. R., & Pal, S. K. (1993). A review on image segmentation techniques. *Pattern Recognition, 26*(9), 1277–1294.

Zhu, S. C., et al. (1996). Region competition: Unifying snakes, region growing, and Bayes/MDL for multiband image segmentation. *IEEE Transactions on Pattern Analysis and Machine Intelligence, 18*(9), 884–900.

Felzenszwalb, P. F., & Huttenlocher, D. P. (2004). Efficient graph-based image segmentation. *International Journal of Computer Vision, 59*(2), 167–181.

Shi, M. J., Li, G. Z., Li, F. F., & Xu, C. (2014). Computerized tongue image segmentation via the double geo-vector flow. *Chinese Medicine, 9*(1), 1–10.

Cui, Z., Zhang, H., Zhang, D., Li, N., & Zuo, W. (2013). Fast marching over the 2D Gabor magnitude domain for tongue body segmentation. *Journal on Advances in Signal Processing, 2013*(1).

Wu, K., & Zhang, D. (2015). Robust tongue segmentation by fusing region-based and edge-based approaches. *Expert Systems with Applications, 42*(21), 8027–8038.

Kass, M., Witkin, A., & Terzopoulos, D. (1988). Snakes: Active contour models. *International Journal of Computer Vision, 1*(4), 321–331.

Wu, J., Zhang, Y., & Bai, J. (2006). Tongue area extraction in tongue diagnosis of traditional Chinese medicine (pp. 4955–4957). IEEE.

Zhang, H., Zuo, W., Wang, K., & Zhang, D. (2006). A snake-based approach to automated segmentation of tongue image using polar edge detector. *International Journal of Imaging Systems and Technology, 16*(4), 103–112.

Pang, B., Zhang, D., & Wang, K. (2005a). The bi-elliptical deformable contour and its application to automated tongue segmentation in Chinese medicine. *IEEE Transactions on Medical Imaging, 24*(8), 946–956.

Pang, B., Wang, K., Zhang, F., & Zhang, F. (2002). On automated tongue image segmentation in Chinese medicine (pp. 616–619). IEEE.

Wang, Y., Zhou, Y., Yang, J., & Wang, Y. (2004). JSEG based color separation of tongue image in traditional Chinese medicine. In *Progress in pattern recognition, image analysis and applications* (pp. 503–508). Springer.

Yu, S., Yang, J., Wang, Y., & Zhang, Y. (2007). Color active contour models based tongue segmentation in traditional Chinese medicine (pp. 1065–1068). IEEE.

Ning, J., Zhang, D., Wu, C., & Yue, F. (2012). Automatic tongue image segmentation based on gradient vector flow and region merging. *Neural Computing and Applications, 21*(8), 1819–1826.
Cui, Y., Liao, S., & Wang, H. (2015). ROC-Boosting: A feature selection method for health identification using tongue image. *Computational & Mathematical Methods in Medicine, 2015* (25), 1–8.
Cui, Y., Liao, S., Wang, H., Liu, H., Wang, W., & Yin, L. (2014). Relationship between Hyperuricemia and Haar-Like Features on Tongue Images. *Biomed Research International, 2015,* 1–10.
Kim, J., Han, G., Ko, S. J., Nam, D. H., Park, J. W., Ryu, B., et al. (2014). Tongue diagnosis system for quantitative assessment of tongue coating in patients with functional dyspepsia: A clinical trial. *Journal of Ethnopharmacology, 155*(1), 709–713.
Li, C. H., & Yuen, P. C. (2002). Tongue image matching using color content. *Pattern Recognition, 35*(2), 407–419.
Li, C. H., & Yuen, P. C. (2000). Regularized color clustering in medical image database. *IEEE Transactions on Medical Imaging, 19*(11), 1150–1155.
Huang, B., & Li, N. (2008). Pixel based tongue color analysis. In *Medical biometrics* (pp. 282–289). Berlin: Springer.
Huang, B., Zhang, D., & Zhang, H., Li, Y., & Li, N. (2011). Tongue color visualization for local pixel (pp. 297–301). IEEE.
Huang, B., Zhang, D., Li, Y., Zhang, H., & Li, N. (2011). Tongue coating image retrieval (pp. 292–296). IEEE.
Rubner, Y., Tomasi, C., & Guibas, L. J. (2000). The earth mover's distance as a metric for image retrieval. *International Journal of Computer Vision, 40*(2), 99–121.
Wang, Y. G., Yang, J., Zhou, Y., & Wang, Y. Z. (2007). Region partition and feature matching based color recognition of tongue image. *Pattern Recognition Letters, 28*(1), 11–19.
Yuen, P. C., Kuang, Z. Y., Wu, W., & Wu, Y. T. (2000). Tongue texture analysis using Gabor Wavelet opponent colour features for tongue diagnosis in traditional Chinese medicine. *Series in Machine Perception and Artificial Intelligence, 40,* 179–188.
Yuen, P. C., Kuang, Z. Y., Wu, W., & Wu, Y. T. (1999). Tongue texture analysis using opponent color features for tongue diagnosis in traditional Chinese medicine. In *Proceedings of TAMV* (pp. 21–27).
Haralick, R. M., Shanmugam, K., & Dinstein, I. H. (1973). Textural features for image classification. *IEEE Transactions on Systems, Man and Cybernetics,* (6), 610–621.
Miao, H. E. (2007). Red-prickled tongue image classification based on Gabor Wavelet and weighed features. *Progress in Modern Biomedicine*.
Huang, B., & Li, N. (2010). Tongue image identification system on congestion of fungiform papillae (CFP). In *Medical biometrics* (pp. 73–82). Berlin: Springer.
Heckerman, D. (1997). Bayesian networks for data mining. *Data Mining and Knowledge Discovery, 1*(1), 79–119.
Wang, H., & Zong, X. (2006). A new computerized method for tongue classification (pp. 508–511). IEEE.
Ikeda, N., & Uozumi, T. (2005). Tongue diagnosis support system. *The Hokkaido Journal of Medical Science* [Hokkaido igaku zasshi], *80*(3), 269–277.
Watsuji, T., Arita, S., Shinohara, S., & Kitade, T. (1999). Medical application of fuzzy theory to the diagnostic system of tongue inspection in traditional Chinese medicine (pp. 145–148). IEEE.
Hui, S. C., He, Y., & Thach, D. T. C. (2007). Machine learning for tongue diagnosis (pp. 1–5). IEEE.
Kim, K. H., Do, J. H., Ryu, H., & Kim, J. Y. (2008). Tongue diagnosis method for extraction of effective region and classification of tongue coating (pp. 1–7). IEEE.
Park, Y. J., Lee, J. M., Yoo, S. Y., & Park, Y. B. (2016). Reliability and validity of tongue color analysis in the prediction of symptom patterns in terms of East Asian Medicine. *Journal of Traditional Chinese Medicine, 36*(2), 165–172.

Chapter 2
Tongue Images Acquisition System Design

Abstract In order to improve the quality and consistency of tongue images acquired by current imaging devices, this research aims to develop a novel imaging system which can faithfully and precisely record human tongue information for medical analysis. A thorough demand analysis is first conducted in this chapter in order to summarize requirements for rendering all possible medical clues, i.e., color, texture, and geometric features. Then a series of system design criteria are illustrated, and following from them three hardware modules of the imaging system, including the illuminant, lighting path, and imaging camera, are optimally proposed. Moreover, one built-in software module, the color correction process, is also provided to compensate for color variations caused by system components. Finally, several important performance indicators, including illumination uniformity, system reproducibility, and accuracy, were tested. Experimental results showed that captured images were of high quality and remained stable when acquisitions are repeated. The largest color difference between the images acquired at different times was 1.6532, which is hardly distinguishable by human observation. Compared to existing devices, the proposed system could provide a much more accurate and stable solution for tongue image acquisition. Furthermore, this developed imaging system has been evaluated by doctors of Traditional Chinese Medicine for almost 3 years and over 9000 tongue images have been collected. Analysis results based on these data also validate the effectiveness of the proposed system.

2.1 Introduction

Visual inspection of the human tongue offers a simple, immediate, inexpensive, and noninvasive solution for various medical applications. However, since the tongue is traditionally observed by the human eye rather than recorded by digital instruments, it is difficult or even impossible to quantitatively store and process tongue images. This intrinsic drawback has seriously impeded the standardization and quantification of tongue inspection for medical applications. Building a high quality and consistent tongue imaging system is essential to promote the modernization and popularization of computerized tongue diagnosis. By the aid of such an imaging

D. Zhang et al., *Tongue Image Analysis*, DOI 10.1007/978-981-10-2167-1_2

system, further applications could also be developed, such as digital data storage, computer-aided image analysis, and data transmission via the Internet for tele-medicine applications.

With the development of digital imaging technology, the use of a digital camera in tongue inspection has been investigated for several years. Ten imaging systems have been implemented and a detailed introduction of these devices is presented in Table 2.1. However, based on much literature, there are two main problems in the current research. First, these systems were designed without following any common criteria, and hence there was no guidance for the design of system components. Thus several obvious design deficiencies can be noted and their recorded images may be of inferior quality. For instance, (Jang et al., 2002; Wong & Huang, 2001; Zhang, Wang, Zhang, Pang, & Huang, 2005) utilized halogen tungsten lamps whose color temperature is too low to render color in high fidelity, and thus their produced images are reddish-biased which lead to inaccurate analysis results. Also, as Fig. 2.1 shows, (Cai, 2002; Chiu, 2000; Pang, Zhang, Li, & Wang, 2004; Jiang, Chen, & Zhang, 2000) the images were captured in a public office environment, which caused the acquired images to be easily affected by the environmental illumination. Furthermore, several systems (He, Liu, & Shen, 2007; Jang et al., 2002; Wong & Huang, 2001) did not involve a color correction procedure which corrects color variations caused by system components, and thus their produced images may be unstable and unreliable. In addition, most of these systems utilized a digital still camera which suffers from blurred motion or inconsistent exposure, and the involvement of a PC for image taking would make this system inconvenient for portable data acquisition. Second, another problem in the current research is that all these devices have not been systematically tested for their accuracy and consistency. From Table 2.1, it can be seen that these developed systems substantially disagree with one another in terms of their system compositions. Various types of imaging cameras and lighting sources with diverse imaging characteristics were utilized. Therefore, the quality of the obtained tongue images considerably varies. This kind of inconsistent image representation makes images capture by different devices incompatible and noninterchangeable. Developed algorithms and obtained results based on these captured images would be unstable and inconvincible. Hence, a comprehensive test of the designed system to ensure their accuracy and stability is necessary. In view of this situation, it is crucial and urgent to develop a high quality and consistent tongue imaging system for computerized tongue image analysis.

This chapter aims to solve problems in the current research of tongue image acquisition, i.e., defective quality and inconsistent image rendering, and thus to propose a new tongue imaging system which can acquire images of high quality and great consistency. First, because the main reason which leads to the present trouble is the lack of design guidance which illustrates critical requirements to ensure accurate and consistent image acquisition, an in-depth requirement analysis of tongue imaging system design is conducted, and then a series of fundamental criteria are established to satisfy these requirements to accurately and consistently extract all possible medical clues, including color, texture, and geometric features for medical analysis. Thereafter, each module of the system, including the illuminant, lighting path, imaging camera, and post-processed color correction procedure,

Table 2.1 Summary of existing tongue image acquisition devices

Year	Illumination	Imaging camera	Color correction	System test	References
2000	Two fluorescent lamps installed in office environment (5400 K)	440 × 400 pixels in a 2/3 CCD camera	Printed color card	No	Chiu (2000)
2000	Daylight-type compact fluorescent lamp (5400 K, Kaiser RB 5000)	Nikon E1, 1280 × 1000	Gray card	No	Jiang et al. (2000)
2001	Halogen tungsten lamps (3100 K)	Olympus DSC camera	N/A	No	Wong and Huang (2001)
2002	Office illumination	Commercial digital still camera, 640 × 480	Munsell Colorchecker	No	Cai (2002)
2002	Optical fiber source (250 W halogen lamp, 4000 K)	Watec WAT-202D CCD camera, 768 × 494	N/A	No	Jang et al. (2002)
2002	OSRAM L18/72-965 fluorescent lamp (6500 K)	Kodak DC 260, 1536 × 1024	Printed color card	No	Wei et al. (2002)
2004	Four standard light sources installed in dark chest (5000 K)	Canon G5, 1024 × 768	Printed color card	No	Wang, Zhou, Yang, and Xu (2004)
2005	Two 70 W cold-light type halogen lamps (4800 K)	Sony 900E video camera, 720 × 576	Printed color card	No	Zhang et al. (2005)
2007	PHILIPS YH22 circular fluorescent lamps (7200 K)	DH-HV3103 CMOS camera, 2048 × 1536	N/A	No	He et al. (2007)
2007–2010	KOHLER illumination light source (wavelength ranges 403–865 nm)	Hitachi KP-F120 CCD camera	N/A	No	Du, Liu, Li, Yan, and Tang, (2007), Li, Wang, Liu, and Sun (2010), Li and Liu (2009), Li, Wang, Liu, Sun, and Liu (2010)

Reprinted from Wang and Zhang (2013b), with permission from Elsevier

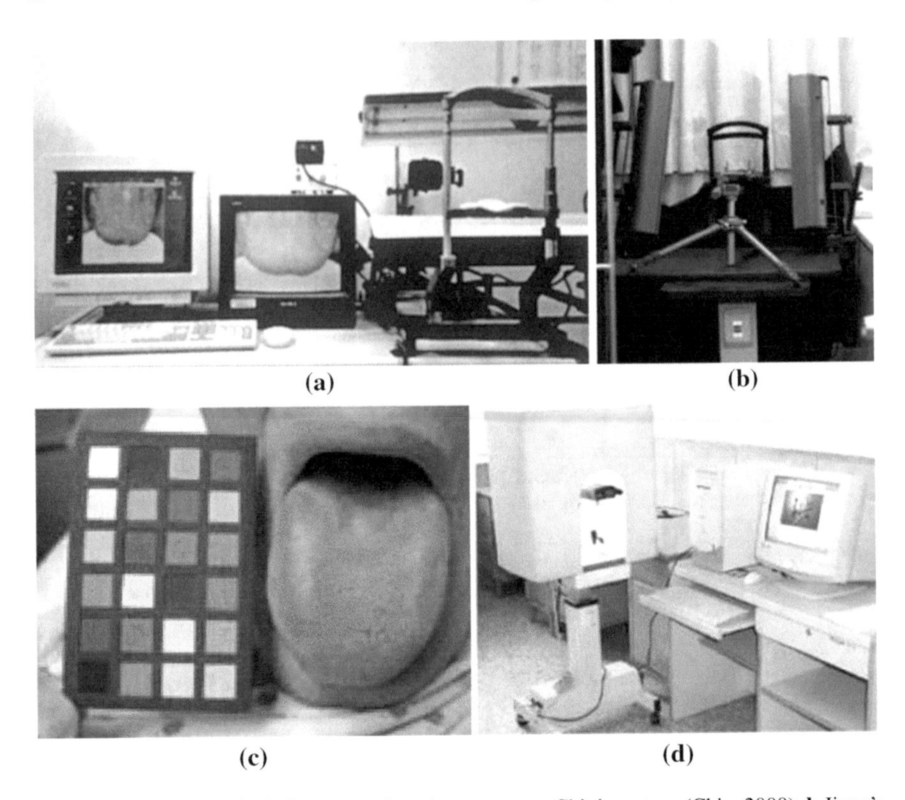

Fig. 2.1 Appearance of existing tongue imaging systems **a** Chiu's system (Chiu, 2000), **b** Jiang's system (Jiang et al., 2000), **c** Cai's device (Cai, 2002), and **d** Wei's imaging device (Wei et al., 2002). All these systems have design deficiencies which lead to production of images with poor quality. Reprinted from Wang and Zhang (2013b), with permission from Elsevier

is optimally designed. Finally, several critical system performance indicators, including illumination uniformity, system reproducibility, and accuracy, are tested to verify the validity of the proposed system.

The remainder of this chapter is organized as follows. Section 2.1 describes the system framework and corresponding requirements for each module to achieve superior quality and consistent tongue image acquisition. The detailed introduction about how each module of the system is optimally implemented is presented in Sect. 2.2. In Sect. 2.3, we conduct a performance evaluation of the proposed system. Finally, the chapter is concluded in Sect. 2.4.

2.2 System Framework and Requirement Analysis

In this section, the framework of the proposed tongue imaging system is introduced and the four principal modules of this system are presented. Then, in order to make sure the human tongue body is accurately and consistently recorded for medical analysis, a thorough requirement analysis is provided to illustrate design criteria for each module of the system.

2.2.1 System Framework

In a typical imaging system, besides the object itself, the other two important factors are illumination and the digital detector. Illumination can be further considered as two independent parts, one is the illuminant which is mainly what types of lighting source should be selected, while the other one is the lighting path which is the design of the optical path and environmental condition. In addition to the above three hardware modules, the color correction process which compensates for variations caused by the system components and to render color images into device-independent color space, is also included in our system as a built-in software module.

Figure 2.2 presents the flowchart of the proposed tongue imaging system. There are four modules in the system: the illuminant, lighting path, imaging camera, and color correction process, are essential for accurate and consistent image acquisition. Illuminated by two carefully selected fluorescent lamps (OSRAM L8W-954), the human tongue is recorded in video file by a 3-CCD video camera (Sony DXC 390P) with a fixed-focal lens (Computer, M0814-MP). Then, the tongue image is extracted and saved by a frame grabber (Euresys Picolo Pro 2). Then, these captured tongue images are sent to the built-in embedded system for the color correction process. In our device, an embedded single board computer (Intel i5 Q1500 2.20 GHz, 2 GB RAM) is used because of its high performance, low power cost, and abundant expansion interfaces. This single board computer was assembled

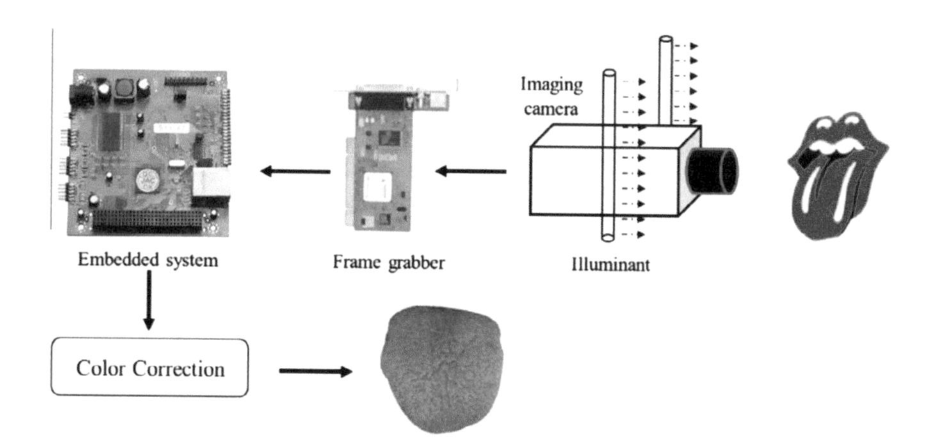

Fig. 2.2 Framework of the proposed tongue imaging system. Reprinted from Wang and Zhang (2013b), with permission from Elsevier

inside the tongue device, and the Windows XP system was installed. Hence, our developed color correction and other related tongue image analysis program could be developed and run on the Windows platform.

The four most critical modules in this system are the illuminant (L), imaging camera (C), lighting path (E), and built-in color correction algorithm (D). If the tongue imaging system is considered as a signal-transfer system which transfers the original tongue signal (denoted by T) to a digital image signal (denoted by I), then characteristics of the four modules can be viewed as significant parameters in the system's transfer function. The relationship between the input signal and output tongue image signal can be formulated as

$$I = T * f(L, C, E, D) \tag{2.1}$$

In this formula, f (L, C, E, D) is the transfer function of the proposed tongue imaging system. L, C, E, and D denote characteristics of four modules which need to be optimized. In order to achieve high quality and consistent tongue image acquisition, these four parameters need to be optimally designed, which is presented in Sect. 2.4.

2.2.2 Requirement Analysis

In TCM the tongue has been considered an essential health index of the human body for a long time, and various types of tongue features have been utilized for medical diagnosis. In order to develop the most suitable and the best quality tongue imaging system for medical analysis, we first summarize all possible features and explore their corresponding requirements on imaging system, and then the system can be easily designed.

According to the principle of tongue diagnosis (Li, 2011; Maciocia, 1987, 2013), three types of features are commonly utilized for medical analysis. The first and most essential one is the tongue color. Figure 2.3 shows four tongue images which present different colors. In the first image the tongue's proper color is red, and the remaining three tongue coating colors are yellow, white, and black respectively. These typical color types are highly correlated to various health statuses of the human body. In order to achieve accurate tongue image analysis, an imaging

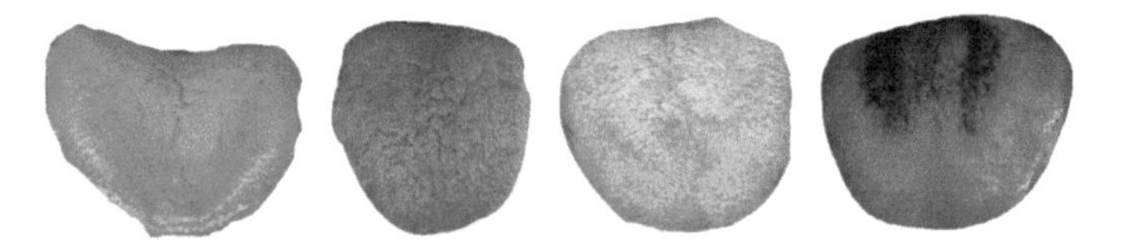

Fig. 2.3 Typical tongue image samples with diverse chromatic characteristics. The main color components of these four images are red, yellow, white, and black from left to right respectively. Reprinted from Wang and Zhang (2013b), with permission from Elsevier

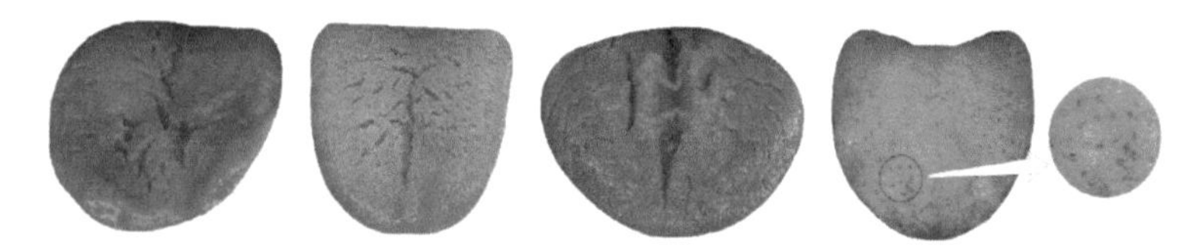

Fig. 2.4 Typical tongue image samples with different texture styles. Reprinted from Wang and Zhang (2013b), with permission from Elsevier

camera needs to faithfully render all types of colors, and thus to record abundant color information of high quality and fidelity in order to distinguish different kinds of diseases. Furthermore, acquired color features should be kept stable among different acquisition sessions in order to achieve a consistent performance.

Besides the color feature, texture features are also frequently utilized for medical diagnosis. Figure 2.4 shows images with typical texture features which include tongue fissure, crack, and local substance. In Fig. 2.4, the first two are images with a tongue fissure. The third one is a tongue crack and the last one is an image with local substance (red point). Different texture styles convey various pathological information of internal organs, for example a red point is usually found on the tongue of a subject with appendicitis. These texture features have distinct spatial dimensions. For example, a tongue crack is often larger than a tongue fissure, and the red point is usually the smallest texture feature style. The fundamental requirement for texture recording is to ensure adequate resolution for distinguishing the smallest texture feature style. Moreover, the obtained texture features should be clear and stable enough, and several deficiencies including motion blur and inconsistent exposure should be avoided.

Another vital feature for tongue diagnosis is the geometric feature (Huang, Wu, Zhang, & Li, 2010). As shown in Fig. 2.5, the tongue length, width, and other

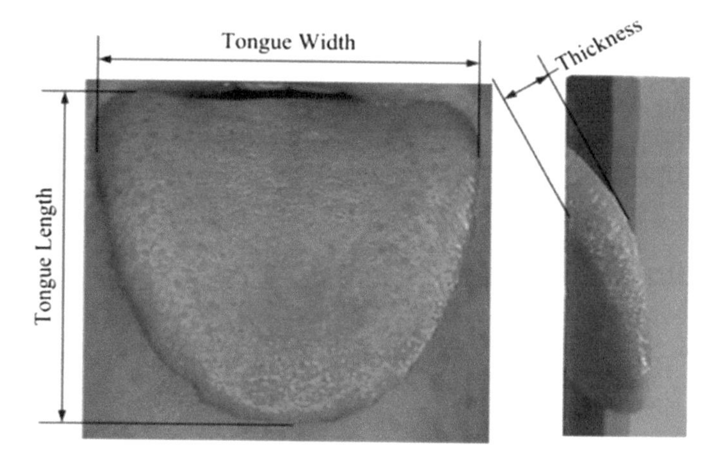

Fig. 2.5 Commonly used tongue geometric features. Reprinted from Wang and Zhang (2013b), with permission from Elsevier

geometric indexes which describe the tongue shape are crucial for diagnosis of several specific diseases (Maciocia, 2013). Also, other kinds of geometric features, including the width–length ratio, area of the tongue body, and inscribed-circle diameter, are frequently used for medical analysis. Moreover, the thickness of the tongue body is similarly found to be useful to reveal pathological changes of internal organs. Thereby, in our proposed system, in addition to a frontal image, a side view image is also captured.

In order to accurately extract all the above tongue features, we link each request with the corresponding system modules in order to establish criteria for the design of the imaging system. For instance, in order to stably and accurately capture tongue color, an illuminant with a high color rendering index should be selected. Also, the color correction procedure should be involved to correct variations caused by system components. Table 2.2 provides a summary of all requirements and possible solutions to fulfill them. Section 2.3 will describe how to design the system in order to meet all these requirements.

Table 2.2 Requirement analysis for tongue imaging system design in order to ensure high-quality and consistent acquisition

Image features	Requirement	Problem domain	Possible solution
Color	High quality and fidelity	Illuminant Imaging camera Lighting path	Select illuminant with: high color rendering index and, full spectral radiation, white color Involve more CCDs (a three-CCD camera is better than a single-CCD camera) Utilize an industrial camera rather than a commercial camera to avoid built-in color enhancement Realized uniform illumination on the capture plane Utilize the lighting and viewing geometry recommended by CIE Capture images in a dark chest, not in open-air
Texture	High stability High clarity	Color correction Imaging camera	Design a color correction algorithm to calibrate acquired tongue images Have enough resolution to distinguish the smallest texture features Avoid motion blur
Geometry	Thickness feature involved	Viewing environment and optical path	Design the imaging path to acquire tongue thickness information
	User-friendly collection	Ease-of-use design	Small size Clean and safe collection Ergonomic interface design

Reprinted from Wang and Zhang (2013b), with permission from Elsevier

2.3 Optimal System Design

Based on the aforementioned proposed framework of a tongue imaging system, this section will design each module to meet all the requirements in order to ensure accurate and consistent image acquisition.

2.3.1 *Illuminant*

The illuminant plays an indispensable role in achieving high performance of tongue image acquisition. If the illuminant changes or has a minor variation, the color perceptions of the same tongue body may differ. Generally, there are two essential parameters needed to select the most suitable illuminant. One is the color rendering index, and the other one is the color temperature.

The color rendering index, or CRI, of a light source describes its capability to accurately render the colors of perceived objects. This index is usually expressed as a number ranging from 0 to 100, where 100 represents the perfect illuminant which can accurately render all colors. As a general rule, the higher the light source's CRI number, the better the lamp will make things appear. This index is the only internationally agreed indicator of the relative color rendering ability which provides some guidance for illuminant assessment. In a tongue imaging system, since the objective is to render tongue colors as accurately as possible, an illuminant with a high color rendering index is needed. According to the international standard on viewing conditions in graphic technology and photography (ISO, 2009), the CRI number of the selected illuminant should be larger than 90 for precise color measurement. Therefore, among all kinds of illuminants, we chose the illuminant which has the largest CRI number (bigger than 90) for tongue imaging.

Another notable characteristic of an illuminant is color temperature. It defines the color appearance of the illuminant, such as its whiteness, yellowness, or blueness. Color temperature is conventionally denoted in the unit of absolute temperature, Kelvin (K). Usually, an illuminant with color temperatures over 7000 K appears bluish, while a low color temperature (2700–3000 K) is yellowish. If an illuminant itself has some color, it cannot accurately render tongue images. Figure 2.6 shows several tongue images which were captured by four illuminants with a distinctive color temperature: an incandescent bulb (3000 K), metal halide lamp (4200 K), fluorescent lamp (5000 K), and fluorescent lamp (6500 K). It should be noted that in the first two images (a and b), the red and yellow component are slightly enhanced, while the last image is somewhat bluish biased. Only Fig. 2.6c shows a balanced color tone to TCM professionals. Thereby, based on the observation of this experiment, an illuminant with a color temperature around 5000 K is suitable for tongue color measurement. Also, according to TCM diagnostic practice, the best illuminant for tongue inspection is sunshine in an open area at 9 a.m. whose color temperature is around 5000–6000 K. This is also in accord

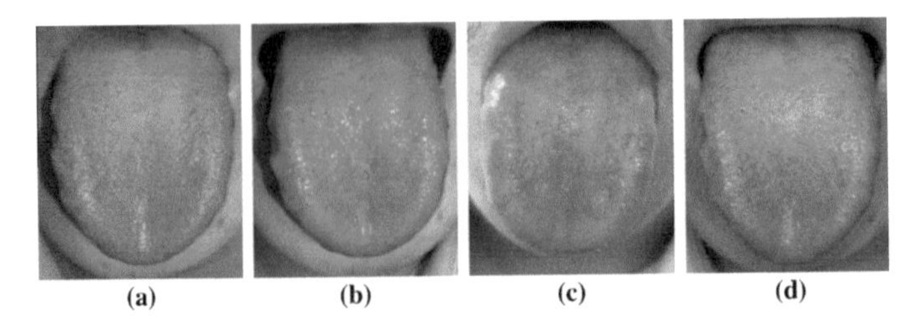

Fig. 2.6 Images of the same tongue body captured under different lighting source. **a** Incandescent bulb (3000 K), **b** metal halide lamp (4200 K), **c** fluorescent lamp (5000 K), and fluorescent lamp (6500 K). Reprinted from Wang and Zhang (2013b), with permission from Elsevier

with the suggestions of ISO3664:2009 (ISO, 2009), in which an illuminant with a color temperature around 5000–6000 K is recommended for unbiased color inspection and measurement. Therefore, based on our experimental findings and ISO standards, an illuminant with a color temperature between 5000 and 6000 K was chosen.

Based on the above analysis of the selection of the most suitable illuminant, and moreover, in order to reduce the dimensions of the imaging device, an OSRAM fluorescent lamp (L8W-954) was finally chosen after comparing a number of products manufactured by lighting companies (OSRAM, Philips, and GE lighting). It is a type of fluorescent lamp which has an extremely strong color rendering ability. Both its color rendering index (P90) and color temperature (5400 K) meet our above criteria (Table 2.2) to guarantee highly accurate tongue color rendering. Moreover, this illuminant is the smallest one (288 mm in length) among all illuminants which have such a high color rendering capability. This small dimension makes it possible to reduce the total size of the imaging device.

2.3.2 Lighting Condition

In addition to selecting the most suitable illuminant for tongue imaging, a lighting path, which includes the optical path and environmental illumination, also plays an essential role in the imaging process.

For the optical path design for precise color measurement, one important concern is how to position the illuminant and imaging camera to achieve a high quality of measurement. CIE (Commission International de L'Eclairage) has provided four standard options for illuminating and viewing geometry (as Fig. 2.7 shows) in reflectance color measurement. These standard illuminating and viewing conditions provide essential geometrical rules to position the illuminant and imaging detector. For example, Fig. 2.7a shows the 45°/0° geometry which recommend illuminating at 45° and viewing at 0°. By following this, reflections caused by a moist tongue surface which significantly affects the color perception of tongue images can be greatly reduced. Thereby, high-quality tongue image acquisition can be assured.

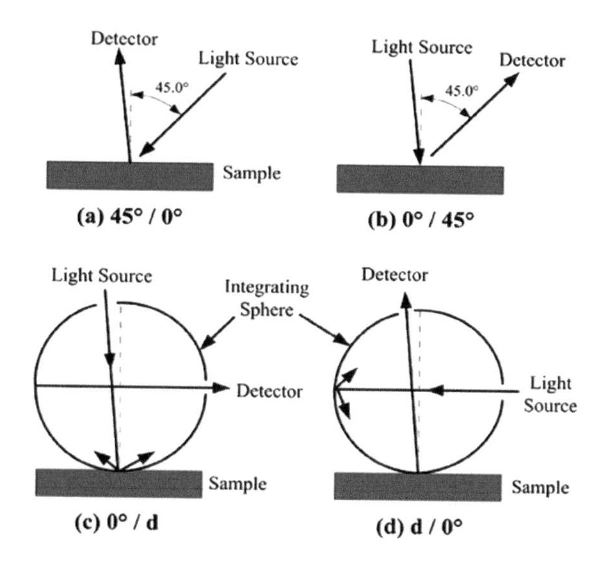

Fig. 2.7 CIE standard illuminating and viewing conditions for precise color measurement. There are four kinds of viewing and illuminating geometries which are recommended by CIE to avoid reflected light. Reprinted from Wang and Zhang (2013b), with permission from Elsevier

Based on the above standard geometry of illuminating and viewing, the optical path proposed in this work is shown in Fig. 2.8. The video camera is placed at the center. The positioning of the illuminant and imaging video camera follows the standard 45°/0° geometry to avoid reflection caused by a moist tongue surface. Moreover, in order to achieve uniform distribution of illumination on the acquisition plane, two lamps are symmetrically placed on either side of the central video camera. In addition, this system is also designed to simultaneously capture the front-view image and the side-view image. A plane mirror is placed beside the acquisition plane to reflect the side-view image into the CCD camera. This plane mirror needs to be finely tuned beforehand to assure the side-view image acquisition.

For the environmental setting in the tongue imaging device, first, in order to reduce the influence of the illumination of where the device is placed, all modules were put inside a nearly closed chest. Only a small acquisition window was left for image acquisition. The dimension of the window was 150 × 100 mm. Furthermore, to avoid the impact of uneven reflection caused by the interior wall,

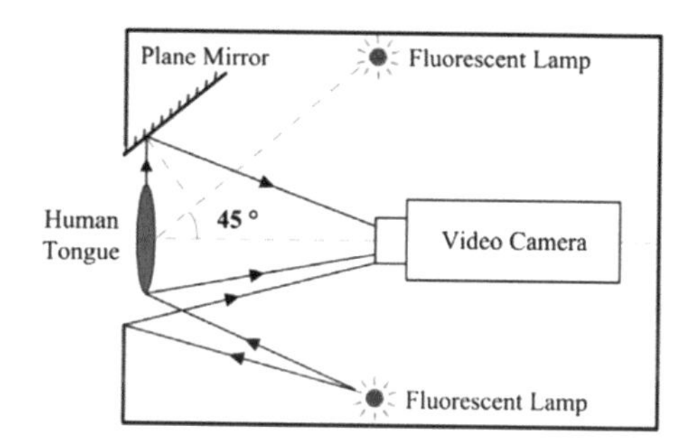

Fig. 2.8 Optical path of the proposed tongue imaging system (*top view*). Reprinted from Wang and Zhang (2013b), with permission from Elsevier

the inside wall was painted with neutral matte grey materials, and thereby the acquired tongue images were robust to illumination variations.

2.3.3 *Imaging Camera*

As Table 2.2 shows, the camera is critical for accurate color and texture rendering. On one hand, its resolution should be high enough to distinguish the smallest texture styles in order to provide images with enough clarity for medical analysis. Additionally, the camera should have a remarkable color rendering capability in order to obtain and classify complex tongue colors. This section will describe how these parameters (resolution and color rendering capability) of an imaging camera were established.

The most important issue for imaging camera selection is to decide what minimum resolution it should have in order to render tongue images with ample clarity. Table 2.1 shows existing utilized cameras with various resolutions, and usually the higher the resolution, the better the tongue texture features. However, the more pixels a tongue image contain, the more computational and storage cost is needed. Thus to discover the minimum resolution for tongue image rendering which is enough to describe the smallest texture feature is essential.

According to oral anatomy (Li, 2011), tongue texture is typically formed by different types of papillae which are microscopic structures on the upper surface of the tongue. As Fig. 2.9 shows, there are four types of papillae presented in a human tongue: filiform, fungiform, foliate, and circumvallate papillae. Among these four kinds of papillae, filiform papillae are the smallest with a dimension around 1–3 mm. Thereby, if the smallest filiform papillae can be distinguished by the imaging camera, all texture styles can be clearly classified.

Suppose the diameter of the smallest filiform papillae is only 1 mm, and there are 3 pixels for each single filiform papilla on average. The resolution would be:

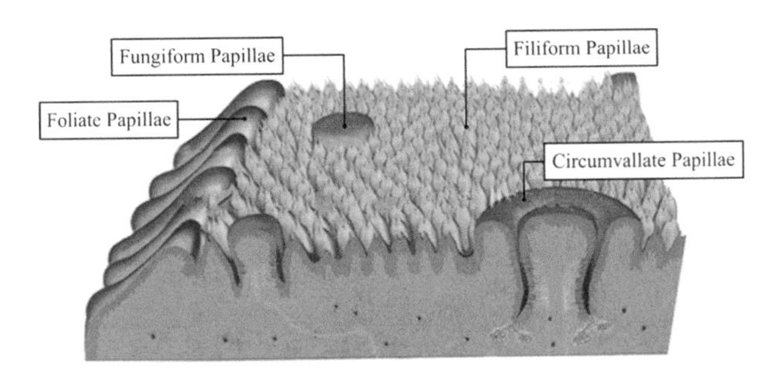

Fig. 2.9 Four types of papillae present in the tongue body which form various kinds of texture types. Reprinted from Wang and Zhang (2013b), with permission from Elsevier

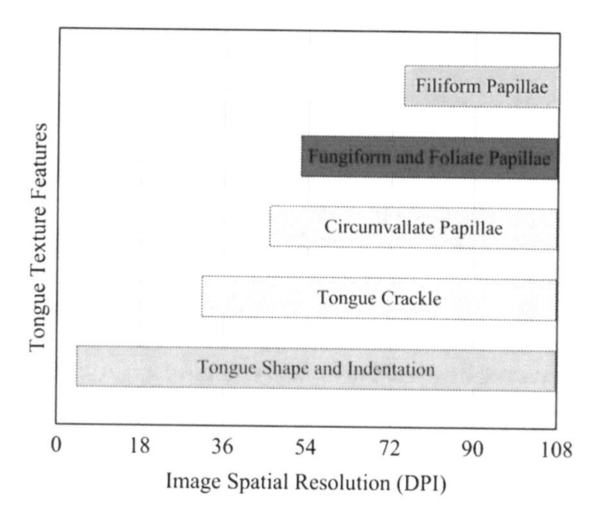

Fig. 2.10 Resolution to ensure sharp tongue texture rendering. The *horizontal axis* represents different imaging resolutions. Each kind of texture can be clearly recorded only when the image resolution reaches the minimum demand. For example, if the image resolution is larger than 30 pixels/in., tongue crackle can be rendered with sufficient clarity. Reprinted from Wang and Zhang (2013b), with permission from Elsevier

$$\mathrm{dpi} = \mathrm{dot}/\mathrm{inch} = 3/(1/25.4) \approx 76 \tag{2.2}$$

In the same way, resolution requirements to clearly render other texture styles can also be achieved, and are presented in Fig. 2.10. When the resolution of the chosen imaging camera is larger than the minimum resolution of 76, all texture styles can be clearly quantized for image analysis.

One more consideration for imaging camera selection is to choose a three-CCD (Charge Coupled Device) camera or a single-CCD camera. A three-CCD camera uses three separate CCDs for the measurement of the three primary colors: red, green, and blue. Generally, it can achieve much better precision and provide superior image quality than a single-CCD camera. As tongue color features plays a crucial role in image analysis for medical application, we need to select three-CCD cameras to acquire high quality tongue images.

Another prominent concern of camera selection is to choose a video camera or a still camera. The tongue is an organ which slightly vibrates all the time. Motion blur is usually observed if a digital still camera is used. Therefore, a video camera is more suitable in order to avoid this situation. Also, using a video camera can overcome other drawbacks of still cameras such as unstable illumination and inconsistent exposure degree. Figure 1.8 shows defective images captured by digital still cameras.

According to the above analysis, a three-CCD video camera, Sony DXC 390P, was selected as the tongue imaging camera. This camera is a high-end industrial camera which can acquire 25 images per second. Its spatial resolution is 768 × 568 pixels. As the size of a human tongue is generally less than 100 × 80 mm, and the field of view in our system is set to 150 × 120 mm, the resolution of our system is around 130 pixels/inch, which is large enough to ensure a clear recording of tongue images.

2.3.4 Color Correction

Color images produced by digital cameras suffer from device-dependent color space rendering, i.e., generated color information is dependent on the imaging characteristics of specific cameras. Furthermore, there are usually noises over the color images due to slight variations of the illumination. Therefore, in order to render the color image in a high-quality way, color correction is necessary for accurate image acquisition and is often regarded as a prerequisite before further image analysis.

The color correction process usually involves deriving a transformation between the device-dependent camera RGB values and device-independent color space attributes by the aid of several reference target samples (Munsell colorchecker 24 as Fig. 2.11b shows or tongue colorchecker (Wang & Zhang, 2013a). In our proposed algorithm, the standard RGB (sRGB) color space was chosen as the target device-independent color space because of its distinctive characteristics such as it is commonly used and has a constant relationship with CIELAB to calculate the color difference. Then, as Fig. 2.11a shows, parameters of the correction model were trained by matching color values of the colorchecker from the source device-dependent RGB color space to the device-independent sRGB color space. Finally, this derived correction model was applied on captured tongue images. A polynomial transform-based color correction algorithm was proposed in this system (Wang & Zhang, 2010). The principle of this algorithm is as follows: Suppose that the reference colorchecker has N color patches. For each patch, its quantized color values generated by digital camera can be represented as a vector V: (R_i, G_i, B_i) $(i = 1, 2, \ldots, 24)$, and the corresponding device independent sRGB tri-stimulus values are S: (SR_i, SG_i, SB_i) $(i = 1, 2, \ldots, 24)$. The idea of the polynomial transform based correction algorithm is to map the matrix generated by combining different polynomial terms of the input vector to the objective sRGB vector and thereby obtain the transformation model. For example, if we use the combination of polynomial x: $[R, G, B, 1]$, the transformation model can be represented as follows:

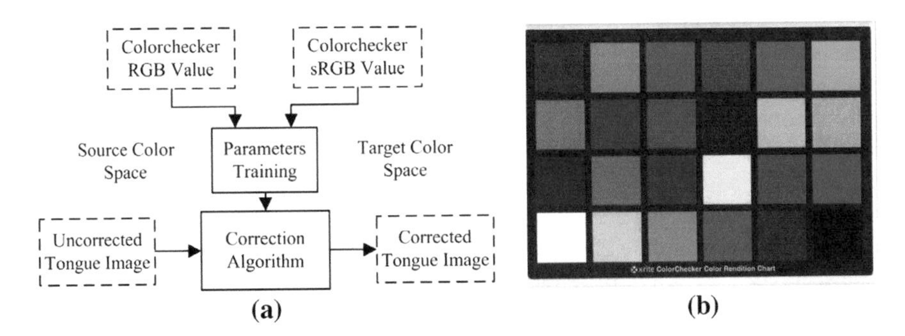

Fig. 2.11 Color correction on tongue images, **a** procedure of the color correction algorithm and **b** Munsell colorchecker 24 was utilized as the reference target for color correction. Reprinted from Wang and Zhang (2013b), with permission from Elsevier

$$\begin{cases} SR_i = a_{11}R_i + a_{12}G_i + a_{13}B_i + a_{14} \\ SG_i = a_{21}R_i + a_{22}G_i + a_{23}B_i + a_{24} \\ SB_i = a_{31}R_i + a_{32}G_i + a_{33}B_i + a_{34} \end{cases} \quad (i = 1, 2, \ldots, 24). \tag{2.3}$$

This equation can also be rewritten in matrix format as

$$\mathbf{S} = \mathbf{A}^{\mathbf{T}} \cdot \mathbf{X} \tag{2.4}$$

where $\boldsymbol{A}$ is the mapping coefficient matrix and $\boldsymbol{X}$ is the matrix generated by different polynomial combinations x. Using the least-square regression method, the solution to (2.4) is as follows:

$$\mathbf{A} = \left(\mathbf{X}^{\mathbf{T}}\mathbf{X}\right)^{-1}\mathbf{X}^{\mathbf{T}}\mathbf{S} \tag{2.5}$$

We can further apply this transform coefficient matrix $\boldsymbol{A}$ to correct tongue images. Suppose the generated polynomial matrix $\boldsymbol{X}$ for tongue image is $\boldsymbol{X}_{\text{in}}$, then the output image matrix $\boldsymbol{X}_{\text{out}}$ is:

$$\mathbf{X} = \mathbf{A} \cdot \mathbf{X}_{\text{in}} \tag{2.6}$$

By comparing different polynomial combinations which have different numbers of polynomial terms, a polynomial which involves 11 terms x: [R, G, B, RG, RB, GB, R, G_2, B_2, RGB, 1] was employed to train parameters of the correction model based on corresponding attributes of the Munsell colorchecker. This derived correction model was then used on acquired tongue images to render them into a device-independent sRGB color space. Moreover, variations of captured tongue images caused by imaging system components were greatly reduced. Experimental result shows that the CIELAB color difference [calculated as (2.7)] between the estimated values with target ground truth values of the Munsell colorchecker was less than 5 ($\Delta E^*_{ab} < 5$).

$$\Delta E^*_{ab} = \sqrt{\left(L^*_1 - L^*_2\right)^2 + \left(a^*_1 - a^*_2\right)^2 + \left(b^*_1 - b^*_2\right)^2} \tag{2.7}$$

2.3.5 System Implementation and Calibration

As the four core modules were designed in the above sections, this subsection discusses how these modules were implemented together to realize a user-friendly image collection. Also, in order to improve the accuracy and reproducibility of the system, we also illustrate the calibration procedure before it is applied in practice.

In order to make the acquisition procedure user-friendly, several ergonomic concerns have been taken into account. Figure 2.12a shows the appearance of the

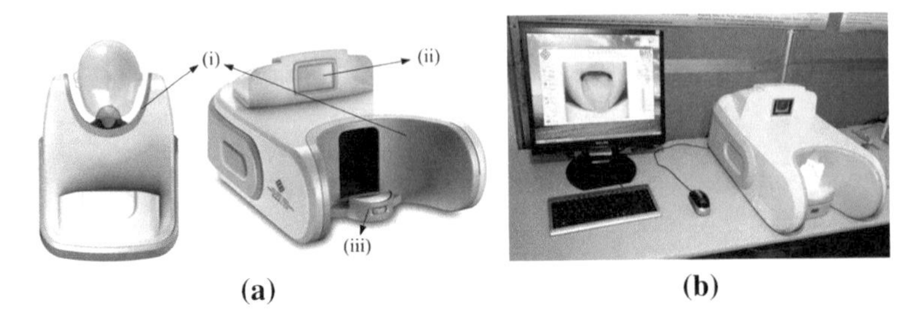

Fig. 2.12 Appearance of the tongue imaging system **a** appearance design and **b** working image of the tongue imaging device. Reprinted from Wang and Zhang (2013b), with permission from Elsevier

tongue imaging system. In order to reduce as much as possible the influence of the environmental illumination, an acquisition interface which perfectly fits the human head model was designed (as (i) in Fig. 2.12a). Furthermore, a small monitor (ii in Fig. 2.12a) was placed at the top of the device to guide users putting their tongue in the appropriate place. Also, a chin rest (iii in Fig. 2.12a) which can hold the user's chin to make them feel comfortable was also added in this device. The working image of this device is shown in Fig. 2.12b. The total dimension of this tongue device is 506 $\times$ 370 $\times$ 307 mm, and the working distance between the acquisition plane to the camera is 140 mm.

System calibration, which is the process of adjusting a system's accuracy to ensure it is within the designer's specifications, is essential to reduce the measurement uncertainty and improve the quality and consistency of a measurement system. In our system, the system calibration was accomplished through three consecutive steps, which, in sequential order, are the determination of the camera lens aperture, the camera color balance, and the color correction transformation from the device-dependent imaging system space to the device-dependent sRGB space. The aim of all steps is to maximize the accuracy and reproducibility of the imaging system.

2.3.5.1 Camera Lens Aperture

The apertures of a camera lens need to be fixed to avoid overexposure. Usually, it is achieved by setting the camera response to the largest value of 255 for a perfectly reflecting object (white board). In our system, the White Balance ColorChecker (X-rite, Inc., USA) was first imaged by the system, and then, the average value of G channel ($\langle G \rangle$) of a single or a group of pixels in the acquired images was checked. If it was lower than 255, the aperture needed to be enlarged, otherwise, it needed to be narrowed. In sum, the goal is to let the value of the G channel be equal to or close to 255 ($\langle G \rangle = 255$). Actually, to avoid overexposure, this number was set to 254 in practice. This step was executed only one time before the first use of this device, and thereafter this aperture needs to be locked to save the setting. Also, if possible, this step needs to be re-executed over a period of time (such as 4 weeks or longer) to avoid fluctuation.

2.3.5.2 Camera Color Balance

Usually due to slight variations among the three CCDs, responses of each color channel for a neutral object would be different from others, and this kind of internal systematic error needs to be reduced beforehand. Therefore, the aim of color balance is to ensure that the camera response is equal on its three channels (R, G, and B) for a perfectly neutral object (X-rite Gray Balance ColorChecker in this system). In a real case, the gray colorchecker is first imaged, and then, the offset for each channel is adjusted to ensure $(R) = (G) = (B)$. In our proposed system, the imaging camera was equipped with a 10-bit digital signal processor (DSP), and thus this offset adjustment could be directly conducted and saved. This procedure only needs to be executed once before the first use of this device, but it needs to be re-checked at regular intervals.

2.3.5.3 Color Correction Model

The proposed polynomial-based color correction algorithm was implemented into the built-in embedded system to correct every tongue image before it is saved into the database. The correction procedure is as follows. First, the Munsell colorchecker 24 was imaged by the camera to get the colorchecker image, then the 24 color values of these colorchecker image were automatically extracted by our implemented extraction program. This program can automatically extract the average value for each color patch. Finally, the color correction matrix was obtained by mapping these extracted 24 color values to their standard values (color attributed in sRGB colors space). This derived correction model was saved in the embedded system and applied for correction of all acquired tongue images in the same session. Also, it is only valid for one session and needs to be executed every time before the system is rebooted or reused.

2.4 Performance Analysis

The proposed system was tested in terms of three aspects: illumination uniformity, accuracy which measures the quality of the acquired image, and consistency which measures the precision or reproducibility among different capture sessions or different devices. These performance analysis results are presented as follows.

2.4.1 *Illumination Uniformity*

Illumination uniformity, which is used to measure the relationship of the spatial distribution of illuminance across the working area, is important for high-quality image rendering (Rea, 2000). Poor uniformity, especially shadows, may distort the visual perception of objects. Based on the statistical analysis of the distribution of illumination, there are several definitions that express uniformity, and the most common one is the min–max ratio (U_1):

$$U_1 = E_{\min}/E_{\max} \tag{2.8}$$

where $E_{\min}$ and $E_{\max}$ are the minimum and maximum illuminance. Another popular one is the contrast ratio: $U_2 = (E_{\max} - E_{\min})/(E_{\max} + E_{\min})$. Additionally, several metrics based on statistics were also proposed, such as the minimum-average ratio: $U_3 = E_{\min}/\overline{E} = E_{\min}\left(\sum_{i=1}^{N} E_i/N\right)^{-1}$, and the ratio of the standard deviation to the mean (also known as coefficient of variation):

$$\mathrm{CV} = \sigma_E/\overline{E} = \left[\sum_{i=1}^{N} \left(E_i/\overline{E} - 1\right)^2/(N-1)\right]^{0.5} \tag{2.9}$$

where $\overline{E}$ and σ_E are the mean and standard deviation of the illuminance respectively.

In this experiment, the Munsell gray colorchecker was first imaged by the designed device, and then, intensity values of all pixels in this image were used to calculate the uniformity of illumination. Based on the above calculation formulas, the uniformity of our proposed imaging system was obtained as Table 2.3 shows. From this table, it can be seen that the min–max ratio was 0.8617. Compared to the minimum uniformity of the standard illumination condition recommended by ISO 3664 which is 0.75, this result shows that the uniformity in our system is much better than recommended the ISO standard. Moreover, the measurement of CV shows that the illuminant slightly changes across the acquisition plane because the standard deviation σ_E is very small. In sum, these results show that the developed device provides a uniform illuminance condition for tongue image acquisition.

Table 2.3 Illumination uniformity of the proposed imaging system

	U_1	U_2	U_3	CV
Uniformity	0.867	0.0743	0.9135	0.0641
Reference value	0.75			

Reprinted from Wang and Zhang (2013b), with permission from Elsevier

2.4.2 System Consistency

Consistency is the precision or the reproducibility of measurement, or the degree of repeated measurements that is close to the average of those measurements which are conducted under different conditions, such as at different time points, in different locations or by different imaging devices. According to various measurements conditions, different types of consistency can be distinguished: consecutive consistency (σ_1), intra-run consistency (σ_2), inter-run consistency (σ_3), and between-device consistency (σ_4). Consistency testing experiments are normally conducted based on a reference target such as a colorchecker which has fixed number of color patches. In this experiment, the Munsell colorchecker 24 (Mccamy, Marcus, & Davidson, 1976; X-Rite, 2012), which is regarded as the de facto standard for visual evaluation, was utilized as the reference object because of its popular usage. It was imaged many times under different conditions. Then, in order to quantitatively calculate the degree of consistency, the average CIE color difference between these 24 color values of the colorchecker was calculated according to (2.7).

Figure 2.13 shows an illustration of these four types of consistency. The consecutive consistency (σ_1) computes the average color difference among five images continuously acquitted within a short time interval (less than 10 s) at a specific time point. This metric describes the minimum difference produced by this device, and it thus can be regarded as a benchmark for the consistency measurement. The intra-run consistency (σ_2), also named as within-run consistency or precision, measures the difference among images acquired at different time points within a single acquisition session. In this experiment, images were captured at 6 different time points, i.e., 0, 1, 2, 3, 5, and 10 min after the system was started. A system needs to be stabilized before it can be applied in practice. Therefore, by computing the color difference among these 6 images, we could not only obtain the value of intra-run consistency but also find how long of this system needed to become stable. Also, by this measurement, we can also evaluate the influence of temperature

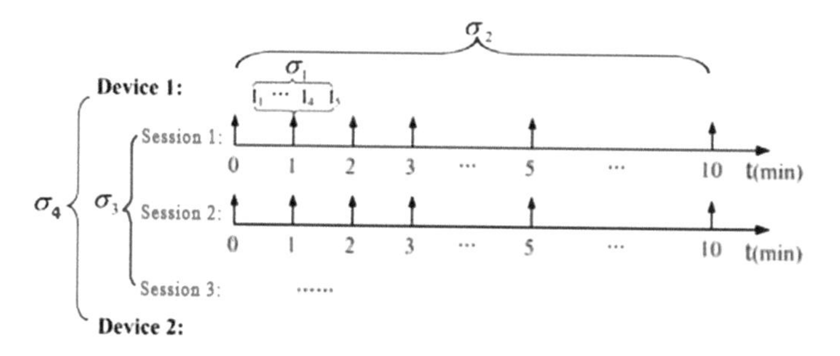

Fig. 2.13 Four kinds of consistency measurements, i.e., consecutive consistency (σ_1), intra-run consistency (σ_2), inter-run consistency (σ_3), and between-device consistency (σ_4). These four metrics are designed to describe the reproducibility of the imaging system

Table 2.4 Experimental result of consecutive consistency σ_1

Time point	t1	t2	t3	t4	t5	t6
Average $\Delta E^*_{ab} < 5$	0.5485	0.5886	0.4708	0.4365	0.4872	0.4343

variation when the system works. The inter-run consistency (σ_3), also named as between-run consistency, measures the degree of closeness among images captured from different capture session with the same imaging device. In order to test the repeatability of the system, especially the time durability, we captured three sessions of the Munsell colorchecker. The first session was captured after the system was just implemented (a brand-new system). Session 2 was conducted half a month after session 1, and images from session 3 were taken one year after the time of session 1. Finally, the between-device consistency (σ_4), shows the degree of reproducibility between two acquisition devices which have the same components and configuration.

2.4.2.1 Consecutive Consistency

Table 2.4 presents the results of consecutive consistency (σ_1) in session 1. We captured 5 images at each time point (t1–t6), and calculated the average color difference among them by first adding the color difference of all 24 color patches and then dividing by 24. From Table 2.4, it can be seen that σ_1 was around 0.4343–0.5886. At the beginning, after the device just started (t1 and t2), the color difference between continuously acquired tongue images was bigger than 0.5485. Then, when the device is stable, this number decreased and stabilized around 0.48. This result also shows that the minimum color difference produced by this developed imaging system was less than 0.5, which is almost indistinguishable by the human eye.

2.4.2.2 Intra-run Consistency

For the intra-run consistency (σ_2), the color difference among images from session 1 was calculated as an example. Also, in order to explore the main cause which leads to this kind of intra-run variation, the intensity difference between images captured from consecutive time points was also calculated to find if these two kinds of differences are correlated. In this experiment, the intensity difference between two colorchecker was obtained by calculating the absolute value of the lightness difference for the same neutral patch. We transferred the image from RGB color space to CIE LAB color space, and the difference on the L component represents the intensity difference. From Table 2.5, it can be seen that both the average color difference and intensity difference gradually decrease, i.e., from 2.6934 to 0.5331 and 3.4247 to 0.5141 respectively. What is more, the same decreasing trend can be

Table 2.5 Experimental result of the intra-run consistency (σ_2)

	t2–t1	t3–t2	t4–t3	t5–t4	t6–t5
Average $\Delta E^*_{ab} < 5$	2.6934	0.7294	0.5465	0.5597	0.5331
Intensity difference	3.4247	0.3316	0.4314	0.3344	0.5141
Correlation coefficient	0.9918				

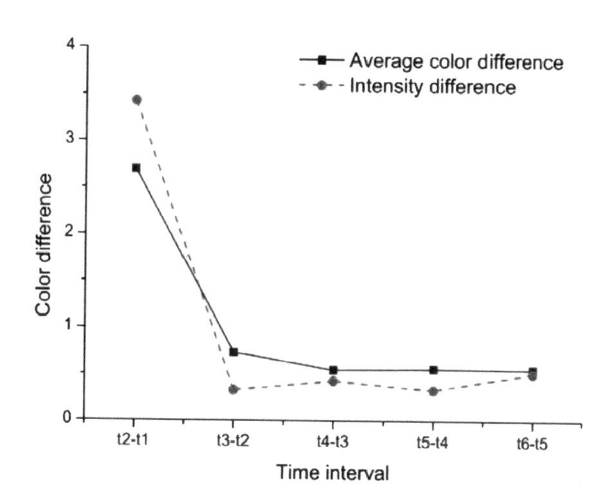

Fig. 2.14 Results of intra-run consistency. The color difference and intensity difference present a similar decreasing trend which illustrates they are highly correlated with each other. Reprinted from Wang and Zhang (2013b), with permission from Elsevier

noticed from Fig. 2.14. Values of color difference dropped dramatically during the first 1–2 min, and then they became stable at a specific level. Moreover, the result of the correlation coefficient which was 0.9918 also illustrates they are highly correlated with each other. From these results, the three findings can be summarized. First, the system needs to be stabilized before real acquisition, and this stabilization usually requires 1–2 min. Second, the intra-run consistency is around 0.55. Although it is larger than the consecutive consistency of 0.48, this color difference is still small enough to be ignored. Third, this kind of intra-run difference is possibly caused by the instability of illumination because the average color difference is highly correlated to the intensity variation (the correlation coefficient is 0.9918).

2.4.2.3 Inter-run Consistency

The inter-run consistency describes the closeness of images captured at different capture sessions. Ordinarily a session here means the time span between the system startup and shutdown. We captured images at three separate sessions after the system was completely stabilized. Session 1 was captured by a brand-new device, session 2 was obtained by the same device half a month later, while session 3 was nearly one year later. The same as for the analysis of intra-run consistency, both the

Table 2.6 Experimental result of the inter-run consistency (r3) among three separate sessions

	(s1, s2)	(s2, s3)	(s1, s3)
Average $\Delta E^*_{ab} < 5$	0.5034	0.5436	0.6389
Intensity difference	0.3956	0.5742	0.6698
Correlation coefficient	0.9196		

Reprinted from Wang and Zhang (2013b), with permission from Elsevier

average color difference and intensity difference are provided in Table 2.6. In this table, (s1, s2) represents the difference between images captured in session 1 and session 2. Surprisingly, it may be noted that the inter-run precision is almost of the same order of magnitude as the intra-run consistency, which is between 0.5034 and 0.6389. This result shows that the system is fairly stable in achieving high-consistent tongue image acquisition. Regarding the time durability, we found that there was no substantial difference among images captured at different times. Despite the fact that the (s1, s3) difference is larger than the other two cases, it is still very small and cannot be noticed by human inspection. This result shows that the device can retain high quality for a very long time. Also, if possible, more experiments need to be conducted to test color difference for a longer time such as two years or five years. The same as for the result of intra-run consistency, we found that this between-run difference is also closely related to intensity difference caused by the fluctuation of illumination because their correlation coefficient is 0.9405.

2.4.2.4 Between-Device Consistency

The above results show that a single well-calibrated imaging device can achieve highly consistent tongue image acquisition. Furthermore, the consistency among different devices which have the same imaging components and configuration, i.e., between-device precision or batch reproducibility, is also crucial for system performance. We developed two imaging systems according to our proposed specification. After calibration, these two devices were supposed to have the same image rendering ability. In this experiment, the same Munsell colorchecker 24 was first imaged by these two devices, and then the color difference was calculated to measure the between-device precision. We captured 5 groups of images for each of these two devices, and calculated color differences between them which are shown in Table 2.7. The results show that the difference between these two devices was between 1.0341 and 1.6532. Obviously, the between-device precision is larger than

Table 2.7 Experimental result of the between-device consistency (σ_4)

Group no.	1	2	3	4	5
Average $\Delta E^*_{ab} < 5$	1.2038	1.6532	1.5982	1.0341	1.3647

Reprinted from Wang and Zhang (2013b), with permission from Elsevier

its inter-device counterpart (including inter-run and intra-run consistency) which is around 0.5. A possible explanation for why the between-device variation is much larger is as follows. The inter-device variation is principally generated because of the fluctuation of illumination which belongs to random error, and this kind of random error cannot be completely eliminated. Moreover, in addition to the random error, another factor which makes the two devices different is the variance of imaging characteristic of the camera. Regardless of the fact that the calibration procedure may reduce this kind of disparity, it belongs to systematic error and cannot be fully eliminated.

2.4.3 Accuracy

Accuracy is the way in which the measurement made by the imaging system is close to its true value which is usually measured by other reference instruments. In this experiment, as the texture information is usually easily acquired in high fidelity, a test on accuracy of chromatic feature rendering was the main objective.

To quantify the accuracy of this imaging system, we computed the average and maximal CIE color difference $\Delta E^*_{ab} < 5$ over a test colorchecker, i.e., the Munsell colorchecker 24. Several colors of this chart were used as a reference target for model training in system calibration. We captured five images of this test colorchecker at different times when the system was stabilized. Table 2.8 shows the results of the accuracy test. It shows that the average color difference between the acquired image when its true value is smaller than 4, is unnoticeable to the human eye. Also, the maximum and minimum color differences show that variations among these 24 tested colors are minor, which illustrates that the imaging system can accurately render all colors.

2.4.4 Typical Tongue Images

The developed tongue imaging system has been utilized in practical image acquisition in a hospital for almost 3 years. Doctors of Traditional Chinese Medicine have also thoroughly evaluated this device during real applications. To date, a large and comprehensive tongue image database has been established. This database includes over 9000 images which were collected from 5222 subjects, in which over

Table 2.8 Accuracy test of the proposed imaging device

Test image no.	Average $\Delta E^*_{ab} < 5$	Max. $\Delta E^*_{ab} < 5$	Min. $\Delta E^*_{ab} < 5$
1	3.9079	8.1551	0.7959
2	3.8652	7.7201	1.1914
3	3.7873	8.2872	1.1385

Reprinted from Wang and Zhang (2013b), with permission from Elsevier

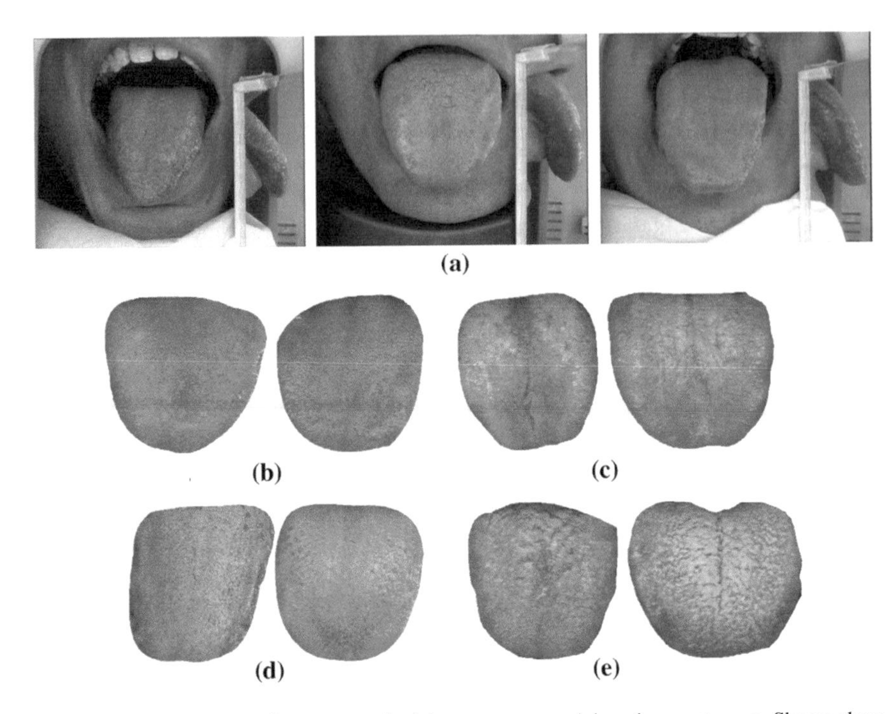

Fig. 2.15 Typical tongue images acquired by our proposed imaging system. **a** Shows three original images which contain side-view images. Other images are the pure tongue body which was extracted from background. They are in different health statuses, including: **b** healthy, **c** pneumonia, **d** chronic kidney disease, and **e** pancreatitis. The proposed system can faithfully render all kinds of colors, textures, and geometric features. Reprinted from Wang and Zhang (2013b), with permission from Elsevier

2780 subjects were patients in almost 200 disease types. Several typical images acquired by this developed system are shown in Fig. 2.15. Obviously, images with different health statuses have different chromatic and texture characteristics. For example, images from people with appendicitis (Fig. 2.15b) are commonly a deep red color and have a lot of red-points, and images from people with chronic kidney disease contain a lot of yellow color components. These obtained images have been applied to medical analysis of disease diagnosis, and preliminary results verify the effectiveness of this system. Furthermore, we are also planning to open this database to other researchers for academic usage in the future.

2.5 Summary

This chapter conducted a thorough and fundamental study on the development of an accurate and consistent tongue imaging device for computerized tongue image analysis. There are mainly two contributions of this study. First, a series of guidelines for a tongue imaging system design were presented. This is the first proposed design guideline in the research community, and it can even be regarded as a design standard because most of the proposed criteria were constructed by international standards on color imaging technology. Second, a new tongue imaging system was presented in this work, and several components were first designed in this system, such as the plane mirror to capture the side-view image, the embedded system to enhance the mobility, and the minimum resolution of a CCD camera for tongue imaging.

Compared to existing devices, this proposed system is more accurate and stable. By following the guideline, all system components have been optimally designed, and hence all possible medical clues including the tongue width can be acquired by this device in high quality. Moreover, with the help of the implemented embedded system, this device is more convenient and portable. This would grant the system a wider and deeper utilization in real computerized tongue diagnosis applications. Unlike other existing devices, this developed system was completely tested for its accuracy and consistency before it was applied in practice. Test results show that captured images remain stable when acquisition is repeated at different time points or by different devices. The biggest observed color difference ($\Delta E^{*}_{ab} < 5$) between two images acquired by two devices is 1.6532, which is hard to be distinguished by the human eye. Besides these kinds of performance evaluation, the proposed system has been utilized to capture over 9000 tongue images in the hospital, and preliminary analysis results also validate the effectiveness and advantages of this system.

Theoretically speaking, all elements in this device have been optimally designed, and an implemented device following these design criteria should have similar high quality.

References

Cai, Y. (2002). A novel imaging system for tongue inspection (pp. 159–164). IEEE, 1999.

Chiu, C. (2000). A novel approach based on computerized image analysis for traditional Chinese medical diagnosis of the tongue. *Computer Methods and Programs in Biomedicine, 61*(2), 77–89.

Du, H., Liu, Z., Li, Q., Yan, J., & Tang, Q. (2007). A novel hyperspectral medical sensor for tongue diagnosis. *Sensor Review, 27*(1), 57–60.

He, Y., Liu, C., & Shen, L. (2007). Digital camera based tongue manifestation acquisition platform. *World Science and Technology-Modernization of Traditional Chinese Medicine and Materia Medica, 5.*

Huang, B., Wu, J., Zhang, D., & Li, N. (2010). Tongue shape classification by geometric features. *Information Sciences, 180*(2), 312–324.

ISO. (2009). Graphic technology and photography—Viewing conditions.

Jang, J. H., Kim, J. E., Park, K. M., Park, S. O., Chang, Y. S., & Kim, B. Y. (2002). Development of the digital tongue inspection system with image analysis (pp. 1033–1034). IEEE.

Jiang, Y. W., Chen, J. Z., & Zhang, H. H. (2000). Computerized system of diagnosis of tongue in Traditional Chinese Medicine. *Chinese Journal of Integrated Traditional and Western Medicine, 20*(2), 145–147.

Li, N. (2011). *Tongue diagnostics*. Cambridge: Academy Press.

Li, Q., & Liu, Z. (2009). Tongue color analysis and discrimination based on hyperspectral images. *Computerized Medical Imaging and Graphics, 33*(3), 217–221.

Li, Q., Wang, Y., Liu, H., & Sun, Z. (2010). AOTF based hyperspectral tongue imaging system and its applications in computer-aided tongue disease diagnosis (pp. 1424–1427).

Li, Q., Wang, Y., Liu, H., Sun, Z., & Liu, Z. (2010b). Tongue fissure extraction and classification using hyperspectral imaging technology. *Applied Optics, 49*(11), 2006–2013.

Maciocia, G. (1987). *Tongue diagnosis in Chinese medicine*. Seattle: Eastland Press.

Maciocia, G. (2013). *Diagnosis in Chinese medicine: A comprehensive guide*. Amsterdam: Elsevier Health Sciences.

Mccamy, C. S., Marcus, H., & Davidson, J. G. (1976). A color-rendition Chart. *Journal of Applied Photographic Engineering, 2*, 95–99.

Pang, B., Zhang, D., Li, N., & Wang, K. 2004. Computerized tongue diagnosis based on Bayesian networks. *IEEE Transactions on Biomedical Engineering, 51*(10), 1803–1810.

Rea, B. M., & Ed. (2000). *Iesna lighting handbook* (9th ed.). Illuminating engineering society of north america.

Wang, X., & Zhang, D. (2010). An optimized tongue image color correction scheme. *IEEE Transactions on Information Technology in Biomedicine, 14*(6), 1355–1364.

Wang, X., & Zhang, D. (2013a). A new tongue colorchecker design by space representation for precise correction. *IEEE Journal of Biomedical and Health Informatics, 17*(2), 381–391.

Wang, X., & Zhang, D. (2013b). A high quality color imaging system for computerized tongue image analysis. *Expert Systems with Applications, 40*(15), 5854–5866.

Wang, Y., Zhou, Y., Yang, J., & Xu, Q. (2004). An image analysis system for tongue diagnosis in traditional Chinese medicine. In *Computational and information science* (pp. 1181–1186). Berlin: Springer.

Wei, B. G., Shen, L. S., Wang, Y. Q., Wang, Y. G., Wang, A. M. & Zhao, Z. X. (2002). A digital tongue image analysis instrument for Traditional Chinese Medicine. *Chinese Journal of Medical Instrumentation* [*Zhongguo yi liao qi xie za zhi*], *26*(3), 164–166.

Wong, W., & Huang, S. (2001). Studies on externalization of application of tongue inspection of TCM. *Engineering Science, 3*(1), 78–82.

X-Rite. (2012). Munsell ColorChecker Classic.

Zhang, H. Z., Wang, K. Q., Zhang, D., Pang, B., & Huang, B. (2005). *Computer aided tongue diagnosis system* (pp. 6754–6757). IEEE.

Part II
Tongue Image Segmentation and Shape Classification

Chapter 3
Tongue Image Segmentation by Bi-elliptical Deformable Contour

Abstract Automated tongue image segmentation, in Chinese medicine, is difficult due to two special factors: (1) there are many pathological details on the surface of the tongue, which have a large influence on edge extraction, and (2) the shapes of the tongue bodies captured from various persons (with different diseases) are quite different, so it is impossible to properly describe them using a predefined deformable template. To address these problems, in this chapter we propose an original technique that is based on a combination of a bi-elliptical deformable template (BEDT) and an active contour model: the bi-elliptical deformable contour (BEDC). The BEDT captures gross shape features using the steepest decent method on its energy function in the parameter space. The BEDC is derived from the BEDT by substituting template forces for classical internal forces, and can deform to fit local details. Our algorithm features the fully automatic interpretation of tongue images and a consistent combination of global and local controls via the template force. We applied the BEDC to a large set of clinical tongue images and present experimental results.

3.1 Introduction

Tongue images can be captured using a specific set of image acquisition devices, including an advanced kernel camera and its corresponding lighting system. A tongue image sample obtained using our device is shown in Fig. 3.1a. Before the process of tongue classification, an exact region of the tongue must be extracted from an image, which almost always includes lips, parts of the face or the teeth. Due to the fragmentary weakness of the tongue's edge and the pathological details on the surface of the tongue, traditional low-level image processing techniques, such as region growing and general edge detection, fail to segment the tongue from its surroundings, as shown in Fig. 3.1b. The reason for this failure is that those methods do not properly take the shape into account, which is an essential feature in such a task.

A model-based segmentation scheme, used in concert with image preprocessing, can overcome many of these limitations, but such a scheme is not a panacea. Due to

D. Zhang et al., *Tongue Image Analysis*, DOI 10.1007/978-981-10-2167-1_3

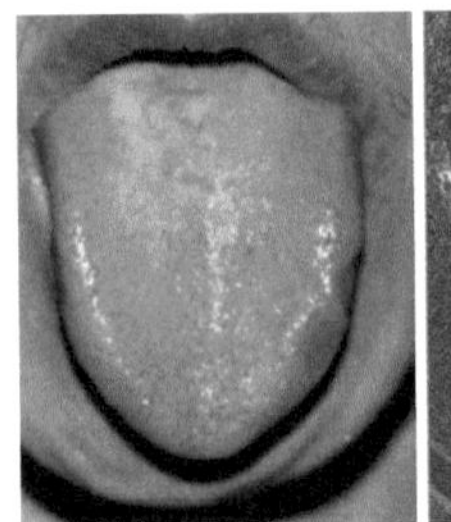
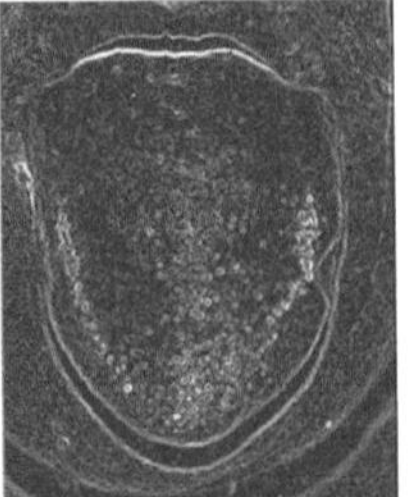

Fig. 3.1 A tongue image sample in our database and the image-enhancing result. **a** A tongue image from a patient suffering pancreatitis, and **b** its enhanced result using the Sobel operator.

shape deformation and variation within object classes, the use of rigid templates, a typical model-based method, cannot in general produce satisfactory results. This realization has led to the use of deformable shape models in image segmentation.

Among model-based techniques, deformable models (McInerney & Terzopoulos, 1996) offer a unique and powerful approach to image analysis that combines geometry, physics, and approximation theory. They exploit (bottom-up) constraints derived from the image data together with (top-down) a priori knowledge about the location, size, and shape of these structures. Deformable models are capable of accommodating the significant variability of biological structures over time and across different individuals.

Active contour models (ACM) or Snakes (Kass, Witkin, & Terzopoulos, 1988), as one of the most important classes of deformable shape models, are a sophisticated method for contour extraction and image interpretation. They advocate the view that the presence of an edge depends not only on the gradient at a specific point, but also on the spatial distribution. Snakes incorporate this global view of edge detection by assessing continuity and curvature combined with the local strength of an edge. The principal advantage of this approach over other feature extraction techniques is the integration of image data, an initial estimate of the contour, the desired contour properties, and knowledge-based constraints in a single extraction process.

Although powerful and effective, the original ACM techniques have their intrinsic limits. First, as a method tailored to semi-automatic applications, the initial contour of the ACM must, in general, be close to the true boundary or it will likely converge to an incorrect result. Second, during deformation, two undesirable effects may occur: shrinking of the contours of closed models due to internal forces, and clustering or gathering of vertices in the corners of a model due to the external forces. Third, in the presence of noise, ACM will find a lot of spurious edges, and in other words, the flexibility of the active contours becomes a drawback. Finally, ACM uses only the information from its local surroundings, and the information about the global shape is missing. Several methods (Cohen, 1991; McInerney & Terzopoulos, 1995; Gunn & Nixon, 1997; Lai & Chin, 1993; Lee, Hamza, & Krim, 2002; Lie & Chuang, 2001; Park, Schoepflin, & Kim, 2001; Caselles, Kimmel, & Sapiro, 1997) were proposed to address these problems, but they can compromise other aspects of performance.

The deformable template (DT) (Terzopoulos, 1980; Yuille, Hallinan, & Cohen, 1992; Cootes, Taylor, Cooper, & Graham, 1995; McInerney & Terzopoulos, 1996; Jain, Zhong, & Lakshmanan, 1996; Mardia, Qian, Shah, & de Souza, 1997; Scaggiante, Frezza, & Zampato, 1999; Hamarneh & Gustavsson, 2000; Valverde et al., 2001; Nikou, Bueno, Heitz, & Armspach, 2001; Joshi et al., 2002) matching scheme, on the other hand, provides an appealing solution to the segmentation tasks because of its capability to model an overall shape while accommodating shape variations. These deformable templates are specified by a set of parameters that enable a priori knowledge about the expected shape of the features to guide the detection process. The templates are flexible enough to be able to change their size, position, and orientation, so as to match themselves to the image data. The inclusion of object-specific knowledge in a model enables the template-based method to be much more robust to occlusion and noise with respect to local deformable models, such as snakes. However, these global templates can neither exercise local control along the contour nor represent local distortion, which results in the loss of possibly meaningful details, such as tooth marks along the rim of the body of the tongue that are used in TCM applications.

Deformable models based on super quadrics (Terzopoulos & Metaxas, 1990; Metaxas & Terzopoulos, 1993) are another example of deformable shape templates that can deform both locally and globally by incorporating the global shape parameters of a super ellipsoid with the local degrees of freedom of a membrane spline in a Lagrangian dynamics formulation. The model's (six) global deformation degrees of freedom capture gross shape features from visual data, while the local deformation parameters reconstruct the details of complex shapes that the global abstraction misses. As a general-purpose model, however, the deformable super quadrics seems too symmetrical to represent tongue shapes that usually take on a shape of "wider upside (the root of the tongue) and narrower downside (the tip of the tongue)."

Cootes et al. (1995) presented a statistically based technique for building deformable shape templates and used these models to segment various organs from medical images. The statistical parameterization provides global shape constraints and allows the model to deform only in ways implied by the training set. The shape models represent objects by sets of landmark points which are manually placed in the same way on an object boundary in each input image. Whereas the idea of restricted elastic deformation of an average shape model is very promising, the parameterization of shapes by displacement of corresponding points on their contours is not a convenient technique, especially for large training sets. Staib and Duncan (1992) cast the shape representation in the elliptic Fourier parameterization framework with probability distributions defined on the parameters of the representation, which biased the model toward an expected range of shapes. Boundary finding was formulated as an optimization problem using a maximum a posteriori objective function. Székely, Kelemen, Brechbühler, and Gerig (1996) combined the power of Fourier parameterization with statistical modal analysis. They proposed Fourier snakes, which are represented by a parameter vector describing the mean contour and by a set of Eigen modes of the parameters characterizing the shape variation. An elastic fit of the mean model in the subspace of Eigen modes restricts possible deformations. Basically, the assumption underlying these approaches is that at some representational level, biological structures have a similar topology and differ only in shape details. This is, however, far from the case for tongue representation, since the tongue is a flexible organ that usually takes on great variability of shape over time and across different individuals. Moreover, the Fourier snakes still requires manual displacement of albeit a small set of stable landmarks for each image under analysis, i.e., it is an interactive methodology.

In this chapter, we combine DT with ACM to solve these problems. First, a deformable template consisting of a double ellipse (bi-elliptical model) is proposed to model a tongue, which gives a rough description of the shape of the tongue body. This model interacts with the edge map, which is a preprocessed result obtained by convoluting the source image with an image-enhancement filter, in a dynamic manner by changing its parameters to alter the position, orientation, size, and other properties until the minimum of a predefined energy function is reached. Energy minimization is directly accomplished in the space of the parameters that are used to describe the bi-elliptical model. Then, the contour of the deformed model is properly sampled to obtain the best initial snake (from the fully automatic initialization point of view), called the bi-elliptical Deformable Contour (BEDC). Different from conventional snakes, the BEDC uses a brand-new term, called the template force, to replace the internal force. The main advantages of using the template force are (1) it can drive the model to locally deform in order to represent the details while maintaining a consideration for the global shape, and (2) the template force, by its nature, provides an effective solution to undesirable deformation effects of traditional snakes, such as shrinking and clustering. Finally, the BEDC can interpret tongue images in a totally automatic manner, which is essential for the automatic tongue diagnosis system.

3.2 Bi-elliptical Deformable Template for the Tongue

3.2.1 Definitions and Notations

In geometry, an ellipse is defined as a curve in a plane, which is composed of all points that are an equal total distance from two fixed points, termed the focuses (or foci). From this point of view, a circle can be viewed as a specific case of an ellipse with two superposed focuses. Therefore, an ellipse can be intuitively viewed as a circle that has been inflated or compressed by a ratio of b/r or a/r, respectively, along the horizontal or vertical axis, as shown in Fig. 3.2. This relationship can be directly derived from the regular equation of an ellipse as follows:

$$x^2/a^2 + y^2/b^2 = 1. \quad (3.1)$$

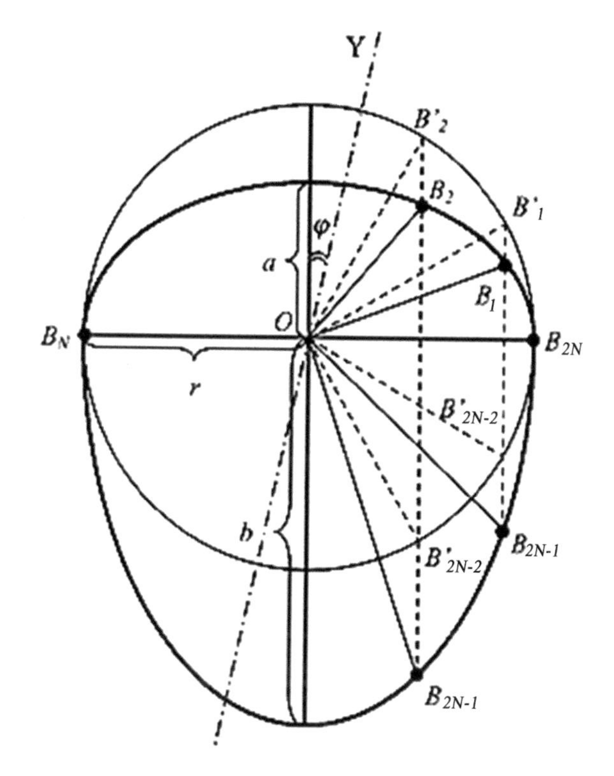

Fig. 3.2 Bi-elliptical tongue template (BEDT, drawn with a *bold line*) interpreted from the geometry point of view; and its root circle (with a *thin line*). © 2016 IEEE. Reprinted, with permission, from Pang et al. (2005)

Then, multiplying both sides by a^2 we obtain

$$x^2 + \left(\frac{y}{b/a}\right)^2 = a^2, \tag{3.2}$$

which can be viewed as the equation of a circle in an uneven space that is being stretched or contracted vertically (i.e., *y*-axis direction) by *b*/*a*. Thus, for each ellipse there is a corresponding circle, called a *root circle*, from which the ellipse originates. From this perspective, a root circle can be used to derive a sequence of ellipses by changing the ratio of compression or inflation along its two axes. Hereinafter, we use capital characters, such as "*A*" and "*B*," to denote nodes on an elliptical segment, and marked capital characters, such as "*A*′" and "*B*′" to denote points on the corresponding root circle.

3.2.2 The Tongue Template

Making use of the above-mentioned description of an ellipse, we present a specific deformable template for the tongue body, called the *Bi-Elliptical Deformable Template*

(BEDT, drawn with a bold line in Fig. 3.2). B_i, B_i (i = 1, 2, …, 2N) indicate nodes sampled on the boundary of the BEDT and their corresponding points on the root circle. It is composed of two elliptical segments—the upper semi-ellipse and lower semi-ellipse, corresponding to the upper and lower boundary of the tongue body, respectively. Both of these segments have an identical root circle, namely circle, O, shown in Fig. 3.2, but they have different ratios: α/γ for the upper arc and b/γ for the lower arc. Depending on the introduction of the root circle, the six parameters used to describe the template are defined as follows:

- The coordinates of the template center, (c_x, c_y), as the center of its root circle, namely point O.
- The length of the template radius, γ, as the radius of its root circle.
- The ratios, (γ_a, γ_b), as measurements of the lengths of the two vertical axes to γ.
- The angle, φ, as the template orientations that are represented. (For a better representation of the template, we use an oblique vertical axis of the coordinate system in Fig. 3.2.)

Using these parameters, each point, $\vec{x}(x, y)$, on the top arc of the template can be represented as

$$\begin{bmatrix} x \\ \hline y \end{bmatrix} = \begin{bmatrix} c_x \\ \hline c_y \end{bmatrix} + \mathrm{rot}(\varphi) \cdot \begin{bmatrix} r \cdot \cos\theta \\ \hline r \cdot \sin\theta \cdot r_a \end{bmatrix} \quad 0 \le \theta \le \pi \tag{3.3}$$

and each point, $\vec{x}(x', y')$, on the bottom boundary of the template can be represented as

$$\begin{bmatrix} x' \\ \hline y' \end{bmatrix} = \begin{bmatrix} c_x \\ \hline c_y \end{bmatrix} + \mathrm{rot}(\varphi) \cdot \begin{bmatrix} r \cdot \cos\theta \\ \hline r \cdot \sin\theta \cdot r_a \end{bmatrix} \quad 0 \le \theta \le 2\pi, \tag{3.4}$$

where θ is the angle between $\vec{x}$ and the positive direction of the horizontal axis, and $\mathrm{rot}(\varphi)$ is the rotation matrix

$$\mathrm{rot}(\varphi) = \begin{bmatrix} \cos\varphi, -\sin\varphi \\ \hline \sin\varphi, \cos\varphi \end{bmatrix}. \tag{3.5}$$

The six parameters are placed together in a vector, $p = (c_x, c_y, r, \gamma_a, \gamma_b, \varphi)$, which can be updated over time by minimizing an energy function that is defined later.

3.2.3 *Energy Function for the Tongue Template*

We now define the potential energy for the BEDT, which is a function of its parameter vector. The minimum of the energy function corresponds to the best fit with the interested features, namely the edges in our application. The parameters of the template can be updated by some rules. This corresponds to following a certain path in the parameter space of the model.

Different from the one used with a snake, such an energy minimizing framework has the positive effect of constraining the motion of every single point on a curve, in each iteration, to the motion of all the other points. The direct consequence is an improvement in the global behavior of the model, where the motion of every single point on a curve is only linked to that of adjacent points and to the local forces arising from the image.

Generally, the energy functions of a model can be divided into two parts: the internal energy and the external energy. The internal energy function stores a priori information about the feature to be extracted, which will take no effect here since the deformation is performed in the parameter space. The external energy function is chosen so that it has its minima on the high contrast regions in the image. Because edges consist of points with high contrast values, the energy will be minimal on those points. Given a gray-level image, *I(x, y)*, the external energy function of the tongue template is given by the following relationship:

$$\begin{gathered} E_{\text{ext}} = \frac{1}{\text{Length}} \int_{\text{Bi-elliptical-curve}} P(\vec{x}) \mathrm{d}s \quad , \\ P(\vec{x}) = -|\nabla I(X, Y)| \quad \text{or} \quad P(\vec{x}) = -|\nabla (G_\sigma * I(x, y)| \end{gathered} \tag{3.6}$$

where G_σ is a two-dimensional Gaussian function with standard deviation σ, ∇ is the gradient operator, and $p(\vec{x})$ is the external force field. It is easy to see from these definitions that larger values will cause the boundaries to become blurrier. Such large values are often necessary, however, to increase the capturable range of the template and reduce noise as well.

The external energy term can also be written as a function of the parameter values (regardless of the orientation parameter) as follows:

$$\begin{aligned} E_{\text{ext}} = & \frac{1}{L_a} \int_{\text{Upper-elliptic-curvd}} P\big(c_x + r \cdot \cos\theta, c_y + r \cdot \sin\theta \cdot r_a\big) \mathrm{d}s \\ & + \frac{1}{L_b} \int_{\text{Lower-elliptic-curve}} P\big(c_x + r \cdot \cos\theta, c_y + r \cdot \sin\theta \cdot r_a\big) \mathrm{d}s, \end{aligned} \tag{3.7}$$

where L_a and L_b correspond to the arc length of the upper and lower elliptical curves, respectively. Note that scale independence is achieved by dividing the curvilinear integrals by the arc length.

The parameters of the deformable template are computed over time by minimizing the energy function, E_{ext}, and by applying the Euler–Lagrange equations. In other words, the minimization is done using the steepest descent method on the energy function in the parameter space. Thus, the update rule of the parameter vector, P, is given by

$$\frac{d_p}{\mathrm{d}t} + \frac{\partial E_{\text{ext}}}{\partial_P} = 0. \tag{3.8}$$

To set up an iterative solution, let the curve be sampled on the variable, θ, as follows:

$$\theta \Rightarrow \theta_i = 2\pi \cdot i/2N. \tag{3.9}$$

It should be noted that θ is the sample step on the root circle of the template. Then, the external energy computed on the set of nodes (B_i, shown in Fig. 3.2) can be written as

$$E_{\text{ext}} = \frac{1}{2N}\sum_{i=1}^{2N} P(x_i, y_i). \tag{3.10}$$

Similarly, (3.7) can be rewritten as follows:

$$\begin{aligned} E_{\text{ext}} &= \frac{1}{N}\sum_{i=1}^{N} P(c_x + r \cdot \cos\theta_i, c_y + r \cdot \sin\theta_i \cdot \gamma_a) \\ &+ \frac{1}{N}\sum_{i=N+1}^{2N} P(c_x + r \cdot \cos\theta_i, c_y + r \cdot \sin\theta_i \cdot \gamma_a). \end{aligned} \tag{3.11}$$

Equation (3.8) evaluated on the set of nodes is

$$\begin{aligned} \frac{d_P}{\mathrm{d}t} &= -\frac{\partial E_{\text{ext}}}{\partial_p} = -\frac{\partial E_{\text{ext}}}{\partial_X} \cdot \frac{\partial_X}{\partial_P} \\ &= -\left(\frac{\partial E_{\text{ext}}}{\partial_X} \cdot \frac{\partial_X}{\partial_P} + \frac{\partial E_{\text{ext}}}{\partial_y} \cdot \frac{\partial_y}{\partial_P}\right) \\ &= -\frac{1}{2N}\sum_{i=1}^{2N}\left(\frac{\partial P(x_i, y_i)}{\partial_x} \cdot \frac{\partial_x}{\partial_p} + \frac{\partial P(x_i, y_i)}{\partial_y} \cdot \frac{\partial_y}{\partial_p}\right), \end{aligned} \tag{3.12}$$

where $X = (x, y)$.

To compute the p time derivatives and the partial derivatives of $P(x, y)$ along the curve, let the index n correspond to t and the time step for each iteration be Δt. Then, the required partial derivatives can be approximated:

$$
\begin{aligned}
P_t &= \frac{1}{\Delta t}\left(P^{n+1}P^{n}\right) \\
\frac{\partial P(x,y)}{\partial_x} &= \frac{P(x+1,y)-P(x-1,y)}{2} \\
\frac{\partial P(x,y)}{\partial_x} &= \frac{P(x,y+1)-P(x,y-1)}{2}.
\end{aligned}
\tag{3.13}
$$

The derivatives $\partial_x/\partial_{\mathbf{P}}$ and $\partial_y/\partial_{\mathbf{P}}$ can be obtained from (3.3) and (3.4), respectively. Finally, these equations give our iterative solution to the BEDT.

The iteration should be stopped when an energy minimum is reached. However, this could lead to the algorithm stopping prematurely due to a local minimum in the energy function, which is caused by noisy data. This problem can be overcome by allowing the algorithm to continue even though the value of the energy function is not decreasing. The stopping criteria may involve interrupting the algorithm if a lower value for the energy function is not found within a certain number of iterations. Simulated annealing (Storvik, 1994) and dynamic programming (Geiger, Gupta, & Costa, 1995) have also been proposed to reduce the problems caused by local minima. In practice, BEDTs always work well using the steepest decent method for the minimization of their energy functions, and we thus do not employ these methods here.

3.3 Combined Model for Tongue Segmentation

Although powerful and robust, the BEDT, as a global DT, has certain intrinsic limitations. For example, it is difficult to represent local details. Locally deformable models such as snakes, which are capable of performing local control along the track of the features, can be used to solve this problem. However, active contour models or snakes usually suffer difficulties in initialization and global shape representation. To address these problems, we intuitively combine the two models. First, we use the BEDT to obtain a rough description of the contour of the tongue body. After the minimum of the BEDT energy function is reached, the resultant contour is then resampled to obtain the best initialization for a subsequent snake (in a fully automated manner). To incorporate global shape constraints and shape information in the model, and to remove the unwanted contraction and clustering forces while retaining the local continuity and smoothness constraints, we introduce an original term called the *template force*, which replaces the conventional internal forces. Then, the dynamic contour model actively modifies its shape, under the influences of both the template force field and an external force field derived from some image feature energy distribution, until it enters a stationary state at the end.

3.3.1 Two Kinds of Template Forces

A traditional snake is a curve, $v(s) = [x(s), y(s)]$, $s \in [0, 1]$, which moves through the spatial domain of an image to minimize the energy function, that is

$$E = \int_0^1 (E_{\text{int}}(v(s)) + E_{\text{ext}}(v(s)))\mathrm{d}s, \tag{3.14}$$

where $E_{\text{int}}(v(s))$ are $E_{\text{ext}}(v(s))$ the internal and external energy functions, respectively, that can be formulated as

$$\begin{aligned} E_{\text{int}}(v(s)) &= \int_0^1 \left(\alpha|v'(s)|^2 + \beta|v''(s)|^2\right)\mathrm{d}s \\ E_{\text{ext}}(v(s)) &= r\int_0^1 P(v(s))\mathrm{d}s, \end{aligned} \tag{3.15}$$

where α and β are weighting parameters that control the snake's tension and rigidity, respectively, $P(v(s)) = P(x, y) = -|\nabla[G_\sigma * I(x, y)]|$ denotes a scalar potential function defined on the image plane, $I(x, y)$ and is a weighting parameter that controls the magnitude of the potential. It can be seen from (3.14) that when $|E_{\text{ext}}(v(s))|$ is small, the energy is dominated by the internal term, that is, the weighted sum of the squares of the first and second derivatives of $v(s)$. This is the origin of the snake's inherent contraction force.

To address this problem, we first sample the resultant contour of the BEDT on the variable, ψ, to obtain a set of nodes, A_i (i = 1,2, …, $2M$). It should be noted that ψ is the sample step on the root circle of the tongue template (drawn with a dashed line in Fig. 3.3). Then, all of the nodes are forced to move radially. That is, when driven by external and template forces, each node A_i will only change its position bi-directionally along the line, OA_i, instead of moving unconstrained in the force fields as the snake allows (Kass et al., 1988). Obviously, such a deformation constraint will remove the tangential shrinking force caused by the traditional internal forces.

To provide a definition for the template forces, we present a concept called "radius" for each node along the contour. Similar to the template radius defined in Sect. 3.2.2, the radius of a node is given by

$$R_i = x_i / \cos(i, \psi), \tag{3.16}$$

where x_i is the x-coordinate of node, A_i. It can be seen from (3.16) that all radiuses of the nodes are initially identical to the template radius, r, and they will take on

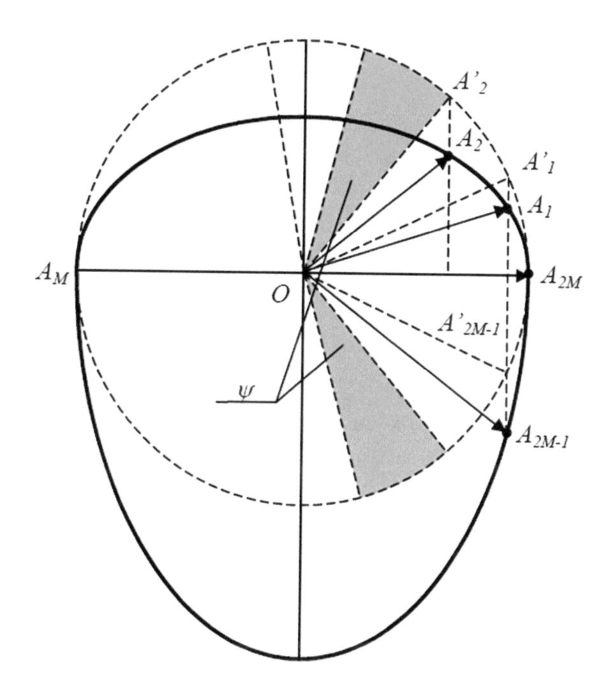

Fig. 3.3 Sampling rule for the combined model. A tongue template and its root circle are drawn in *bold* and *dashed lines*, respectively (sampling interval, ψ, is a constant angle on the root circle). A_i, A_i^r $(i = 1, 2, \ldots, 2M)$ denote nodes on the boundary of the BEDT and corresponding points on the root circle. © 2016 IEEE. Reprinted, with permission, from Pang et al. (2005)

various values as the contour modifies its shape. To describe the average dimensions of the deformable contour, we introduce a variable, R_{avg}, as follows:

$$R_{\text{avg}} = \frac{1}{2M} \sum_{i=1}^{2M} R_i. \tag{3.17}$$

3.3.1.1 Linear Template Force (LTF)

Similar to the rigidity term in the internal energy function in (3.15), the linear template energy can be written as follows:

$$E_{\text{tmp}}^{(1)} = \frac{1}{2M} \sum_{i=1}^{2M} \left(1 + \frac{\overrightarrow{A_iA_{i-1}} \cdot \overrightarrow{A_iA_{i+1}}}{\left| \overrightarrow{A_iA_{i-1}} \right| \cdot \overrightarrow{A_iA_{i+1}}} \right). \tag{3.18}$$

We wish to stress here that, in a global sense, a linear template force will exhibit concave potentials when applied to the energy minimization of a closed convex contour, thus it is also called the concave template force. Even with that restriction, a linear template force is extremely useful in many applications since it can exercise unbiased local control along the contour, which is a significant characteristic in the absence of a priori information about the shape.

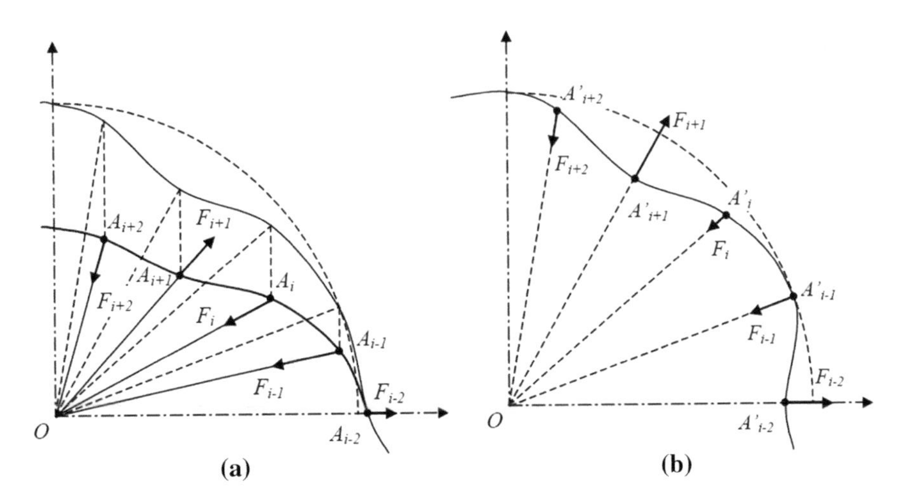

Fig. 3.4 Two kinds of the template force for the BEDC. **a** Linear template force and **b** elliptical template force. © 2016 IEEE. Reprinted, with permission, from Pang et al. (2005)

The linear template force, $\widehat{F}_{\text{tmp}-l}, i$, which is illustrated in Fig. 3.4a as F_i, is therefore formulated as

$$\widehat{F}_{\text{tmp}-l}, i = \left|\overrightarrow{OA_{i+1}} + \overrightarrow{OA_{i-1}} - \overrightarrow{2OA_i}\right| \hat{e}_i, \tag{3.19}$$

where $c_i > 0$ is the weighting parameter and $\hat{e}_i$ is the unit vector in the direction of $\overrightarrow{OA_i}$, as shown in Fig. 3.4a. In Fig. 3.4, the initial root circle is marked as a dashed line, an intermediate figure of the deformed root circle. The corresponding contour segment is a thin and bold line, respectively. Note that the contour segment of the BEDC is not drawn in (b) since elliptical template forces directly act on nodes along the root circle.

3.3.1.2 Elliptical Template Force (ETF)

The elliptical template energy is calculated by making use of a relationship between the length of the radiuses of each node and its adjacent neighbors, as follows:

$$E_{\text{tmp}}^{(2)} = \frac{1}{2M} \sum_{i=1}^{2M} \left| \frac{R_{i-1} + R_{i-1}}{2} - R_i \right|. \tag{3.20}$$

The corresponding elliptical template force, $\widehat{F}_{\text{tmp}-l}, i$, shown in Fig. 3.4b as F_i, can be written as

$$\widehat{F}_{\text{tmp}-e,i} = d_i |R_{i+1} + R_{i+1} - 2R_i| \hat{e}_i, \tag{3.21}$$

where $d_i > 0$ is the weighting coefficient, R_i is the radius [referring to (3.16)] and is the unit vector in the direction of $\overrightarrow{OA_i}$ as shown in Fig. 3.4b. Note that in (3.18)–(3.21), "−" and "+" in the subscripts are both operators modulo 1/2 M, and the factor 1/2 M is added to make the template energies independent of the number of sampled nodes along the contour.

Unlike the linear template force, the elliptical template force will drive the contour to take on a regular shape where the external force field is weak or zero. Furthermore, the final shape of the active contour in such a force field can be the BEDT itself provided there is no image data anywhere. Note that the way the elliptical template force acts on a node is indirect. In other words, it modifies the position of a node by changing the length of the radius of that node. A very important characteristic of the ETF is that, when it is combined with template constraints, the locally defined formulation can simultaneously represent the global shape and impose local control. Therefore, the elliptical template energy could have a special advantage if information about the shape is available.

3.3.2 Bi-elliptical Deformable Contours

We introduce a new snake, called the bi-elliptical Deformable Contours (BEDC), by replacing the internal energy term with the template energy functions defined in the previous section. The new active contour is defined as a set of mass-less nodes and is driven by both template and external forces that originate from the template and external potential energies, respectively. Shape constraints and information are incorporated into the term for the template forces. The discrete energy function of the BEDC can be written as

$$E^{(1)} = \frac{1}{2M} \sum_{i=1}^{2M} \left(\omega_{\text{ext}} P(x_i, y_i) + \omega_{\text{tmp}} \left(1 + \frac{\overrightarrow{A_iA_{i-1}} \cdot \overrightarrow{A_iA_{i+1}}}{\left|\overrightarrow{A_iA_{i-1}}\right| \cdot \left|\overrightarrow{A_iA_{i+1}}\right|} \right) \right) \tag{3.22}$$

or

$$E^{(2)} = \frac{1}{2M} \left(\sum_{i=1}^{2M} (\omega_{\text{ext}} P(x_i, y_i) + \omega_{\text{tmp}} \left| \frac{R_{i-1} + R_{i+1}}{2} \right| - R_i \right), \tag{3.23}$$

where $2M$ denotes the number of nodes sampled along the contour and $P(x_i, y_i)$ is the external force field defined in (3.6). The weighting factors, ω_{ext} and ω_{tmp}, control the trade-off between the external and template forces and may have default values for each application, but they allow modification by the operator. By emphasizing the external forces, one can make the model more precisely follow the extracted image features, whereas placing emphasis on the template forces will smooth out the path of the contour.

To eliminate the problem of shrinking in traditional snakes, we made some modifications to the term for the external forces. In fact, vertex displacement along the path of the contour model does not make any contribution to the deformation of the model and it is even a defect. Therefore, the external force $\widehat{F}_{\text{ext}}$ itself is not used, but instead it is decomposed into its local radial and tangential components, and only the local radial component is used to drive the vertices of the contour model. If we denote the local radial component of $\widehat{F}_{\text{ext},i}$ by $\widehat{F}_{\text{ext,ri}}$, it can be calculated as a dot product by

$$\widehat{F}_{\text{ext}} = \left(\widehat{F}_{\text{ext}},\ i \cdot \hat{e}_i\right)\hat{e}_i, \tag{3.24}$$

where is the unit vector in the local radial direction of the ellipse (for the linear template model in Fig. 3.4a) or the root circle (for the elliptical template model in Fig. 3.4b). The local radial forces, $\widehat{F}_{\text{ext,Ti}}$ and $\widehat{F}_{\text{tmp},i}$ $\widehat{F}_{\text{tmp}-l,i}$ or $\widehat{F}_{\text{tmp}-e,i,}$, provide a resulting driving force on a vertex of the contour model that is purely devoted to deformation of the model without moving the vertex along the path of the contour.

As a result of the forces that act on a vertex, this vertex will start to move and change its position until it enters an equilibrium position. Such a process will be performed for each node along the contour in a single iteration. When all nodes come to a resting position in the force field, the resultant contour gives the final solution. The actual deformation procedure is implemented as a so-called numerical time integration process in which the complete state of the contour model is calculated at a sequence of discrete positions in time.

3.3.2.1 Tongue Segmentation Algorithm

The overall approach for tongue segmentation is composed of two main procedures: minimization of the energy functions of the BEDT and BEDC, as illustrated in Fig. 3.5. Three main points should be emphasized. First, the calculations of both energy functions are based on a predefined *edge map*, $h(x, y)$, that is derived from a gray-level channel, $I(x, y)$, of a true color tongue image, which has the property that it is larger near the edges of the image. To make the external energy function take on its smallest values at the boundaries, we define the external force field as

$$P(x,y) = -h(x,y). \tag{3.25}$$

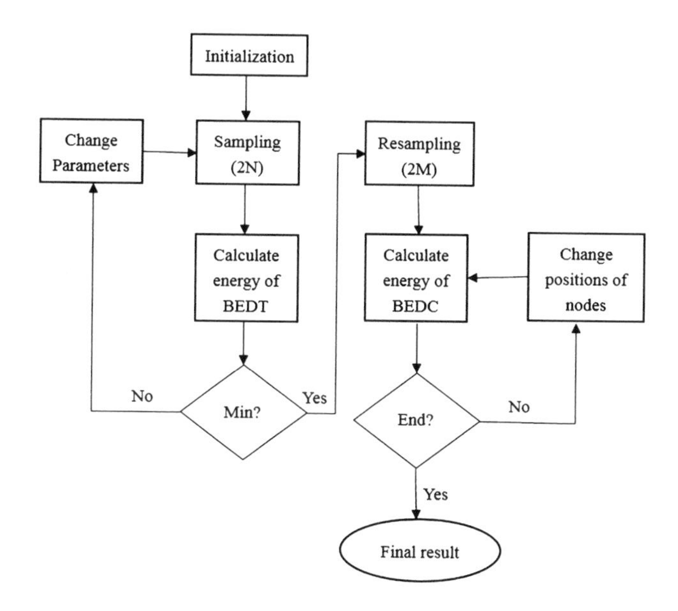

Fig. 3.5 Flowchart of the tongue segmentation procedure using the BEDC. © 2016 IEEE. Reprinted, with permission, from Pang et al. (2005)

Second, the external force fields for the BEDT and BEDC are actually different since they are calculated based on different levels in a scale space. It is the dissimilar purposes of the BEDT and BEDC that lead to such a difference. In fact, the BEDT is applied to roughly locate the boundary starting from an arbitrary initial position, which might be far from the true edges, in an edge map full of noise and fragmentary weakness. Therefore, for the BEDT, emphasis should be placed on the robustness and the relatively large capturable range. Accordingly, larger values of σ for edge-enhancing operators, such as the Laplacian of Gaussian operation, are usually used to compute the edge map, so as to remove the noise and enlarge the capturable range of the model. In contrast, the BEDC is used to refine the intermediate resultant contour, given by the BEDT, within a relatively small distance near the true boundary. In this case, a smaller value of σ is often employed to obtain better local control.

Finally, the sampling intervals in the BEDT and BEDC can also be different, and they are usually evaluated so that M>N. The reason for this is similar to that stated above: the intention of the BEDT process, performed in the parameter space, is to roughly locate the boundary. Thus, a reasonably small number of sampling points will be enough, and furthermore, it can significantly reduce the computation time. However, the BEDC process is used to represent local features, and consequently a relatively large number of sampling nodes could be more helpful.

3.4 Experiment Results and Analysis

We developed a prototype implementation of the described approach and applied the BEDC to a total of 3572 samples that were purposely chosen (for diagnosis) from our database, which contains over 12,000 clinical tongue images. In this section, we will present some useful results.

In the following experiments, we used the red channel of the original tongue image as the test sample, which is actually a gray-level image, so as to highlight the tongue domain because red is usually the dominant color within tongue body images. To compute the energy functions, we first need to calculate the edge map. The two possibilities are $h^{(1)}(x, y) = |\nabla I(x, y)|$ and $h^{(2)}(x, y) = \nabla(G_{\sigma}(x, y) * I(x, y))$, where the latter is more robust in the presence of noise and it can enlarge the capturable range of the models. Moreover, Gaussian filters with a time-varying standard deviation can be used to further improve the performance with respect to both stability and accuracy (Pang, Wang, & Zhang, 2000). Other more complicated noise-removal techniques, such as median filtering and morphological filtering, could also be applied to improve the underlying edge map. For all of the experiments, we used $\omega_{\text{ext}} = 1.0$ and $\omega_{\text{tmp}} = 0.8$.

The first example is illustrated in Fig. 3.6, which shows the results of applying the BEDC as well as original snakes to a real tongue image (640×480 pixels, each 24 bits). Because of the limited capturable range of traditional snakes, the initial contours (two connected parabolic segments shown with black-dashed lines in Fig. 3.6a, b) are placed near the real edge of the tongue body. We made a modification to both snakes. The parameters were evaluated as $\alpha > > \beta, \gamma$ [see (3.15)], which are the weighting parameters of the internal and external terms, respectively (Kass et al., 1988), so as to remove the shrinking force. It can be seen from Fig. 3.6a, b that, in both cases, the traditional snake failed to locate the real edges due to their flexibility and sensitivity to noises (pay attention to the upper resulting contour near the teeth in both figures, the first snake with a smaller beta value was entrapped into several spurious edges caused by reflecting points). The reason for the failure of a traditional snake is that there are lots of pathological details and glistening points on the tongue's surface. These details have turned into noise points when filtered by the edge-enhancing templates, as shown in Fig. 3.6f. In contrast, the initial contour for the BEDT can be set far from the true contour, as illustrated in Fig. 3.6c, since the search approach of the BEDT can provide a large capturable range. Thanks to its global control as the energy minimization progresses as it acts like a DT and its robustness to noise, the BEDT can give a rather good representation to the boundary of the tongue, as shown in Fig. 3.6d, without becoming entrapped in spurious edges. Finally, Fig. 3.6e shows the resulting contour using the BEDC that performs a posterior local refinement based on the resultant model. It is clear that the BEDC exhibits better performance than traditional snakes in dealing with noises.

Figure 3.7 illustrates the BEDC's capability for local control as compared with the DT method. In this example, the BEDT was first utilized to model the tongue

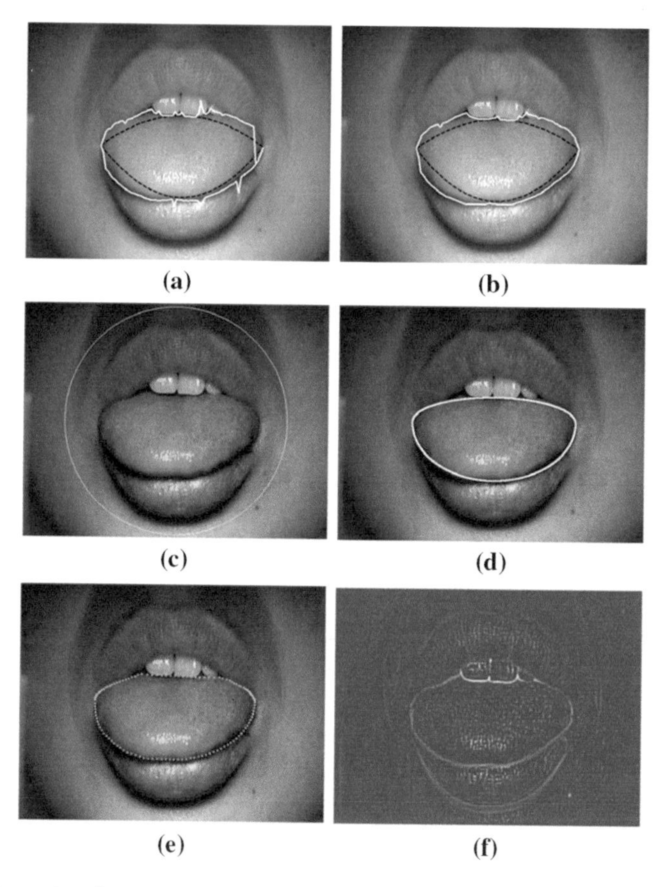

Fig. 3.6 Comparison between a snake and the BEDC. Edge extraction using a traditional snake with **a** $\beta = 0.2$ and **b** $\beta = 0.8$. **c** An initial contour for the BEDT. **d** The resulting template of the BEDT. **e** The final resulting contour using the BEDC. **f** An edge map, $|\nabla(G_\sigma * I|$, with $\sigma = 3$.

body. Different from any local models, such as snakes, deformable templates incorporate global shape information into their parameter vectors, and thus they have better stability in the presence of noise. However, they are usually only able to give a rough description of the features and they encounter difficulties in an exact local search, as shown in Fig. 3.7c, d, which means they are far from meeting the requirements for tongue diagnosis in Chinese medicine. The reasons can be explained as follows. First, tongues of different people always present a variety of different shapes as a result of dissimilar physiological structures. Even a series of captured sample images of the tongue from the same person can take on different shapes since the tongue is a movable apparatus. Therefore, no single predefined DT can model all of the possible shapes of tongue bodies. Second, the examination of

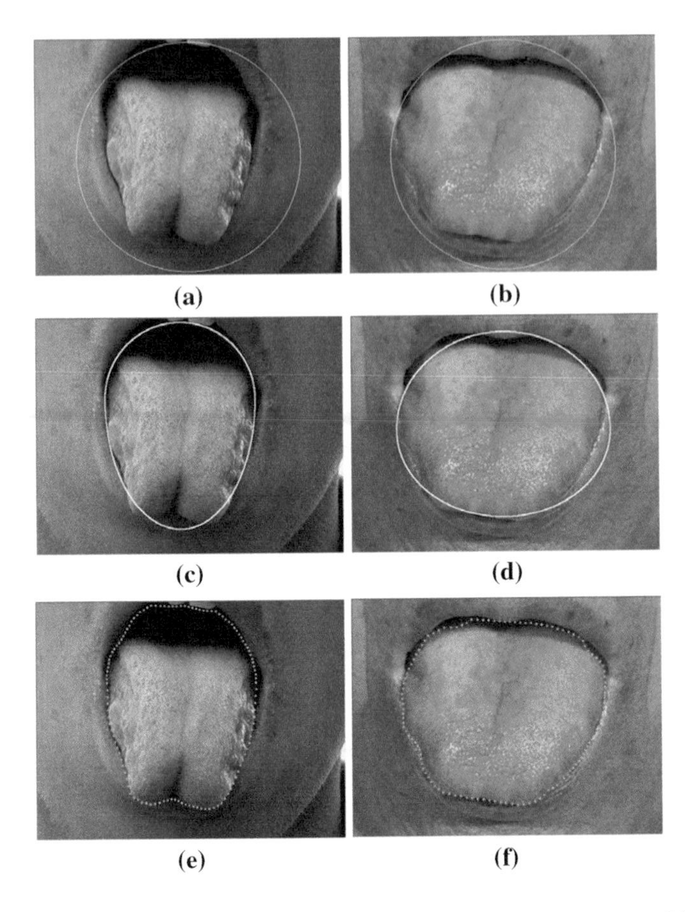

Fig. 3.7 Comparison between the DT and BEDC. **a** An initial curve on a captured image of a tongue with a long, deep vertical crack in the midline reaching to the tip. **b** An initial curve on a captured image of a partial swollen tongue on the half edge. **c**, **d** The intermediate contours obtained using the DT. **e**, **f** The final contours by applying the BEDC. © 2016 IEEE. Reprinted, with permission, from Pang et al. (2005)

the shape of the tongue body is one of the most important aspects of tongue diagnosis, where the physical contour of the tongue plays a significant role. Although many medical disorders generally appear as a variation in the shape of the tongue body, (such as thin or swollen, long or short, etc.) local distortions along the contour of the tongue, such as tooth marks and partial swelling (see Fig. 3.7b), are usually more meaningful hints for diagnosis.

Figure 3.7a, b presents two typical tongue bodies. One tongue has a long, deep vertical crack in the midline reaching to the tip, while the other is partially swollen on the right edge and is accompanied by light tooth marks. The resulting contours of these tongues are shown in Fig. 3.7e, f using a combined model that is composed of a BEDT and its derived BEDC. Both results clearly demonstrate the effective local control of our approach.

We next discuss the sensitivity of the final result to the shape of the initial contour. In other words, how reproducible is the result when we start from different initial contours? The following example demonstrates two significant advantages of the BEDC: insensitivity to the initial position of the contour and a large capturable range. Figure 3.8 shows the different initial contours (as solid pale lines) that were used in our experiments: (1) far outside the tongue's boundary [Fig. 3.8a], (2) inside the tongue's boundary (Fig. 3.8b), and (3) overlapping with the upper and lower edges of the tongue (Fig. 3.8c, d, respectively). In all cases, the traditional snake stops in a very undesirable configuration due to its limited capturable range and its poor robustness to noise (although the results are not shown here). In the model developed by Cohen (1991), potential forces are directly imposed on a snake, thus it may allow some partial segments of the contour to become trapped in spurious edges due to its flexibility. However, the BEDC utilizes a DT to search for the location of the tongue's boundary in the external potential force field so that a much better representation, from a global point of view, is obtained. It can be seen that the results do not depend strongly on the location of the initial contour, which is actually one of the reasons for using a DT model instead of drawing the contours manually. In a number of well-defined applications, it seems feasible to generate the initial contour

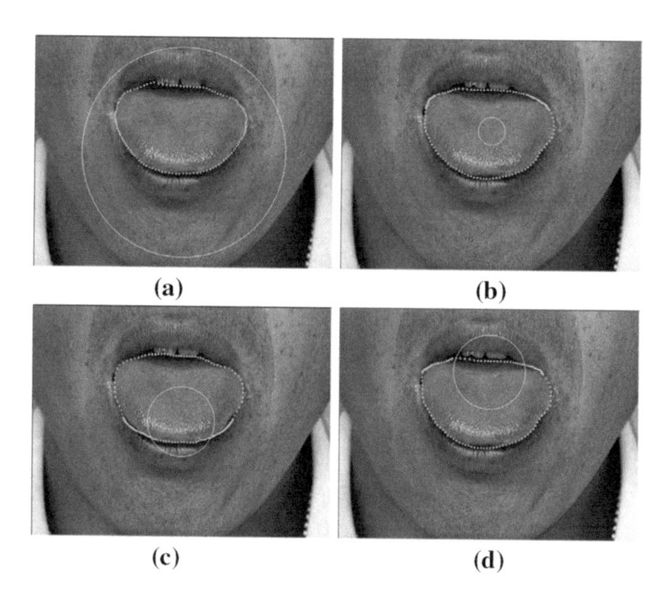

Fig. 3.8 Two significant improvements of the BEDC: insensitivity to the initial location of the contour and having a large capturable range. Convergence of the BEDC starting from different initial positions: **a** outside the tongue's boundary, **b** inside the tongue's boundary, and **c**, **d** overlapping with the *upper* and *lower edges* of the tongue, respectively. Interaction thereby makes the entire approach automatic and reproducible. © 2016 IEEE. Reprinted, with permission, from Pang et al. (2005)

without any user interaction, thereby making the entire approach automatic and reproducible.

The last clinical example is presented in Fig. 3.9, where our attention now turns to the particular effectiveness of the template forces of the BEDC. There are many pathological features on the surface of the tongue, such as points, spots, and thorns or prickles. When filtered by certain edge-enhancing operators, these features may be transformed to such strong edges that they can even overwhelm the information about the tongue's boundary. This obviously adds difficulties to the problem of tongue segmentation and common edge detection methods become useless in such a situation. One possible solution is to over-filter the original images, such as by applying a Laplacian of Gaussian operator with a large σ, to smooth out the troublesome pathological features. However, such an approach only solves one

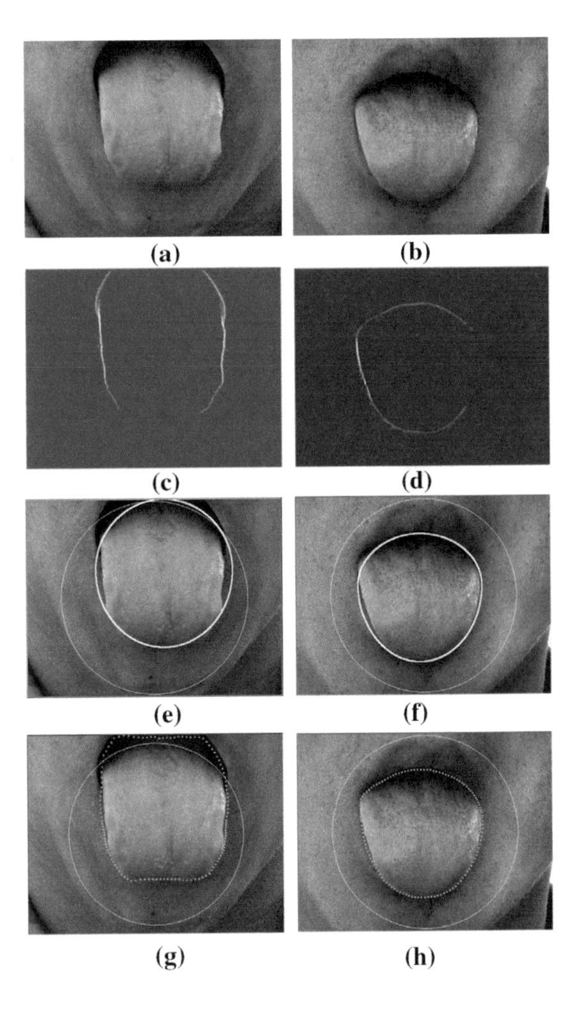

Fig. 3.9 Two examples showing the particular effectiveness of the template force of the BEDC. **a**, **b** Two original clinical images; **c**, **d** Over-filtered edge maps using a LoG with $\sigma = 5$ and $\sigma = 3$, respectively; **e**, **f** The resulting contours (shown with a *bold solid line*) using the BEDT starting from an initial contour (drawn with a *thin solid line*); and **g**, **h** The final resulting contours using the BEDC with an elliptical template force

problem while it creates another: the boundary of the tongue body exhibits fragmentary weakness in the over-filtered edge map, as shown in Fig. 3.9c, d. Nevertheless, the BEDC model can address this problem, thanks to the template forces creating the potentials that make the model take on a specific shape.

Figure 3.9a, b shows the original images whose over-filtered edge maps were created by applying a Laplacian of Gaussian filter with $\sigma = 5$ and $\sigma = 3$, respectively (see Fig. 3.9c, d). It can be seen that the resultant boundaries become fragmentary and weak, and they are even blank on the upper and lower edges of the tongue for Fig. 3.9c and on the right edges for Fig. 3.9d. The resulting models of the BEDT are displayed in Fig. 3.9e, f with bold solid lines, which apparently give a coarse representation of the boundaries of the tongue bodies. The final results, depicted in Fig. 3.9g, h, reveal that by substituting the elliptical template force for both the tensile and rigid internal forces, the BEDC would prefer to take on a regular shape (elliptical curves in this case) and it provides a good estimation for the real edges in the regions with zero potential forces, rather than contracting together as a conventional snake usually does. The reason for such a characteristic in the BEDC is that the elliptical template force, as a whole, can exercise global control due to the root circle, although it has a local formulation.

We applied the BEDC to a total of 3572 clinical tongue images, out of which 3405 samples (about 95.3% of the total number) were successfully segmented. Note that all the experimental samples are gray-level images (red color plane of true color bitmaps), and therefore we did not quantitatively assess the performance of our algorithm. Instead, we used qualitative indices “success” and “failure,” where “success” indicates a satisfactory result for the follow-up feature analysis process in the automatic tongue diagnosis system (see Fig. 3.10) and “failure” otherwise.

This impressive degree of success of the algorithm stems from its robustness to noises and sparse data, and its ability to conduct local and global controls in a consistent way. Generally, deformable models experience difficulties in dealing with noisy data, and in other words, the flexibility becomes a drawback. Solutions to this problem include the incorporation of shape constraints, exploiting global

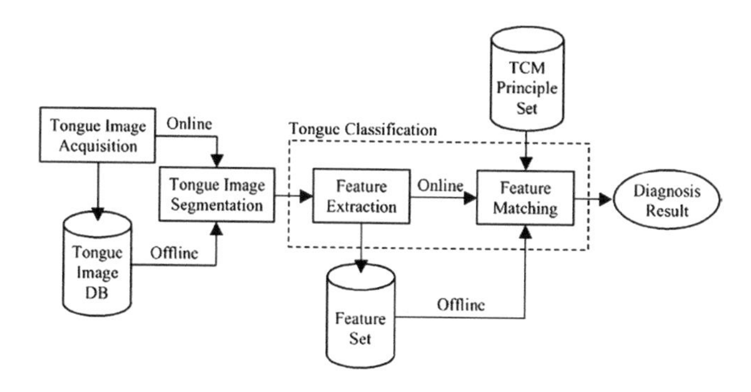

Fig. 3.10 Flowchart of a biometrics-based automatic tongue diagnosis system in TCM. © 2016 IEEE. Reprinted, with permission, from Pang et al. (2005)

information, or the use of multiscale techniques. These methods, however, usually employ separate local and global controls, resulting in the incapability of dealing with sparse data. The main reason for this kind of weakness is the complete ignorance of the global shape representation when the model is conducting the local deformation. Therefore, the model can seldom make valid assumption of the missing contour segments via local control. The BEDC, on the contrary, can overcome this limitation by applying the template force, which can drive the contour to take on regular shapes according to current global representation in the absence of edge data points. Finally, the insensitivity of the BEDC to initial position makes the initialization step totally unnecessary (we can use fixed parameters for all samples), which exactly fills the need for automatic tongue segmentation.

In some cases, however, the BEDC fails to find the correct tongue contour (about 4.7% of the 3572 samples produced wrong results). Figure 3.11 shows a typical example of unsuccessful segmentation. Analysis of the results has shown that the tongue and its surroundings may occasionally take on similar values on the red color plane, especially around the tip of the tongue (see Fig. 3.11). Therein, the edges become very vague or even totally missing, which is mainly responsible for the failure. A potential solution is to develop color-enhancing techniques rendering the tongues prominent from their surroundings.

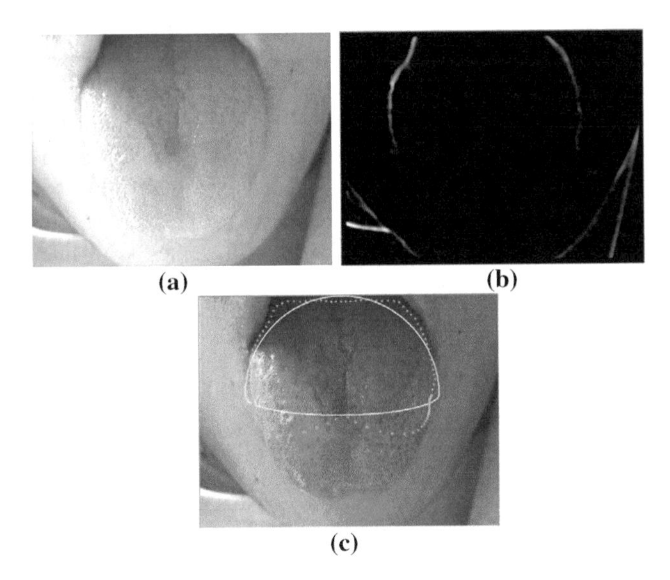

Fig. 3.11 Typical example illustrating segmentation failure of the BEDC. **a** Gray-level image showing the *red color* plane of a tongue image, **b** the corresponding edge map, and **c** the resultant BEDT (in *bold solid line*) and BEDC. © 2016 IEEE. Reprinted, with permission, from Pang et al. (2005)

3.5 Summary

In this chapter, we elaborate a new deformable contour approach, the BEDC, for automated tongue edge extraction in the tongue diagnosis system. Based on a combination of the BEDT and ACM, our proposed approach can exercise both local and global controls in a consistent way by introducing a template force, originating from the BEDT, into the energy function of the BEDC to replace the traditional internal force terms. Experimental results from 3572 clinical tongue images demonstrate that our new approach is able to interpret tongue images in a fully automatic manner due to its insensitivity to initial positions and robustness to noises and sparse data. Moreover, the main idea in the BEDC, namely realizing a global shape representation only through local control, might also be useful in other edge detection applications provided a specific template force could be suitably defined.

References

Caselles, V., Kimmel, R., & Sapiro, G. (1997). Geodesic active contours. *International Journal of Computer Vision, 22*(1), 61–79.
Cohen, L. D. (1991). On active contour models and balloons. *CVGIP: Image Understanding, 53*(2), 211–218.
Cootes, T. F., Taylor, C. J., Cooper, D. H., & Graham, J. (1995). Active shape models-their training and application. *Computer Vision and Image Understanding, 61*(1), 38–59.
Geiger, D., Gupta, A., & Costa, L. A. (1995). Dynamic programming for detecting, tracking, and matching deformable contours. *IEEE Transactions on Pattern Analysis and Machine Intelligence, 17*(3), 294–302.
Gunn, S. R., & Nixon, M. S. (1997). A robust snake implementation; a dual active contour. *IEEE Transactions on Pattern Analysis and Machine Intelligence, 19*(1), 63–68.
Hamarneh, G., & Gustavsson, T. (2000). Combining snakes and active shape models for segmenting the human left ventricle in echocardiographic images (pp. 115–118). IEEE.
Jain, A. K., Zhong, Y., & Lakshmanan, S. (1996). Object matching using deformable templates. *IEEE Transactions on Pattern Analysis and Machine Intelligence, 18*(3), 267–278.
Joshi, S., Pizer, S., Fletcher, P. T., Yushkevich, P., Thall, A., & Marron, J. S. (2002). Multiscale deformable model segmentation and statistical shape analysis using medial descriptions. *IEEE Transactions on Medical Imaging, 21*(5), 538–550.
Kass, M., Witkin, A., & Terzopoulos, D. (1988). Snakes: active contour models. *International Journal of Computer Vision, 1*(4), 321–331.
Lai, K. F., & Chin R. T. (1993). On regularization, formulation and initialization of the active contour models (snakes) (pp. 542–545). Citeseer.
Lee, B. R., Hamza, A. B., & Krim, H. (2002). An active contour model for image segmentation: A variational perspective (pp. 1585). IEEE.
Lie, W., & Chuang, C. (2001). Fast and accurate snake model for object contour detection. *Electronics Letters, 37*(10), 624–626.
Mardia, K. V., Qian, W., Shah, D., & de Souza, K. M. (1997). Deformable template recognition of multiple occluded objects. *IEEE Transactions on Pattern Analysis & Machine Intelligence* (9), 1035–1042.
McInerney, T., & Terzopoulos, D. (1995). Topologically adaptable snakes (pp. 840–845). IEEE.

McInerney, T., & Terzopoulos, D. (1996). Deformable models in medical image analysis: A survey. *Medical Image Analysis, 1*(2), 91–108.

Metaxas, D., Terzopoulos, D. (1993). Shape and nonrigid motion estimation through physics-based synthesis. *IEEE Transactions on Pattern Analysis and Machine Intelligence, 15*(6), 580-591.

Nikou, C., Bueno, G., Heitz, F., & Armspach, J. (2001). A joint physics-based statistical deformable model for multimodal brain image analysis. *IEEE Transactions on Medical Imaging, 20*(10), 1026–1037.

Pang, B., Wang, K., & Zhang, D. (2000). Time-adaptive Snakes for tongue segmentation.

Pang, B., Zhang, D., & Wang, K. (2005). The bi-elliptical deformable contour and its application to automated tongue segmentation in Chinese medicine. *IEEE Transactions on Medical Imaging, 24*(8), 946–956.

Park, H., Schoepflin, T., & Kim, Y. (2001). Active contour model with gradient directional information: directional snake. *Circuits and Systems for Video Technology, IEEE Transactions on, 11*(2), 252–256.

Scaggiante, A., Frezza, R., & Zampato, M. (1999). Identifying and tracking ellipses: A technique based on elliptical deformable templates (pp. 582–587): IEEE.

Staib, L. H., & Duncan, J. S. (1992). Boundary finding with parametrically deformable models. *IEEE Transactions on Pattern Analysis & Machine Intelligence* (11), 1061–1075.

Storvik, G. (1994). A Bayesian approach to dynamic contours through stochastic sampling and simulated annealing. *Pattern Analysis and Machine Intelligence, IEEE Transactions on, 16*(10), 976–986.

Székely, G. A. B., Kelemen, A. A. S., Brechbühler, C., & Gerig, G. (1996). Segmentation of 2-D and 3-D objects from MRI volume data using constrained elastic deformations of flexible Fourier contour and surface models. *Medical Image Analysis, 1*(1), 19–34.

Terzopoulos, D. (1980). Matching deformable models to images: direct and iterative solutions (pp. 164–167).

Terzopoulos, D., & Metaxas, D. (1990). Dynamic 3D models with local and global deformations: Deformable superquadrics (pp. 606–615). IEEE.

Valverde, F. L., Guil, N., Munoz, J. E., Li, Q., Aoyama, M., et al. (2001). A deformable model for image segmentation in noisy medical images (pp. 82–85). IEEE.

Yuille, A. L., Hallinan, P. W., & Cohen, D. S. (1992). Feature extraction from faces using deformable templates. *International Journal of Computer Vision, 8*(2), 99–111.

Chapter 4
A Snake-Based Approach to Automated Tongue Image Segmentation

Abstract Tongue diagnosis, one of the most important diagnosis methods of Traditional Chinese Medicine, is considered a very good candidate for remote diagnosis methods because of its simplicity and noninvasiveness. Recently, considerable research interests have been given to the development of automated tongue segmentation technologies, which is difficult due to the complexity of the pathological tongue, variance of the tongue shape, and interference of the lips. In this chapter, we propose a novel automated tongue segmentation method via combining a polar edge detector and active contour model (ACM) technique. First, a polar edge detector is presented to effectively extract the edge of the tongue body. Then we design an edge filtering scheme to avoid the adverse interference from the nontongue boundary. After edge filtering, a local adaptive edge bi-thresholding algorithm is introduced to perform the edge binarization. Finally, a heuristic initialization and an ACM are proposed to segment the tongue body from the image. The experimental results demonstrate that the proposed method can accurately and effectively segment the tongue body. A quantitative evaluation on 200 images indicates that the normalized mean distance to the closest point is 0.48%, and the average true positive percent of our method is 97.1%.

4.1 Introduction

As previously stated, adverse factors, such as noise, diffuse boundaries, and redundant edges, seriously affect the effectiveness of the segmentation algorithm. For example, boundaries may be blurred due to the movement of the target, miss-focus of camera, the low signal-to-noise ratio of the capture device, or the similarity of the surrounding tissues. In such cases, performance of the regular image segmentation techniques would be greatly degraded, and prior knowledge would be very effective in circumventing the underdetermined nature of the automatic segmentation process.

D. Zhang et al., *Tongue Image Analysis*, DOI 10.1007/978-981-10-2167-1_4

The active contour model (ACM), characterized by shape initialization, representation, and the evolution rule, has been very successful in medical image segmentation. The performance of the regular ACM, however, is seriously affected by the result obtained using edge detection. Usually, edge detection has a great effect on the shape initialization and evolution of the edge-based active contour technique. If the edge maps are very noisy or are contaminated with spurious edges, false initialization or error segmentation are then obtained. For example, previous works (Cai, 2002; Pang, Wang, Zhang, & Zhang, 2002) on tongue segmentation usually used the classical gradient operators to detect the boundary of tongue body, and then utilized an ACM to crop the tongue area. The gradient on parts of the tongue boundary was sometimes very weak and inconsecutive, which made it difficult to be distinguished from the other disturbing edges, resulting in an adverse effect on the segmentation result.

Recently, polar transformation, especially log-polar transformation, has been introduced in image analysis research. The log-polar transformation is based on the neural-physiological findings that the information received by the cortex is a log-polar mapping of the retinal stimulus. Log-polar mapping has been adopted in face detection and recognition, feature extraction, and edge detection (Gomes, & Fisher, 2003; Koh, Ranganath, & Venkatesh, 2002; Smeraldi, & Bigun, 2002; Wallace, & McLaren, 2003).

Tongue segmentation is one of the most prerequisite and difficult steps in an automated tongue diagnosis system. The result of tongue segmentation directly influences the performance of the entire system. However, the complexity of the pathological tongue, variance of the tongue shape, and interference of the lips make automated tongue segmentation very challenging.

In this chapter, we introduce a novel automated tongue segmentation method, which combines the polar edge detector, edge filtering, adaptive edge binarization, and an ACM to automatically segment the tongue body from an image. First, we present a novel polar edge detector which utilizes the physical character of the boundary of the tongue body. Physically, the tongue, face, and lips are different organs of the body, and it is obvious that the boundary of the tongue body and its neighboring parts (such as the lips) are not continuous, where usually a hollow or gap can be found. This characteristic makes the illumination of the tongue boundary lower than the tongue body and its neighboring parts, and thus can be used to discriminate the edge of the tongue body. Second, we introduce an edge filtering method to weaken the adverse effects caused by the tongue's color, texture, and coating, and a local adaptive bi-thresholding algorithm to binarize the edge image. Finally, we use an ACM to complete the automated segmentation of the tongue image.

The organization of this chapter is as follows. Sect. 4.2 presents the framework of our automated tongue segmentation algorithm. Sect. 4.3 experimentally evaluates the performance of the proposed method. Sect. 4.4 provides a summary of the proposed method.

4.2 Automated Segmentation Algorithm for Tongue Images

The difficulty of tongue segmentation makes it unrealistic to extract only the tongue area with one kind of traditional segmentation method, such as the deformable template and ACM. One possible solution is to integrate both low-level and high-level domain knowledge for automated image segmentation (Xue, Pizurica, Philips, Kerre, Van De Walle, & Lemahieu, 2003). In tongue segmentation, (Pang et al., 2002) intuitively combined deformable templates and ACM, but the problem of automated tongue segmentation was still not well solved. This method, however, seriously suffers from the result of edge detection, which is usually very poor, inconsecutive, and difficult to be distinguished from the other interference edges.

In the following, we first propose a polar edge detection method to effectively enhance the edge of the tongue body in Sect. 4.2.1. Then, we introduce an empirical edge filtering process and local adaptive edge binarization method in Sect. 4.2.2. We also present an initialization and ACM to automatically segment the tongue in Sect. 4.2.3. The process of the proposed segmentation method is finally presented in Sect. 4.2.4.

4.2.1 Polar Edge Detection of Tongue Image

Physically, the tongue body and its neighboring parts (such as the lips) are not on a continuous surface, and thus the illumination of the tongue boundary usually is lower than the tongue body and its neighboring parts. This characteristic is very valuable and can be used to direct the design of a detector to properly enhance the true edge of the tongue body from disturbing ones.

A typical tongue image from our database is shown in Fig. 4.1a, and the intensities in six directions are shown in Fig. 4.1b. The edges of the tongue body in these directions are also labeled in Fig. 4.1b. It can be indicated that the intensities of tongue boundary are usually a local minimum in the radial direction. This phenomenon motivates us to present a novel tongue boundary detection method, the polar edge detector.

In polar edge detection, the original tongue image I is transformed to the corresponding polar image $I'(r, \theta)$. Let (x_0, y_0) be the image center of the polar coordinates, then each pixel $I'(r, \theta)$ in the polar image can be computed by

$$I'(r,\theta) = I(r \sin\theta + x_0, r \cos\theta + y_0), \tag{4.1}$$

where the value of $I(r \sin\theta + x_0, r \cos\theta + y_0)$ is computed using bilinear interpolation or bicubic interpolation in the original image. When the boundary of the target has a distinct pattern in the radial direction, polar transformation is expected

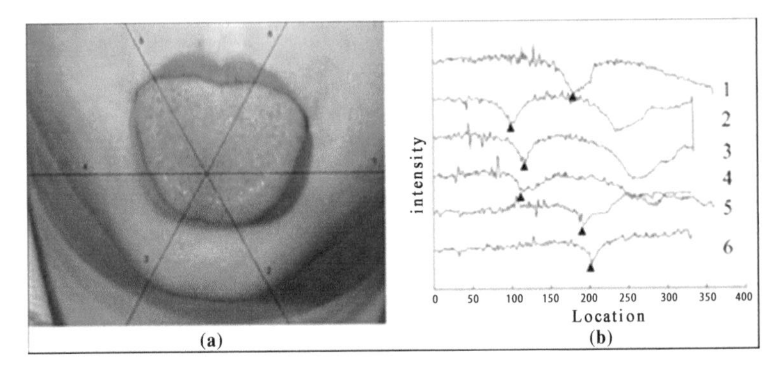

Fig. 4.1 **a** Original image; **b** Variations of intensity in six different directions. Copyright © 2016 Wiley. Used with permission from Zhang, Zuo, Wang, and Zhang (2006)

to be more efficient than a regular edge enhancer (Morelande, Iskander, Collins, & Franklin, 2002). Analogously, the inverse transform is defined as

$$I(x, y) = I'\left(\sqrt{(x - x_0)^2 + (y - y_0)^2}, \operatorname{arctg}\left(\frac{x - x_0}{y - y_0}\right)\right) \tag{4.2}$$

After polar transform, we can use the line detection technique to enhance the boundary of the tongue body. Usually, the standard second derivative of Gaussian filter is used for dark line detection (Steger, 1998). When using this method, we should previously determine the value of the standard deviation r based on the line width to be detected. If the line width is uncertain or not unique, the determination of the r value is still a nontrivial task. In tongue boundary detection, what we care most is the location of the line, not the line width. Thus, we used a much simple operator to enhance the boundary to be detected. In our tongue boundary detector, we first used a horizontal Gaussian smoothing operator with windows $N \times 1$ and standard deviation σ to smooth the polar image. Then we proposed a $1 \times (2k + 1)$ horizontal edge detector $[1, 1, \ldots, 1, -2k, 1, \ldots, 1, 1]$ to enhance the edge in the polar image:

$$E(i,j) = \sum_{i=1}^{k} (I(i,j+k) + I(i,j-k) - 2I(i,j)), \tag{4.3}$$

where $I(i, j)$ is a pixel of the polar image, and $E(i, j)$ is the corresponding intensity of the polar edge image. If we set the value of k higher than the maximum line width, the proposed operator can be used to effectively enhance all the lines to be detected.

The locations of the image centers also affect the performance of edge detection. If they are out of the tongue region, the locations of image centers seriously affect the performance of the segmentation method. If the locations of image centers are in the tongue region, the proposed tongue segmentation method would be robust to the variations of the locations of image centers. We adopt the following method to roughly determine the location of the image center:

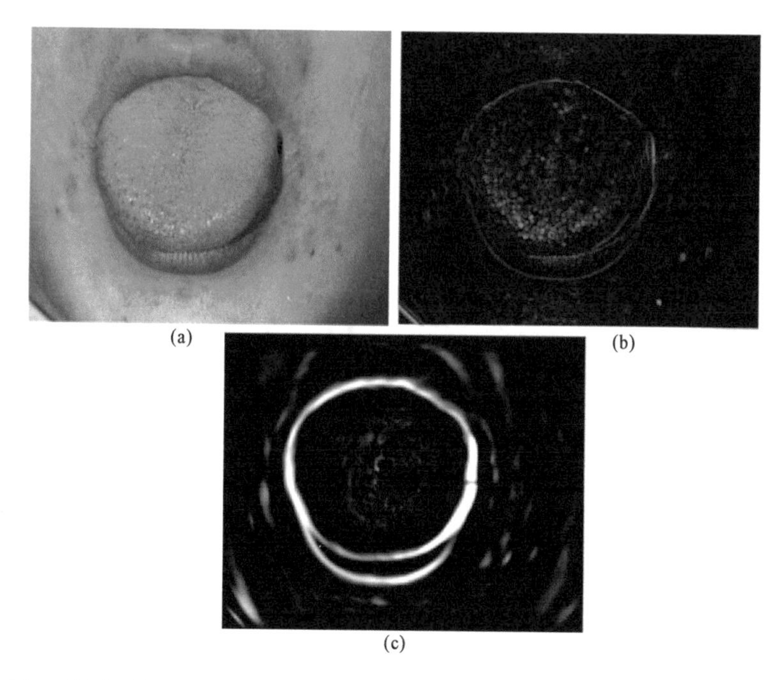

Fig. 4.2 **a** Original image; **b** Edge image detected by the Sobel operator; **c** Edge image detected by the polar edge detector. Copyright © 2016 Wiley. Used with permission from Zhang et al. (2006)

1. Transform the RGB color image to the YIQ color space.
2. Use the histogram stretch method to expand the histogram of the Q component to fill the entire available grayscale range.
3. Compute the image threshold T using Otsu's method.
4. Image thresholding: $Q(i, j) = 1$, if $Q(i, j) > T$; $Q(i, j) = 0$, if $Q(i, j) \leq T$.
5. Rough estimation of the image center (x_c, y_c). Define (x_c, y_c) as the mean of all the (i, j) with $Q(i, j) = 1$.

The edge images of Fig. 4.2a detected using the Sobel and the proposed operator are shown in Fig. 4.2b, c. In Fig. 4.2b, the Sobel operator detects many redundant and useless edges. It is obvious that the polar edge detector can eliminate most local spurious edges and is consistently superior to the Sobel detector.

4.2.2 *Filtering and Binarization of the Edge Image*

The aim of edge filtering is to eliminate or weaken the effect of the textures and the coatings of the tongue. If the intensity in the tongue area is uniform or the variation of intensity is small enough, textures and coatings would have little effect on the result of edge detection. If the variation of intensity in the tongue area is high, the density of the edge of the tongue would also be high. Here we adopt this property for edge filtering.

A standard Sobel operator is used to filter out the useless edges for tongue segmentation. After Sobel edge detection, we first compute the standard deviation of the edge image σ^2, and then use the threshold 2σ to binarize the Sobel edge image. We further use an $N \times N$ Gaussian operator with deviation σ to smooth the edge image and subsequently a threshold T to binarize the image. Finally, a morphological method is adopted to discard the blocks with small size.

After edge filtering, we introduce a local adaptive bi-thresholding method to binarize the polar edge image. Unlike global bi-thresholding, which uses a uniform threshold value to binarize the image, every K line of the polar edge image has its own local threshold value in our local adaptive bi-thresholding method. The details of the local adaptive bi-thresholding algorithm are stated as follows:

Step 1. For the binarization of the ith row of the edge image $E(i, j)$, define the ith local subimage $E_i(i_1, j)(i - K \leq i_1 \leq i + K)$, where K is half of the height of the local subimage. In our method, $K = 1$.
Step 2. Use Otsu's method (Ohtsu 1979) to determine the threshold T_O.
Step 3. Determine the threshold T_p as the maximum level of intensity which satisfies that the proportion of pixels when $E_i(i_1, j) > T_p$ is higher than a predefined proportion $p(p = 0.05)$.
Step 4. Use the threshold $T = \max(T_O, T_p)$ to binarize the polar edge image.

After edge filtering and binarization, a morphological method is further used to post filter an edge without enough length.

Figure 4.3 presents an example to show the function of the filtering and binarization. A color tongue image is shown in Fig. 4.3a and the corresponding edge image is illustrated in Fig. 4.3b. The binary edge images of Fig. 4.3a obtained using the global bi-thresholding and the local adaptive bi-thresholding methods are shown in Fig. 4.3c, d, respectively. As Fig. 4.3 indicates that the edge filtering scheme is effective in weakening the adverse effect of the tongue textures and coatings, and the local adaptive bi-thresholding method is more suitable to obtain a continuous edge of the tongue body.

4.2.3 *Initialization and ACM*

The snake, or active contour model (ACM), has been widely applied in image segmentation (Kass, Witkin, & Terzopoulos, 1988), especially in medical image segmentation. The snake should be initialized close to the boundary of the target to be segmented. Otherwise the ACM is inclined to converge to local minima. To avoid this problem, an interactive user interface or an appropriate initialization close to the ground truth is very necessary.

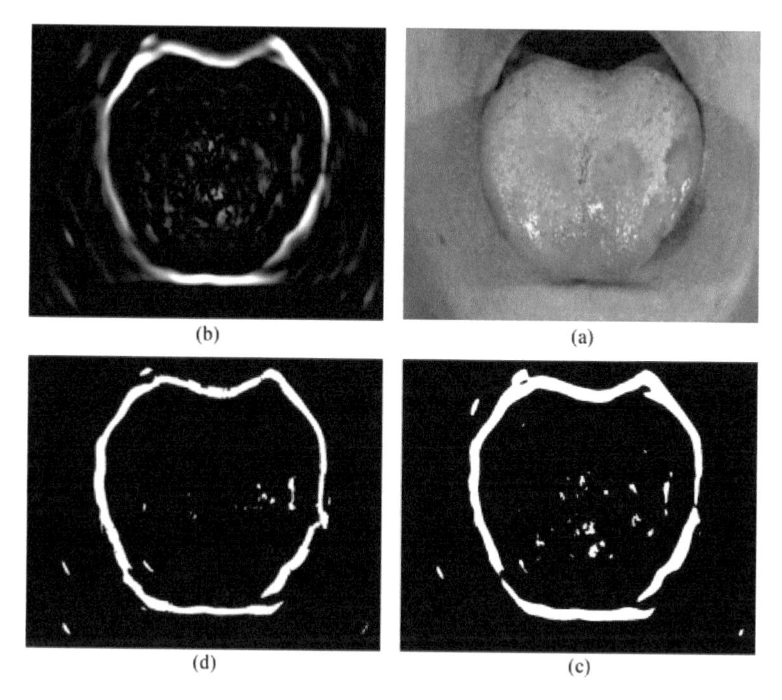

Fig. 4.3 **a** Original image; **b** Edge image detected by the polar edge detector; **c** Global binarization; **d** Local adaptive binarization. Copyright © 2016 Wiley. Used with permission from Zhang et al. (2006)

A snake model can be represented as a curve $v(s) = (x(s), y(s), s \in [0,1])$, which moves through the spatial domain of an image to minimize the energy function:

$$\begin{aligned} E^{*}_{\text{toyal}} &= \int_{0}^{1} E(v(s))ds \\ &= \int_{0}^{1} E_{\text{int}}(v(s)) + E_{\text{image}}(v(s)) + E_{\text{con}}(v_{\text{ss}}(s))ds \end{aligned} \tag{4.4}$$

The internal energy E_{int} is used to constrain the model to be smooth, which is defined as,

$$E_{\text{int}}(v(s)) = (\alpha(s)|v_s(s)|^2 + (s)|v_{ss}(s)|^2), \tag{4.5}$$

where $\alpha(s)$ and $\beta(s)$ are weighting parameters that control the snake's tension and rigidity, respectively, and $v_s(s)$ and $v_{ss}(s)$ denote the first and second derivatives of $v(s)$ with respect to s. The first-order term makes the snake act like a membrane and the second-order term makes it act like a thin plate.

The image energy function E_{image} is a weighted combination of three components, the line energy E_{line}, the edge energy E_{edge}, and the termination energy E_{term}

$$E_{\text{image}}(v(s)) = w_{\text{line}}E_{\text{line}}(v(s)) + w_{\text{edge}}E_{\text{edge}}(v(s)) + w_{\text{term}}E_{\text{term}}(v(s)), \tag{4.6}$$

where w_{img}, w_{edge}, and w_{term} are the weights of these three kinds of energies. The line energy $E_{\text{line}} = I(x, y)$ is used to simply attract the contour to lower or higher intensity values. The edge energy $E_{\text{edge}} = -|(\nabla I(x, y))|^2$ is used to attract the contour to the location with a high gradient. The termination energy E_{term} is the curvature of the level contour in a Gaussian smoothed image, attracting the contour to line terminations.

The constraint energy E_{con}, defined by,

$$E_{\text{con}}(v(s)) = -k(x_1 - x_2)^2 \tag{4.7}$$

is used to attract points on the contour to points in the plane, where x_1 and x_2 are the points on the contour and in the plane, respectively, and k is the spring constant.

With the definition of the energy functions, we use the time-delayed discrete dynamic programming method proposed by (Amini, Weymouth, & Jain, 1990) to solve the energy minimization problem defined by the ACM. The Amini method first discretizes the energy term, reformulates the problem into the solution of a sequence of optimization problems of one variable, and then uses the dynamic programming scheme to obtain an optimal solution.

In this chapter, a heuristic snake initialization method is introduced. First, we choose the nearest edge point from the origin as the tongue boundary in each direction. Next we choose the longest continuous edge segment as one part of the tongue boundary. Finally, we use the chosen tongue boundary segment and the continuity property to direct the heuristic initialization of the tongue boundary in each direction.

We use the ACM to determine the final segmentation result. Specifically, we explain how to use the gray-level image and the edge image to calculate the line energy E_{line} and the edge energy E_{edge}. In the definition of the line energy, $E_{\text{line}} = I(x, y)$, $I(x, y)$ is the intensity of the gray tongue image. In the definition of the edge energy, $E_{\text{edge}} = -| E(x, y) |^2$, $E(x, y)$ is defined as the intensity of the edge image after polar edge detection.

Figure 4.4a shows a color tongue image. Figure 4.4b, c illustrate the initialization and final segmentation result on Fig. 4.4a, respectively. Although there is serious interference produced by the tongue coating, the proposed method, as Fig. 4.4 shows, correctly initializes the tongue boundary and the active contour converges to the boundary of the tongue body.

4.2.4 Summary of the Automated Tongue Segmentation Method

Figure 4.5 is a flowchart of the proposed automated tongue segmentation method. The input image is first transformed to the corresponding polar image, and then a

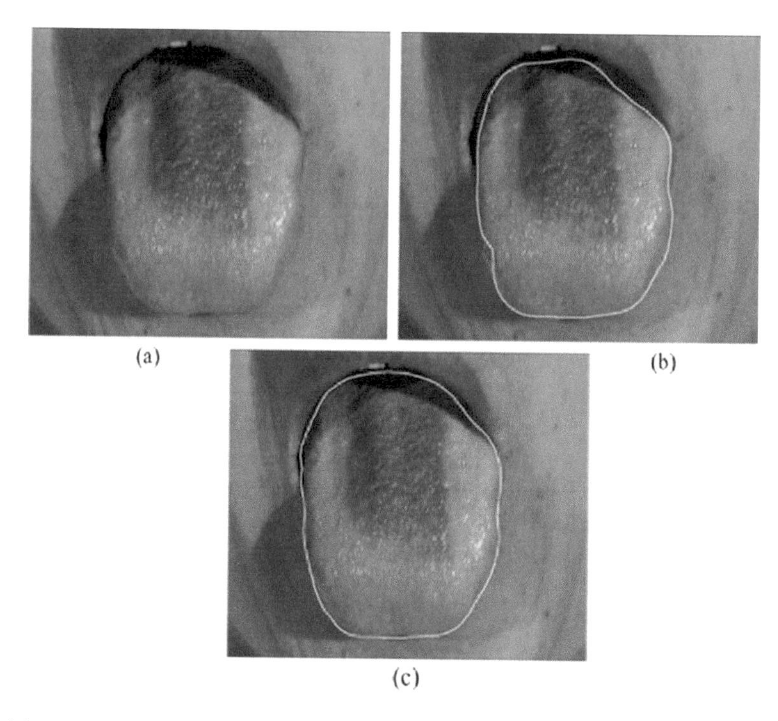

Fig. 4.4 **a** Original image; **b** Initialization of active contour; **c** Final output. Copyright © 2016 Wiley. Used with permission from Zhang et al. (2006)

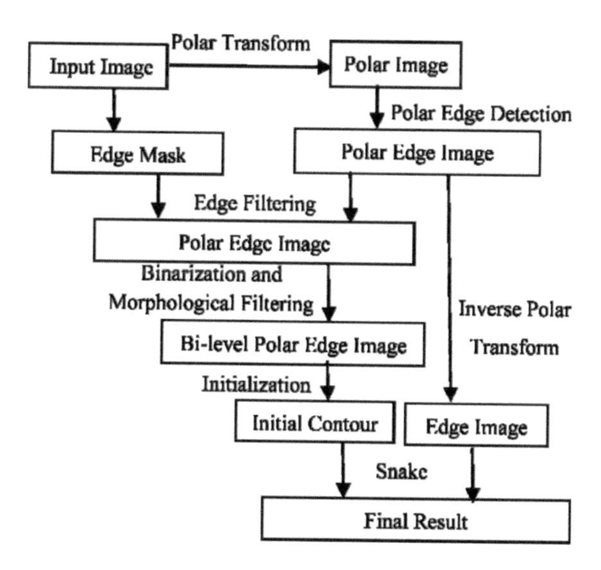

Fig. 4.5 Flowchart of the proposed automated tongue segmentation method. Copyright © 2016 Wiley. Used with permission from Zhang et al. (2006)

polar edge detector operates on the polar image. Then the input image is used to construct an edge mask which is to filter the polar edge image. The filtered polar edge image is then binarized using a local adaptive bi-thresholding method. We use the binary edge image to initialize the ACM. Finally, a discrete dynamic programming snake model is used to evolve the contour to the boundary of the tongue body.

4.3 Experiments and Discussion

In this section, 200 tongue images from our database were used to evaluate the performance of the proposed method. We first tested the efficiency of the edge filtering method. Then, both qualitative and quantitative evaluation methods were used to evaluate the performance of the automated tongue segmentation method. To quantitatively evaluate the result, each tongue boundary was manually delineated by five individuals as the ground truths of the image.

4.3.1 *Evaluation on the Edge Filtering Algorithm*

To evaluate the edge filtering algorithm, two aspects should be considered. One is whether it can effectively filter out the redundant and spurious edges produced by the pathological substance and lips. The other is whether it has little effect on the true boundary of the tongue body. The edge filtering algorithm can be evaluated in two ways, directly and indirectly. Direct evaluation is based on the intuitive illustration of the edge filtering result, while indirect evaluation can be carried out by the final performance of the whole segmentation method.

Here we only adopt the first way to evaluate the proposed edge filtering algorithm. Figure 4.6a–d illustrate the original image, the edge mask, and the edge images before and after edge filtering. As Fig. 4.6 shows, the proposed method can filter out most redundant and spurious edges while preserving the useful tongue boundary candidate.

4.3.2 *Qualitative Evaluation*

To demonstrate the performance of the automated tongue segmentation method in segmenting tongue images with rich pathological textures, complex color blocks, irregular shapes, and a poor-quality boundary, four different tongue images were used to qualitatively evaluate the proposed segmentation method.

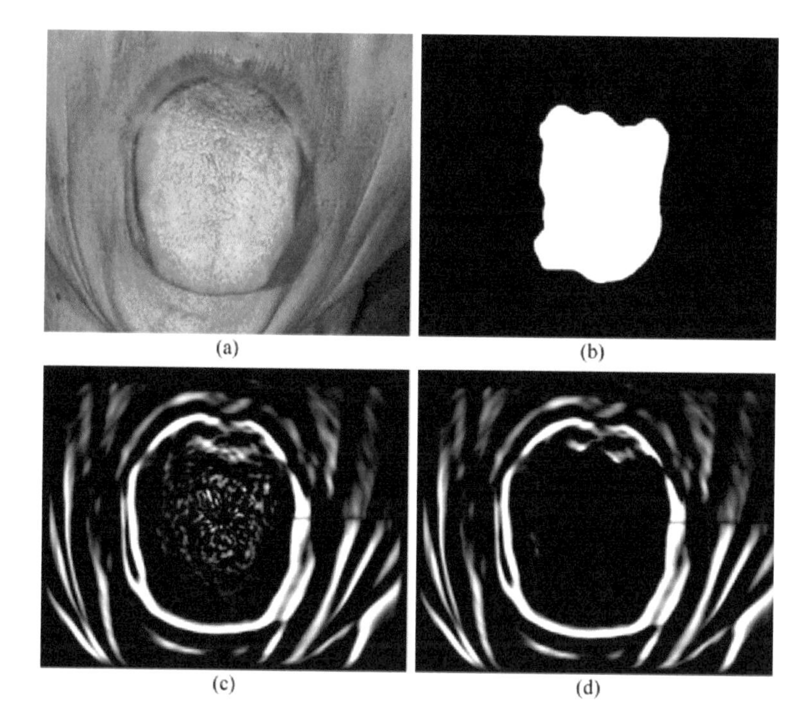

Fig. 4.6 **a** Original image; **b** Edge mask; **c** Edge image before filtering; **d** Edge image after filtering. Copyright © 2016 Wiley. Used with permission from Zhang et al. (2006)

Figure 4.7 shows a tongue image with small color variation and distinct tongue boundary. Figure 4.8 shows a tongue image with rich texture structure, Fig. 4.9 shows an image of a fissure and blood stasis tongue, and Fig. 4.10 shows a tongue with a slippery coating. For each of these four images, the proposed tongue segmentation method is able to correctly and accurately extract the tongue area.

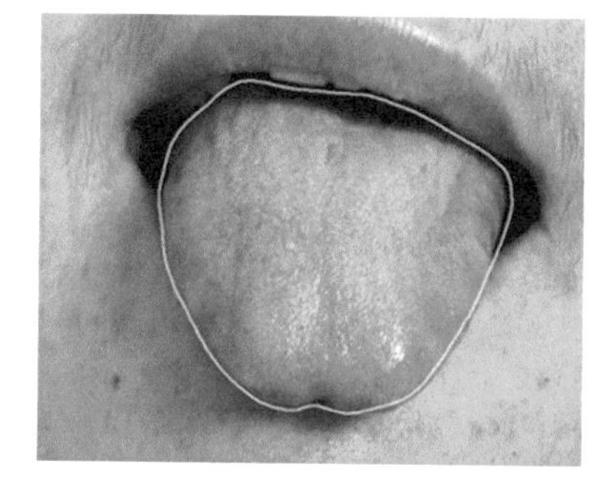

Fig. 4.7 Final Segmentation result of the tongue image with small color variation and a distinct tongue boundary. Copyright © 2016 Wiley. Used with permission from Zhang et al. (2006)

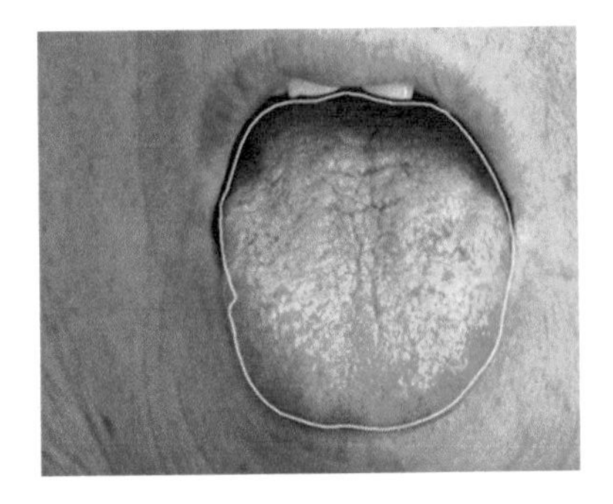

Fig. 4.8 Final Segmentation result of the tongue image with rich texture structure. Copyright © 2016 Wiley. Used with permission from Zhang et al. (2006)

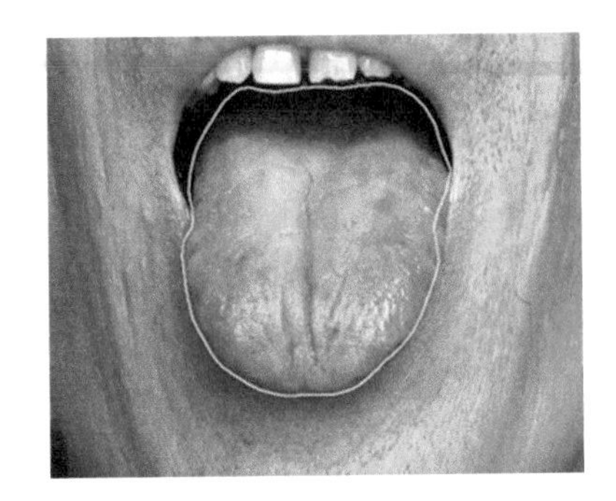

Fig. 4.9 Final Segmentation result of the fissure and blood stasis tongue image. Copyright © 2016 Wiley. Used with permission from Zhang et al. (2006)

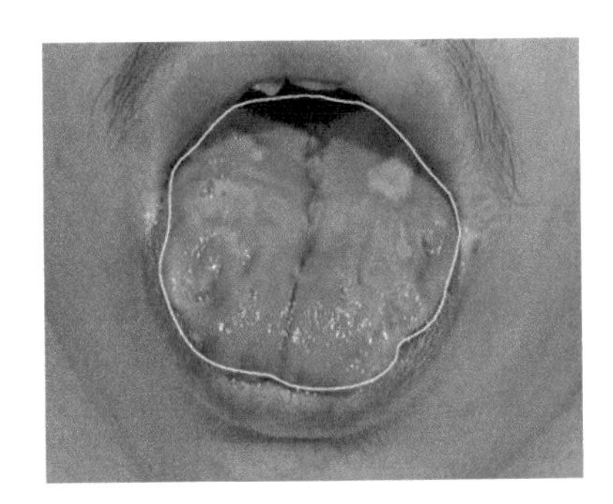

Fig. 4.10 Final Segmentation result of the tongue image with a slippery coating. Copyright © 2016 Wiley. Used with permission from Zhang et al. (2006)

4.3.3 Quantitative Evaluation

Quantitative evaluation of medical image segmentation algorithm is a nontrivial job. The complexity and difficulty of medical image segmentation make it impossible to have a definitive gold standard. In practice, researchers usually adopt the manual segmentation result as an estimation of the gold standard. Manual results, however, vary with different observers and the collection of them is very tedious and time consuming. Besides, to evaluate the algorithm, definitive metrics are necessary to compare the automated segmentation results and the manual results. In this section, we use the manual delineations of the tongue boundary as the gold standard and quantitatively compare the automated segmentation results of the proposed method with the ground truth to obtain an objective evaluation of the segmentation accuracy.

To evaluate the accuracy of the automated segmentation method, Chalana and Kim proposed using the boundary error metrics (Chalana, Linker, Haynor, & Kim, 1996; Chalana, & Kim, 1997), while (Udupa et al., 2002) proposed using the area error measures. We adopted the following process to evaluate the proposed segmentation method:

1. We used 200 typical tongue images from our database to evaluate the segmentation results.
2. For each tongue image, we had five individuals, including three doctors and two programmers, independently delineate the boundary of the tongue body. The automated segmentation result was then compared with these five manually detected contours. We used two kinds of metrics, the mean and the standard deviation of the performance metrics over different manually detected contours, to objectively evaluate the segmentation results.
3. To present an overall evaluation of the segmentation methods, we further calculated the average metric and the average standard deviation over all test images.

4.3.3.1 Boundary Error Metrics

Let $A = \{a_1, a_2, \ldots, a_m\}$ denotes the automated segmentation results by the proposed algorithm, and $M = \{m_1, m_2, \ldots, m_n\}$ denotes the manual contour, where each $a_i = (x_{ai}, y_{ai})$ or $m_i = (x_{mi}, y_{mi})$ is a point on the corresponding contour. We used two boundary error metrics, the Hausdorff distance(HD) and the mean distance to the closest point (DCP), to quantitatively evaluate the automated segmentation algorithm. The DCP for a_i to M is defined as:

$$d(a_1, M) = \min_j(\|m_i - a_i\|_2), \tag{4.8}$$

where $\|\bullet\|_2$ represents the Euclidean norm. The Hausdorff distance between two curves A and M is defined as:

$$hd(A, M) = \max\left(\min_j\{d(a_i, M)\}, \max_j\left\{d\left(m_j, A\right)\right\}\right) \tag{4.9}$$

The mean DCP distance (MD) of two curves A and M can then be defined as:

$$md(A, M) = \frac{1}{m+n}\left(\sum_i d(a_i, M) + \sum_j d(m_j, A)\right) \tag{4.10}$$

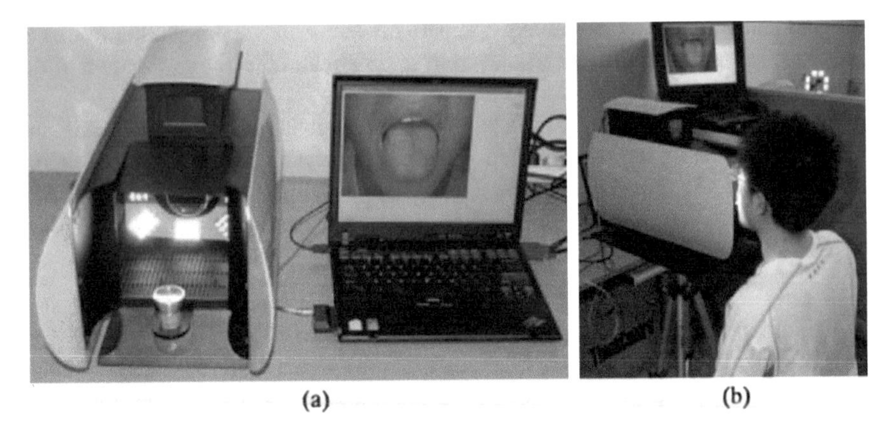

Fig. 4.11 **a** Tongue image acquisition device; **b** Tongue image capture. Copyright © 2016 Wiley. Used with permission from Zhang et al. (2006)

Table 4.1 Evaluation on the mean and standard deviation (SD) of the boundary error metrics

		Methods
	Normalized HD (%)	Normalized MD (%)
Mean ± SD	1.98 ± 0.48	0.06 ± 0.04

Copyright © 2016 Wiley. Used with permission from Zhang et al. (2006)

Using the boundary error metric, we evaluated the performance of the proposed segmentation method from three aspects. First, the distance based on pixels may be less meaningful. But in tongue image capture, we used a self-designed acquisition device (as shown in Fig. 4.11) where the relative location between the camera and tongue is fixed, and the tongue body is approximately in a plane. Since the camera parameters, such as focal length, are fixed for our device, we can roughly estimate the physical distance from the image distance (400 pixels = 50 mm).

Second, we tested the mean and standard deviation of the boundary metrics among all test images, as shown in Table 4.1. The normalized HD and MD, defined by dividing HD or MD by the number of pixels of manual contours, were 1.96 and 0.48%. From Table 4.1, the average standard deviation of the boundary metrics is very small, which indicates that the proposed method can achieve a robust performance when compared with different manual detected contours.

Third, we compared the performance of the proposed method and the bielliptical deformable contour (BEDC) method (Pang et al., 2002), as shown in Table 4.2. The average Hausdorff distance and mean DCP distance on the 200 test images were 24.43 and 5.86 pixels, respectively. From this table, we can see that the proposed method is consistently superior to BEDC based on the boundary metrics.

Table 4.2 Quantitative evaluation of the tongue segmentation methods based on the boundary error metrics

	Methods	
	Normalized HD (%)	Normalized MD (%)
Mean ± SD	1.98 ± 0.48	0.06 ± 0.04

4.3.3.2 Area Error Metrics

Three different area error metrics, the false negative volume fraction (FN), the false positive volume fraction (FP), and the true positive volume fraction (TP), were used to measure the accuracy of the automated segmentation method. We define these three area error metrics, FN, FP, and TP, as follows:

$$FN = \frac{|A_a - A_a \cap A_m|}{A_a}, \tag{4.11}$$

$$FP = \frac{|A_m - A_a \cap A_m|}{A_a}, \tag{4.12}$$

$$TP = \frac{|A_a \cap A_m|}{A_a}, \tag{4.13}$$

where A_m represents the area of the tongue body determined by manual delineations and A_a represents the area of the tongue body determined by the proposed method.

Using the area metrics, we evaluated the performance of the proposed segmentation method from two aspects. First, we tested the mean and standard deviation of the area metrics among all test images, as shown in Table 4.3. The average percentage of pixels which were misclassified as tongue body was 4.6%, while the average percent of tongue body pixels which were not correctly detected by our method was 2.9%. The average true positive percentage was 97.1%. From Table 4.3, the average standard deviation of the area metrics is very small, which indicates that the proposed method can achieve a robust performance compared with different manual detected contours.

Second, we compared the performance of the proposed method and BEDC (Pang et al., 2002), as shown in Table 4.4. From this table, it can be seen that the proposed method consistently outperformed BEDC based on the area metrics.

Finally, we tested the robustness of the proposed method against the location of the image center. By adding a Gaussian noise with $m = [0, 0]$, $\sigma = p \times [50; 50]$ ($p = 0, 1, 2$) on the location of the image center, we recomputed the segmentation

Table 4.3 Evaluation on the mean and standard deviation of the area metrics

	FP (%)	FN (%)	TP (%)
Mean ± SD	4.6 ± 0.22	2.9 ± 0.16	97.1 ± 0.16

Table 4.4 Quantitative evaluation of the tongue segmentation methods based on the area metric

	FP (%)	FN (%)	TP (%)
BEDC	11.2	8.7	91.3
Proposed	4.6	2.9	97.1

results on all the test images, as shown in Table 4.5. From this table, it can be seen that small variations of the image center would have very little effect on the performance of the proposed segmentation method.

Moreover, two test images with greater FN or FP percent are shown in Fig. 4.12a, b. In Fig. 4.12a, the greater FN percent can be attributed to the inherent characteristic of the polar edge detector, which is apt to extract the margin between

Table 4.5 Effect of the locations of image centers on the performance metrics

Degree of noise (p)	Normalized HD (%)	Normalized MD (%)	FP (%)	FN (%)	TP (%)
0	1.98	0.48	4.6	2.9	97.1
1	1.98	0.49	4.7	2.9	97.1
2	2.01	0.52	4.8	3.2	96.8

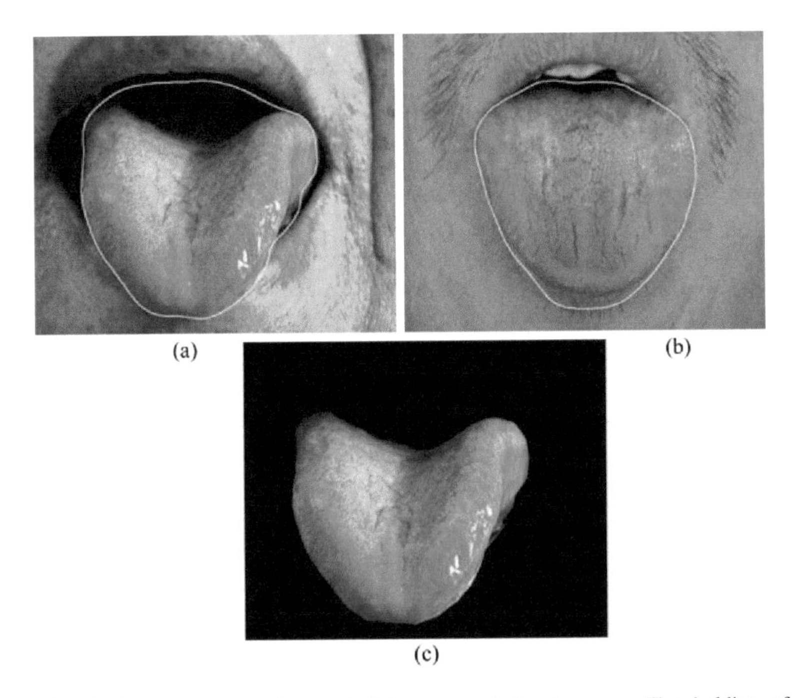

Fig. 4.12 **a** False segmentation image; **b** False segmentation image; **c** Thresholding of (**a**). Copyright © 2016 Wiley. Used with permission from Zhang et al. (2006)

the tongue body and its neighboring parts, not the true boundary of the tongue. Thus, a post processing thresholding can be used to weaken this effect, as shown in Fig. 4.12c. For Fig. 4.12b, the effect of the lower lip and the poor intensity of the true tongue boundary caused the false segmentation on the bottom of the tongue body. This problem will be further studied by the improvement on the initialization and implementation of ACM.

4.4 Summary

In this chapter, we introduce an integrated method of polar edge detection and ACM for automated tongue segmentation. The main steps of the proposed method are as follows:

(1) Polar edge detection. We proposed a novel polar edge detector to effectively enhance the boundary of tongue body.
(2) Edge filtering and bilevel thresholding. Edge filtering and local adaptive bilevel thresholding steps are used to preserve the tongue boundary and binarize the edge image.
(3) ACM. A heuristic initialization and an ACM are introduced to achieve the final result of the proposed segmentation method.

Using the boundary error metrics and the area metrics, a series of experiments was carried out, based on 200 tongue images, to quantitatively evaluate the performance of the proposed tongue segmentation method. The normalized mean DCP distance is 0.48%, and the true positive percent of the proposed method is 97.1%. The results of the experiment indicate that the proposed method can accurately and effectively extract the tongue body area from the tongue image, and will lay the foundations of the subsequent feature extraction of the color, texture, and coating features in the automated tongue diagnosis system.

References

Amini, A. A., Weymouth, T. E., & Jain, R. C. (1990). Using dynamic programming for solving variational problems in vision. *IEEE Transactions on Pattern Analysis and Machine Intelligence, 12*(9), 855–867.

Cai, Y. (2002). *A novel imaging system for tongue inspection* (pp. 159–164). IEEE, 1999.

Chalana, V., & Kim, Y. (1997). A methodology for evaluation of boundary detection algorithms on medical images. *IEEE Transactions on Medical Imaging, 16*(5), 642–652.

Chalana, V., Linker, D. T., Haynor, D. R., & Kim, Y. (1996). A multiple active contour model for cardiac boundary detection on echocardiographic sequences. *IEEE Transactions on Medical Imaging, 15*(3), 290–298.

Gomes, H. M., & Fisher, R. B. (2003). Primal sketch feature extraction from a log-polar image. *Pattern Recognition Letters, 24*(7), 983–992.

Kass, M., Witkin, A., & Terzopoulos, D. (1988). Snakes: Active contour models. *International Journal of Computer Vision, 1*(4), 321–331.

Koh, L. H., Ranganath, S., & Venkatesh, Y. V. (2002). An integrated automatic face detection and recognition system. *Pattern Recognition, 35*(6), 1259–1273.

Morelande, M. R., Iskander, D. R., Collins, M. J., & Franklin, R. (2002). Automatic estimation of the corneal limbus in videokeratoscopy. *IEEE Transactions on Biomedical Engineering, 49* (12), 1617–1625.

Ohtsu, N. (1979). A threshold selection method from gray-level histograms. *IEEE Transactions on Systems Man & Cybernetics, 9*(1), 62–66.

Pang, B., Wang, K., Zhang, D., & Zhang, F. (2002). *On automated tongue image segmentation in Chinese medicine* (pp. 616–619). IEEE.

Smeraldi, F., & Bigun, J. (2002). Retinal vision applied to facial features detection and face authentication. *Pattern Recognition Letters, 23*(4), 463–475.

Steger, C. (1998). An unbiased detector of curvilinear structures. *IEEE Transactions on Pattern Analysis and Machine Intelligence, 20*(2), 113–125.

Udupa, J. K., LaBlanc, V. R., Schmidt, H., Imielinska, C., Saha, P. K., & Grevera, G. J., et al. (2002). *Methodology for evaluating image-segmentation algorithms* (pp. 266–277). International Society for Optics and Photonics.

Wallace, A. M., & McLaren, D. J. (2003). Gradient detection in discrete log-polar images. *Pattern Recognition Letters, 24*(14), 2463–2470.

Xue, J., Pizurica, A., Philips, W., Kerre, E., Van De Walle, R., & Lemahieu, I. (2003). An integrated method of adaptive enhancement for unsupervised segmentation of MRI brain images. *Pattern Recognition Letters, 24*(15), 2549–2560.

Zhang, H., Zuo, W., Wang, K., & Zhang, D. (2006). A snake-based approach to automated segmentation of tongue image using polar edge detector. *International Journal of Imaging Systems & Technology, 16*(4), 103–112.

Chapter 5
Tongue Segmentation in Hyperspectral Images

Abstract Automatic tongue area segmentation is crucial for computer-aided tongue diagnosis, but traditional intensity-based segmentation methods that make use of monochromatic images cannot provide accurate and robust results. We propose a novel tongue segmentation method that uses hyperspectral images and the support vector machine. This method combines spatial and spectral information to analyze the medical tongue image and can provide much better tongue segmentation results. Promising experimental results and quantitative evaluations demonstrate that our method can provide much better performance than the traditional method.

5.1 Introduction

Because of the physiological properties of the human tongue, automatic tongue segmentation is a challenging task in computer-aided diagnosis. The existing methods are not always effective (Pang, Zhang, & Wang, 2005), especially when the surface color of the tongue is similar to its ambient tissue. The reason for this limitation is mainly that all methods are based on the analysis of intensity difference in monochromatic images, which inspires us to continue the study on other more effective methods by exploring not only new algorithms, but also different types of imaging schemes.

The increasing requirement for accurate noninvasive diagnosis and treatment promotes the application of optical technologies in this field. Optical techniques have the ability to perform a diagnosis on tissues without the need for sample excision. Another advantage of optical diagnosis is that the resulting information can be visually available. Current optical diagnostic technologies can be categorized into three broad categories. The first, which records a two-dimensional (2D) image of an area of the sample of interest at one specific wavelength, can be called an optical image (OI). The second, which obtains an entire spectrum of a single tissue within a wavelength region of interest, can be called a spectral image (SI). The third, which is relatively new, combines the two modalities mentioned above, and is often referred to as hyperspectral imaging (HSI) (Vo-Dinh, 2004).

D. Zhang et al., *Tongue Image Analysis*, DOI 10.1007/978-981-10-2167-1_5

Use of HSI for biomedical applications is attractive, since it records the entire emission for every pixel on the entire image in the field of view (Magotra, Wu, Soliz, Truitt, Gelabert, & Stetzler, 1999). The interaction of light with human tissue varies, and has been extensively studied (Tuchin, & Tuchin, 2007; Anderson, & Parrish, 1981). Small changes in the distribution of pigments such as melanin, hemoglobin, bilirubin, and β-carotene in the epidermal and dermal layers of the human skin can produce significant changes in the skin's spectral reflectance (Edwards, & Duntley, 1939). Some researchers (Pan, Healey, Prasad, & Tromberg, 2003; Angelopoulo, Molana, & Daniilidis, 2001) measured skin reflectance spectra over the visible wavelengths and modeled them. For instance, Angelopoulo et al. (2001) used a skin reflectance model to propose a method for skin detection under varying lighting conditions.

As can be seen from the previous chapters, the automatic segmentation of anatomical structures in traditional monochromatic images is often performed using model-based non-rigid registration methods. That is to say, an automatic segmentation of a certain structure can be obtained by registering a labeled model, typically generated in a manual segmentation process, to another data set containing the structure of interest. This registration is difficult and laborious (Crum, Hartkens, & Hill, 2014). This is a problem that might be solved if the variability in the spectra of different tissue types could be used to distinguish between the human tongue and the non-tongue biological substances in hyperspectral image space.

Many supervised methods have been developed to classify multispectral data. Some of the successful approaches to multispectral data classification have used artificial neural networks, such as multilayer perceptions (MLPs) (Bischof, & Leonardis, 1998) and radial basis function neural networks (RBFNNs) (Bruzzone, & Prieto, 1999). However, these approaches are not effective when dealing with a large number of spectral bands since they are highly sensitive to the Hughes phenomenon (Hughes, 1968) known as the curse of dimensionality. That is, for a fixed and finite number of training samples, with an increasing number of features, the classification accuracy first improves to a peak value and then declines. The decline is due to limitations on the precision of class statistics estimation resulting from limited training data. Fortunately, support vector machines (SVM) (Hughes, 1968) can conquer the curse of dimensionality. In recent years, SVM has been successfully used for the classification of hyperspectral data (Melgani, & Bruzzone, 2004). It has three advantages: (1) large input spaces are available for SVM, (2) SVM is robust against noise, and (3) SVM generates sparse solutions, which are subsets of training samples.

In this chapter, we provide a novel framework for tongue area segmentation that uses hyperspectral images acquired with our special device and the supervised SVM classifier. This approach combines the spectral and special information of the tongue surface and presents promising results for further analysis. The remainder of the chapter is organized as follows. We describe the setup of the device in Sect. 5.2 and briefly introduce SVMs in Sect. 5.3. We describe the segmentation framework in Sect. 5.3 and the experimental results and quantitative evaluations in Sect. 5.4. Our conclusions are presented in Sect. 5.5.

5.2 Setup of the Hyperspectral Device

To obtain the hyperspectral image data, a device based on the theory of the pushbroom hyperspectral imager (PHI) (Mouroulis, Green, & Chrien, 2000; Sinclair, Timlin, Haaland, & Werner-Washburne, 2004) was used, whose main modules are illustrated in Fig. 5.1. It consists of a spectrometer, a matrix CCD, an instrument translation module, and a data collection module. This device has the ability to acquire a complete spatial–spectral image cube in 180 ms from 400 to 1000 nm, which basically eliminates motion artifacts. We built a studio with two constant light sources for this capture device so that the illumination is constant. Each of the light sources is a 100 W halogen lamp with a white diffuser screen. The two sources provide approximately uniform illumination on the subject. Also, the camera was calibrated and fixed on the frame. The distance between the lens and the tongue is constant, and the head of the patient can be constrained by a framework (shown in Fig. 5.6). Therefore, the illumination can be considered to be constant in our study.

This device provides a sequence of images in different spectral bands. In other words, the HSI approach provides a "data cube" of spectral information, which consists of a series of optical images recorded at various wavelengths of interest. An example of the image cube is illustrated in Fig. 5.2. Each pixel of the image has two properties: the spectrum property and the intensity property. Based on analyzing the "image cube," it can be seen that different object surfaces can be represented by

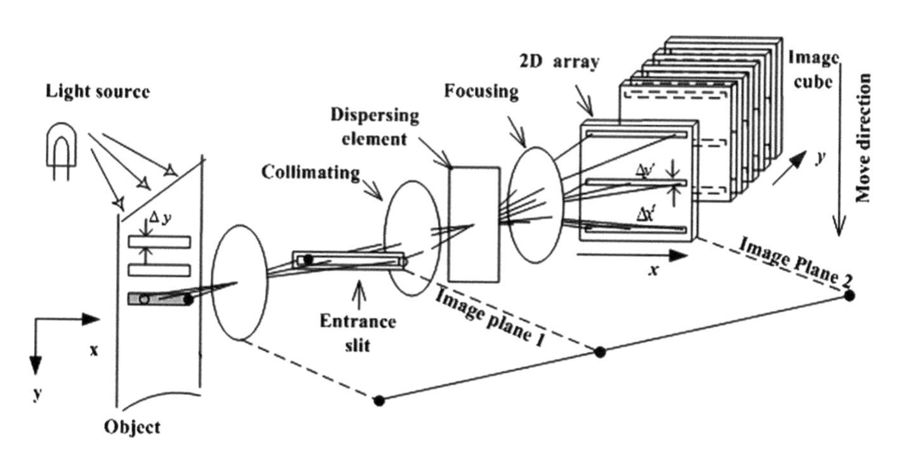

Fig. 5.1 Schematic of hyperspectral imaging sensor system. Reprinted from Liu, Yan, Zhang, & Li, (2007). Copyright (2016), with permission from OSA

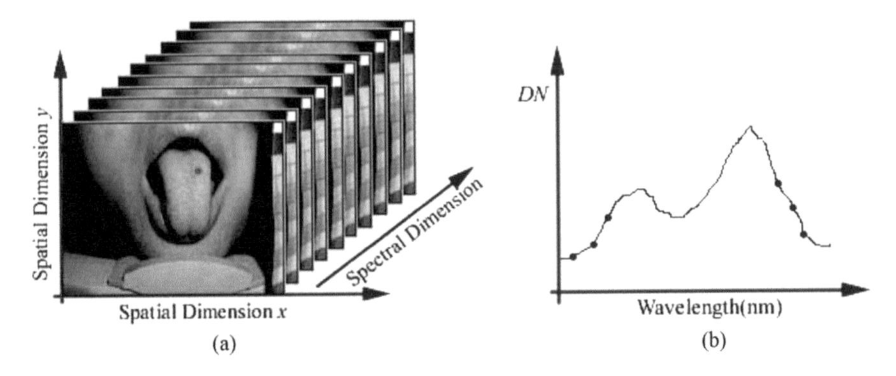

Fig. 5.2 **a** HSI cube and **b** spectrum corresponding to the point in (**a**). Reprinted from Liu et al. (2007). Copyright (2016), with permission from OSA

different band curves. Thus, using these special tongue images, we can do tongue area segmentation according to the difference in spectral curves between the tongue and its ambient organs.

5.3 Segmentation Framework

The SVM is a popular classifier based on statistical learning theory as proposed by Vapnik (2013). The training phase of SVMs is to find a linear optimal separating hyperplane as a maximum margin classifier with respect to the training data. In SVMs, support vectors, which are critical for classification, are obtained in a learning phase that uses training samples. In the test phase for classification, class labels are found for the new (i.e., unknown) feature vectors using support vectors. When the training data are not linearly separable, kernel methods (Camps-Valls, & Bruzzone, 2005) are used in SVMs. These kernel methods map data from the original input space to a kernel feature space of higher dimensionality. The parameters of the kernels are important for the classification results. In contrast to the traditional learning methods, a SVM does not explicitly depend on the dimensionality of input spaces so it is a good candidate for a supervised classification of hyperspectral images. Some references (Hughes, 1968; Vapnik, 2013; Camps-Valls, & Bruzzone, 2005) detailed the information about SVM.

As hyperspectral images can provide both spectral and spatial information to identify and distinguish specific materials, our method integrates HSI with SVM for tongue area segmentation. The process begins with the calibration for hyperspectral images, and then the region of interest is determined. After the input data are normalized, the SVM is used for classification. At last, according to the results of classification, we obtain the contour of the tongue. The pipeline of the procedure is illustrated in Fig. 5.3, and its main modules are described in the following.

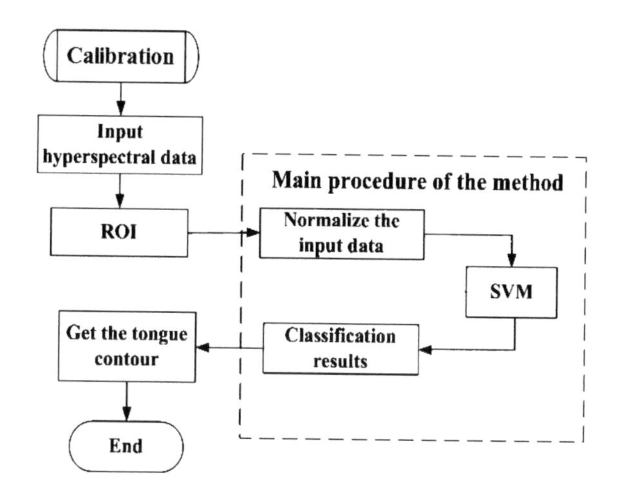

Fig. 5.3 Flow chart of the hyperspectral tongue image segmentation procedure. Reprinted from Liu et al. (2007). Copyright (2016), with permission from OSA

5.3.1 *Hyperspectral Image Calibration*

To obtain the unified representation of the reflectance values for computing, it is necessary to first calibrate the raw hyperspectral images. An effective method for calibration was presented by Pan and Healey (Pan et al., 2003), which we describe briefly as follows.

This method acquires two additional images in black and white. The black image, which has near 0% reflectance, can be obtained by covering the lens. The white image refers to near totally reflected image and is acquired with a white panel in front of the camera at the same distance as for human tongue acquisition. The calibration is traceable to the U.S. National Institute of Standards and Technology (NIST) (Pan et al., 2003).

The image intensity at the spatial coordinate (x, y) for a wavelength can be modeled as

$$I(x,y,\lambda_i) = L(x,y,\lambda_i)S(x,y,\lambda_i)R(x,y,\lambda_i) + O(x,y,\lambda_i) \tag{5.1}$$

where $L(x, y, \lambda_i)$ refers to the illumination, $S(x, y, \lambda_i)$ refers to the system spectral response, $R(x, y, \lambda_i)$ refers to the reflectance of the viewed surface, and $O(x, y, \lambda_i)$ refers to the offset, which includes dark current and stray light. $i = \{1, 2, ..., b\}$, b is the number of spectral bands (in our study, $b = 120$).

For a white image, the intensity of coordinate (x, y) for wavelength λ_i can be modeled as

$$I_W(x,y,\lambda_i) = L(x,y,\lambda_i)S(x,y,\lambda_i)R_W(x,y,\lambda_i) + O(x,y,\lambda_i) \tag{5.2}$$

and for a black image, the intensity of coordinate (x, y) for wavelength λ_i can be modeled as

$$I_B(x,y,\lambda_i) = L(x,y,\lambda_i)S(x,y,\lambda_i)R_B(x,y,\lambda_i) + O(x,y,\lambda_i), \tag{5.3}$$

where $R_w(x, y, \lambda_i)$ and $R_B(x, y, \lambda_i)$ are reflectance functions of the white image and the black image, respectively. Since the viewed surfaces have the same reflectance property for all image pixels, $R_w(x, y, \lambda_i)$ and $R_B(x, y, \lambda_i)$ are theoretically independent of (x, y) and can be denoted as $R_w(\lambda_i)$ and $R_B(\lambda_i)$.

Combining Eqs. (5.2) and (5.3), we can estimate $L(x, y, \lambda_i)$ $S(x, y, \lambda_i)$ as

$$L(x,y,\lambda_i)S(x,y,\lambda) = \frac{I_W(x,y,\lambda_i) - I_B(x,y,\lambda_i)}{R_W(\lambda_i) - R_B(\lambda_i)}. \tag{5.4}$$

When Eq. (5.4) is substituted into Eq. (5.3), $O(x, y, \lambda_i)$ can be estimated as

$$O(x,y,\lambda_i) = I_B(x,y,\lambda_i) \times R_B(\lambda_i) - \frac{I_W(x,y,\lambda_i) - I_B(x,y,\lambda_i)}{R_W(\lambda_i) - R_B(\lambda_i)}. \tag{5.5}$$

With Eqs. (5.4) and (5.5), we obtain the calibration equation provided below:

$$\begin{aligned} R(x,y,\lambda_i) = & \frac{I(x,y,\lambda_i) - I_B(x,y,\lambda_i)}{I_W(x,y,\lambda_i) - I_B(x,y,\lambda_i)} R_W(\lambda_i) \\ & + \frac{I_w(x,y,\lambda_i) - I_B(x,y,\lambda_i)}{I_W(x,y,\lambda_i) - I_B(x,y,\lambda_i)} R_B(\lambda_i). \end{aligned} \tag{5.6}$$

5.3.2 *Segmentation*

The process of segmentation begins by selecting the region of interest (ROI), which eliminates the background from the original images (shown in Fig. 5.4). Thus, the primary sources of variance in the input data, which are the intensity and spectral curve shape, are limited to five classes, i.e., the tongue, the face, the lip, the teeth, and the tissues of the inner mouth. We represent each tongue image using the feature

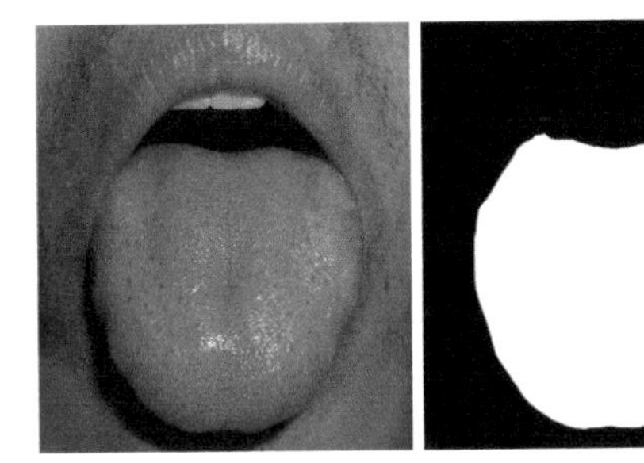

Fig. 5.4 ROI in the captured image (the *left*) and the binary image representing the detected tongue area (the *right*). Reprinted from Liu et al. (2007). Copyright (2016), with permission from OSA

vectors that are extracted from the ROI. The feature vector at coordinate (x, y) can be denoted as $R = [r(x, y, \lambda_1), r(x, y, \lambda_2), \ldots, r(x, y, \lambda_i)]^T$, where $r(x, y, \lambda_i)$ denotes the reflectance at λ_i, and b is the number of spectral bands (in our study, $b = 120$). Then, the normalized spectral reflectance vector R is defined by

$$\tilde{R} = R/\|R\|, \tag{5.7}$$

where $\|\cdot\|$ means the L_2 norm.

Here we should note that in this study the feature vectors are composed of the reflectance values at all wavelength bands. This is because the SVM that we used for classification is different from traditional classifiers that suffer from the curse of dimensionality (Hughes, 1968), such as MLP (Bischof, & Leonardis, 1998) and RBFNN (Bruzzone, & Prieto, 1999). As a superior classification algorithm, SVM works well on hyperspectral data and does not require preprocessing to reduce data dimensionality for conquering the curse of dimensionality (Melgani, & Bruzzone, 2004). In fact, we have found that the accuracy of SVM deteriorates with the application of feature extraction techniques (Shah, Watanachaturaporn, Varshney, & Arora, 2003). This demonstrates that for SVM classification, the possibility of finding an optimum hyperplane for separating the classes is higher in the high-dimensional data set than in the reduced-dimensional data set. Therefore, unlike other classifiers, SVM classifiers may be adopted when the entire data set is required to be used, and so, in our study, we selected all the wave bands as the input features for classification.

The next step is to use the SVM to classify the tongue and non-tongue areas. To do this, the input feature space is first mapped by a kernel transformation into a higher dimensional space, where it is expected to find a linear separation that maximizes the margin between the two classes. In the hyperspectral space, a normally distributed model is a reasonable assumption for optical human organ detection data. A number of kernels have been discussed for the SVM, but it is not clear how to choose one that gives the best generalization for a particular problem. The type of kernel that is chosen and the values of the parameters associated with the kernel both affect the classification accuracy. In our study, the popular Gaussian kernel is exploited for the SVM, and the multiclass strategy for the SVM (Crum et al., 2014) is used to classify the various tissues. SVM labels the separated parts as the tongue, face, lip, teeth, and inner tissue of the mouth. Then the pixel of the tongue area is represented by "1" and that of the non-tongue area is represented by "0" in a corresponding binary image of the same size (Fig. 5.4) extracting the contour of the tongue. Finally, we map the results into the color tongue images (see Fig. 5.5). Note these color images are in red–green–blue (RGB) color space and can be integrated using three frames from a hyperspectral image cube corresponding to 650 nm (red), 510 nm (green), and 475 nm (blue).

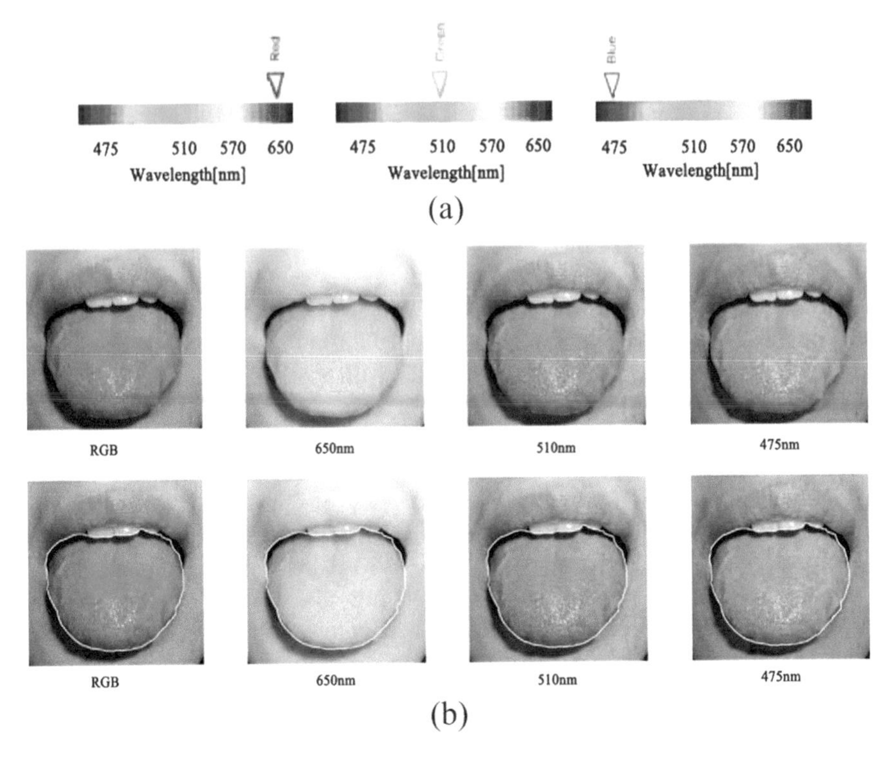

Fig. 5.5 **a** Spectrum of the visible light. **b** *Top row* RGB tongue image synthesized by three spectral images. *Bottom row* segmentation results in hyperspectral images and mapping them directly into the RGB tongue image. Reprinted from Liu et al. (2007). Copyright (2016), with permission from OSA

5.4 Experiments and Comparisons

We used our hyperspectral image capture device to obtain a series of tongue images with efficient pixels of 652 × 488. The device was operated in a spectral wavelength range of 400–1000 nm with two distinct spectra regimes, visible (400 and 720 nm) and near infrared (720 and 1000 nm). One hundred and fifty-two volunteers were sampled for this experiment. Figure 5.6 shows some examples of the captured images from the visible wavelength range at different bands, and Fig. 5.7 illustrates the differences in the spectral curves of different tissues. Eighty samples were randomly chosen from the 152 volunteers and were used to train SVMs, and the remainders were used for testing. In this experiment, for training, we manually extracted from the training sample set samples of the tongue, face, teeth, lip, and the tissue of the inner mouth. We used a "one-against-all" multiclass strategy (Melgani, & Bruzzone, 2004). This very common approach is based on a parallel architecture made up of T ($T = 5$ in our study) SVMs. Each SVM solves a two-class problem defined by one class against all the others. The "winner-takes-all" rule is used for the final decision.

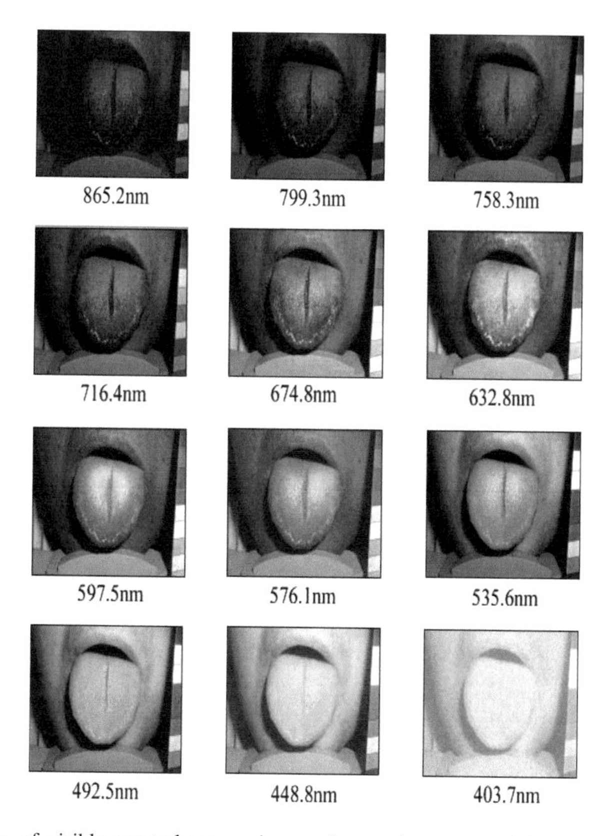

Fig. 5.6 Series of visible spectral tongue images from a hyperspectral image cube. Reprinted from Liu et al. (2007). Copyright (2016), with permission from OSA

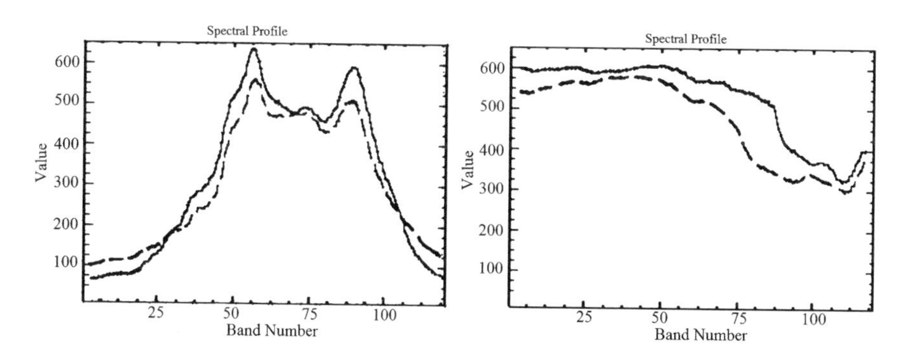

Fig. 5.7 Spectral curves of the tongue and the skin of the face from two subjects. Reprinted from Liu et al. (2007). Copyright (2016), with permission from OSA

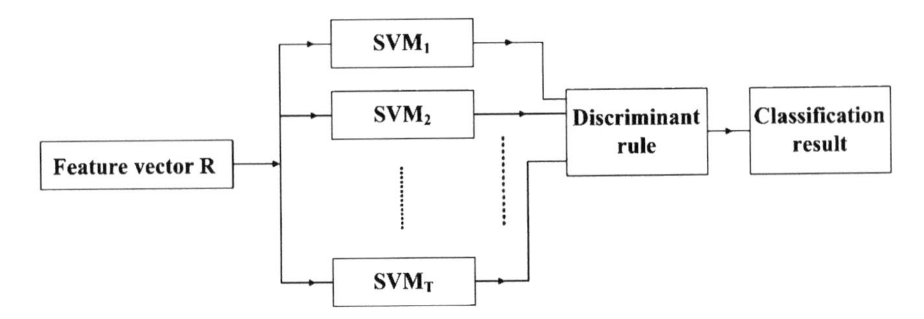

Fig. 5.8 Block diagram of the architecture for solving multiclass problems with SVMs Reprinted from Liu et al. (2007). Copyright (2016), with permission from OSA

That is, the winning class is the one corresponding to the SVM with the highest output (discriminant function value). The architecture of this strategy can be seen in Fig. 5.8.

In the following subsections, we propose the criteria of evaluation and compare our approach with a popular method called the bi-elliptical deformable contour (BEDC).

5.4.1 Criteria of Evaluation

It is necessary to quantitatively evaluate the performance of the segmentation. Chalana and Kim (2002) suggested the use of boundary error metrics to evaluate segmentation performance. Let $A = \{a_1, a_2, \ldots, a_m\}$ and $B = \{b_1, b_2, \ldots, b_n\}$ denote the automatic segmentation result and manual segmentation result, respectively, where $a_1, a_2, \ldots, a_m$ and $b_1, b_2, \ldots, b_n$ are points on the corresponding boundary curve. Define the distance to the closest point (DCP) for a_t, to curve B as

$$d(a_i, B) = \min_j \left\| b_j - a_i \right\|. \tag{5.8}$$

Then, the Hausdorff distance *(HD)* between the two curves is defined as the maximum of the DCP between the two curves. This can be formularized as

$$HD(A, B) = \max(\max_i \{d(a_i, B)\}, \max_i \{b_j, A\}). \tag{5.9}$$

The mean DCP distance (*MD*) of two curves A and B can be defined as

$$MD(A, B) = \frac{1}{m+n}\left(\sum_i d(a_i, B) + \sum_J d((b_j, A))\right). \tag{5.10}$$

5.4.2 Comparison with the BEDC

To the best of our knowledge, the BEDC proposed by Pang et al. (2005) is currently the most effective method for use in tongue segmentation applications. BEDC combines a bi-elliptical deformable template (BEDT) and an active contour model. The BEDT captures gross shape features using the steepest descent method on its energy function in the parameter space. The BEDC is derived from the BEDT by substituting template forces for classical internal forces and can deform to fit local details. However, this method is based on the intensity of images and cannot obtain satisfactory results when the intensity values of the tongue and its ambient tissues are close (Pang et al., 2005). Our HSI + SVM method combines the hyperspectral image spectral features and the effective classifier, SVM, to segment the tongue area, which is immune to the factors that affect the performance of BEDC. Figure 5.9 shows some results of segmentation using our method and BEDC. The results of HSI + SVM are shown in Fig. 5.9b, d, f. We implemented the BEDC algorithm with the images at the spectral band whose central wavelength was 492.5 nm. The results of BEDC can be seen in Fig. 5.9a, c, e.

We evaluated the segmentation performance of HSI + SVM and BEDC using the distance measurement mentioned in Subsection 5.1. To calculate the distance, we manually extracted the ground truths (i.e., the accurate boundaries of the tongue) from the images. We then calculated the distance between the ground truth and the results using HSI + SVM and BEDC, respectively. For the distance measure, we used *HD* and *MD* defined by Eqs. (5.9) and (5.10). *HD* and *MD* as shown in Table 5.1 are both the average of the testing results, which can be formularized as

$$\overline{HD} = \sum_{i}^{N} HD/N\overline{MD} = \sum_{i}^{N} MA/N, \tag{5.11}$$

where N is the number of the testing examples (in our study, N = 152 − 80 = 72). Furthermore, we show the standard error (S_E) of *HD* and *MD* that we used in comparing our method and BEDC. The standard error can be computed as

$$S_E = \frac{s}{\sqrt{N}}, s = \sqrt{\frac{1}{N-1}\sum_{i=1}^{N}(x_i - \bar{x})^2}, \tag{5.12}$$

where s is the sample standard deviation.

Table 5.1 and Fig. 5.10 show the results of the comparison of our method and BEDC. It can be seen that the values of *HD* and *MD* with our method are 11 and 6.23, respectively. In contrast, the two values of BEDC are 27 and 10.14, respectively. It is obvious that our method produces more accurate results than BEDC. Furthermore, the standard errors of *HD* and *MD* when we use our method are both much smaller than those of BEDC. This shows that our method can obtain more stable segmentation results than BEDC.

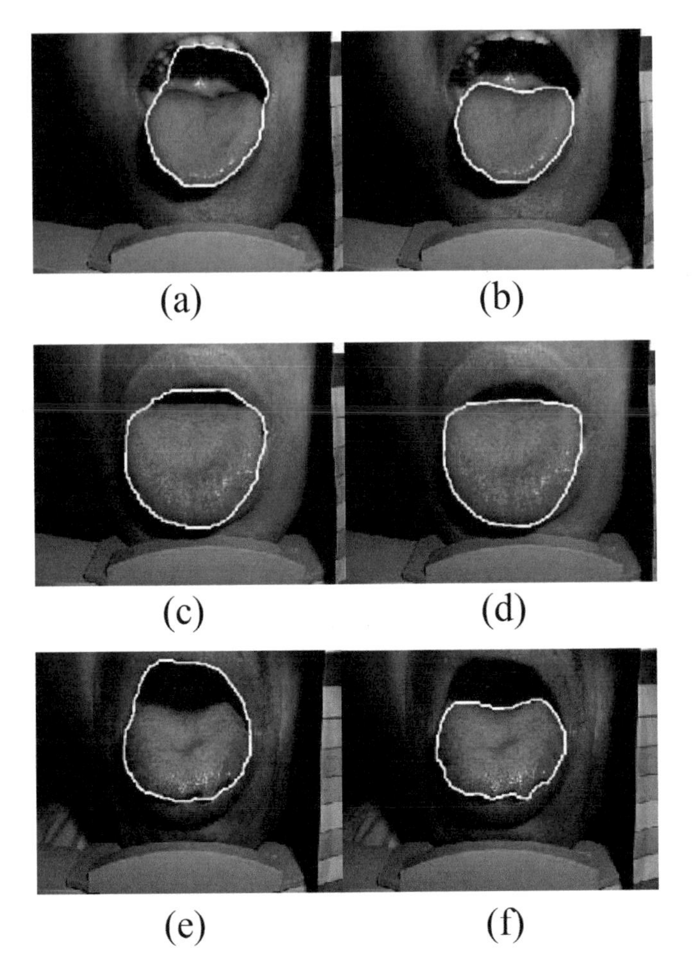

Fig. 5.9 Comparison of tongue segmentation results (**a**). **c** and **e** are the results of the BEDC method (Pang et al., 2005). **b**, **d**, and **f** are the results of our proposed HSI + SVM method. Reprinted from Liu et al. (2007). Copyright (2016), with permission from OSA

Table 5.1 Comparison of the HSI + SVM method and the BEDC method (Pang et al., 2005) tongue segmentation results in terms of boundary metrics

	HD (in pixels)	$S_{E(HD)}$	*MD* (in pixels)	$S_{E(MD)}$
HSI + SVM	11	0.278	6.23	0.233
BEDC	27	0.567	10.14	0.481

Reprinted from Liu et al. (2007). Copyright (2016), with permission from OSA

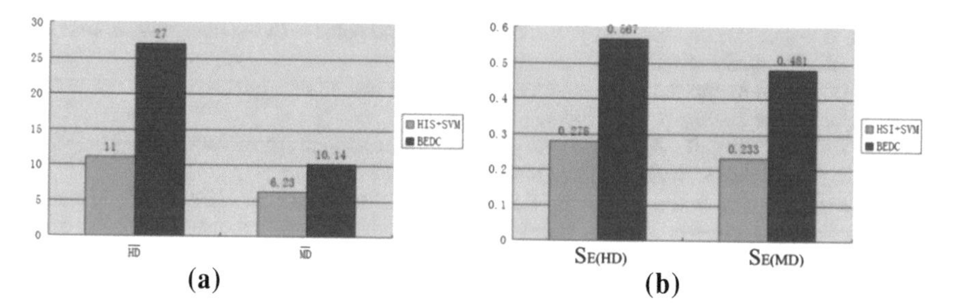

Fig. 5.10 Histogram of the comparison of our method and BEDC: **a** HD and MD and **b** SEHD and SEMD. Reprinted from Liu et al. (2007). Copyright (2016), with permission from OSA

5.5 Summary

In the field of human tongue segmentation, traditional deformable template methods are popular. However, these intensity-based algorithms are not always robust, as in a monochromatic image, the intensity of the surface of the tongue may be similar to that of surrounding tissue. In this chapter, we present a new method for segmenting medical images of the tongue using hyperspectral equipment. The method (HSI + SVM) uses hyperspectral images to differentiate between the tongue and the surrounding tissue by exploiting the spectral variability of different tissue types and combines it with support vector machines, a popular classifier that does not explicitly depend on the dimensionality of input spaces and has a good generalization performance. The experimental result and the corresponding quantitative evaluation demonstrate that the proposed hybrid HSI + SVM approach can provide more effective and robust performance than the traditional method.

References

Anderson, R. R., & Parrish, J. A. (1981). The optics of human skin. *Journal of Investigative Dermatology, 77*(1), 13–19.

Angelopoulo, E., Molana, R., & Daniilidis, K. (2001). Multispectral skin color modeling (pp. 635). IEEE.

Bischof, H., & Leonardis, A. (1998). Finding optimal neural networks for land use classification. *IEEE Transactions on Geoscience and Remote Sensing, 36*(1), 337–341.

Bruzzone, L., & Prieto, D. F. A. N. (1999). A technique for the selection of kernel-function parameters in RBF neural networks for classification of remote-sensing images. *IEEE Transactions on Geoscience and Remote Sensing, 37*(2), 1179–1184.

Camps-Valls, G., & Bruzzone, L. (2005). Kernel-based methods for hyperspectral image classification. *IEEE Transactions on Geoscience and Remote Sensing, 43*(6), 1351–1362.

Chalana, V., & Kim, Y. (2002). A methodology for evaluation of boundary detection algorithms on medical images. *Biomaterials, 23*(19), 3985–3990.

Crum, W. R., Hartkens, T., & Hill, D. (2014). Non-rigid image registration: theory and practice. *The British Journal of Radiology*.

Edwards, E. A., & Duntley, S. Q. (1939). The pigments and color of living human skin. *American Journal of Anatomy, 65*(1), 1–33.

Hughes, G. P. (1968). On the mean accuracy of statistical pattern recognizers. *IEEE Transactions on Information Theory, 14*(1), 55–63.

Liu, Z., Yan, J., Zhang, D., & Li, Q. L. (2007). Automated tongue segmentation in hyperspectral images for medicine. *Applied Optics, 46*(34), 8328–8334.

Magotra, N., Wu, E., Soliz, P., Truitt, P., Gelabert, P., & Stetzler, T. (1999). *Hyperspectral biomedical image formation* (pp. 462–465). IEEE.

Melgani, F., & Bruzzone, L. (2004). Classification of hyperspectral remote sensing images with support vector machines. *IEEE Transactions on Geoscience and Remote Sensing, 42*(8), 1778–1790.

Mouroulis, P., Green, R. O., & Chrien, T. G. (2000). Design of pushbroom imaging spectrometers for optimum recovery of spectroscopic and spatial information. *Applied Optics, 39*(13), 2210–2220.

Pan, Z., Healey, G., Prasad, M., & Tromberg, B. (2003). Face recognition in hyperspectral images. *IEEE Transactions on Pattern Analysis and Machine Intelligence, 25*(12), 1552–1560.

Pang, B., Zhang, D., & Wang, K. (2005). The bi-elliptical deformable contour and its application to automated tongue segmentation in Chinese medicine. *IEEE Transactions on Medical Imaging, 24*(8), 946–956.

Shah, C. A., Watanachaturaporn, P., Varshney, P. K., & Arora, M. K. (2003). Some recent results on hyperspectral image classification (pp. 346–353). IEEE.

Sinclair, M. B., Timlin, J. A., Haaland, D. M., & Werner-Washburne, M. (2004). Design, construction, characterization, and application of a hyperspectral microarray scanner. *Applied Optics, 43*(10), 2079–2088.

Tuchin, V. U. I. V., & Tuchin, V. (2007). *Tissue optics: Light scattering methods and instruments for medical diagnosis* (Vol. 13). SPIE press Bellingham.

Vapnik, V. (2013). *The nature of statistical learning theory*. Springer Science & Business Media.

Vo-Dinh, T. (2004). A hyperspectral imaging system for in vivo optical diagnostics. *IEEE Engineering in Medicine and Biology Magazine, 23*(5), 40–49.

Chapter 6
Tongue Segmentation by Gradient Vector Flow and Region Merging

Abstract This chapter presents a region merging-based automatic tongue segmentation method. First, gradient vector flow is modified as a scalar diffusion equation to diffuse the tongue image while preserving the edge structures of the tongue body. Then the diffused tongue image is segmented into many small regions by using the watershed algorithm. Third, maximal similarity-based region merging is used to extract the tongue body area under the control of the tongue marker. Finally, the snake algorithm is used to refine the region merging result by setting the extracted tongue contour as the initial curve. The proposed method was qualitatively tested on 200 images by Traditional Chinese Medicine practitioners and quantitatively tested on 50 tongue images using the receiver operating characteristic analysis. Compared with the previous active contour model-based bi-elliptical deformable contour algorithm, the proposed method greatly enhances the segmentation performance, and it can reliably extract the tongue body from different types of tongue images.

6.1 Introduction

From the previous chapters, it can be seen that an accurate segmentation of the tongue body from the tongue image is a crucial step in computer-aided tongue diagnosis. Many methods have been proposed to segment the structure of interest for medical images. For example, active contour models (ACM) (Kass, Witkin, & Terzopoulos, 1988; Zhang, Zhang, Song, & Zhou, 2010a, b), also known as "snakes".

However, the above methods are not well suited for tongue body segmentation due to the particular features of tongue images (Pang, Zhang, & Wang, 2005). In general, the tongue body has an approximately ellipse contour, and it is located in the center of the tongue image. In (Pang et al., 2005), Pang et al. proposed the bi-elliptical deformable contour (BEDC) algorithm, which is a type of ACM-based method. However, ACM is very sensitive to the initial curve.

When objects such as the face, lips, neck, wrinkles, and cloth appear around the tongue body, there are often many strong edges inside the initial curves so that

D. Zhang et al., *Tongue Image Analysis*, DOI 10.1007/978-981-10-2167-1_6

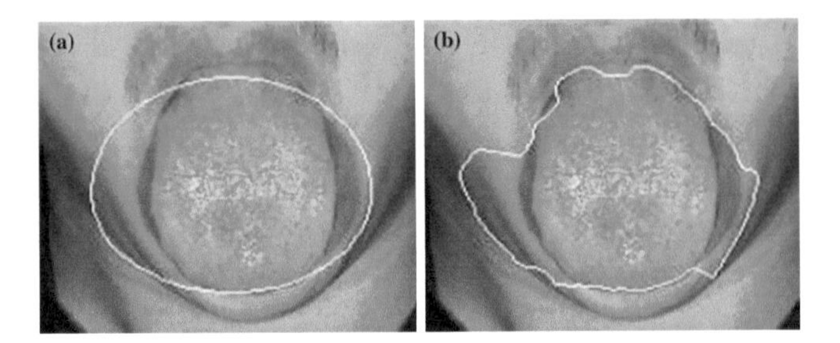

Fig. 6.1 An example of tongue image segmentation by using the BEDC method. **a** Initial bi-elliptical curve obtained by a deformable template and **b** the final segmentation result by BEDC. Reprinted from Ning et al. (2012), with permission of Springer

BEDC has difficulty converging to the true tongue contour. Figure 6.1 shows an example of the tongue segmentation result by using the BEDC algorithm. Because the initial bi-elliptical curve obtained by a deformable template in Fig. 6.1a has strong edge structures of cheek and the tongue shadow inside it, the BEDC method fails to segment the contour of the tongue body (Fig. 6.1b).

To overcome the problems of ACM-based methods, in this chapter we present an automatic tongue segmentation method by using a recently proposed region merging strategy called as maximal similarity-based region merging (MSRM) (Ning, Zhang, Zhang, & Wu, 2010) with initial watershed segmentation. MSRM is an interactive region merging method based on the maximal similarity mechanism and guides the merging process with the help of a marker indicated by the user. The region merging process of MSRM is adaptive to the image content, and the similarity threshold does not need to be set in advance.

In the proposed method, the tongue gradient image (in red channel) is first preprocessed by the modified gradient vector flow (GVF) (Xu & Prince, 1998) to reduce the oversegmentation in the watershed method while preserving the edge structures in tongue images. Second, the MSRM algorithm is used to automatically extract the tongue body area by analyzing the structure of the tongue image. Finally, ACM is used to refine the result by taking the extracted tongue contour as the initial curve.

The rest of the chapter is organized as follows. Section 6.2 describes the initial tongue image segmentation by watershed segmentation after GVF preprocessing. In Sect. 6.3, we use the MSRM algorithm and active contour models to extract the tongue contour. Section 6.4 presents extensive experimental results, and Sect. 6.5 concludes the chapter.

6.2 Initial Segmentation

The captured tongue image is in RGB color space, i.e. at each location, the pixel is composed of red, green, and blue color components. Because red is usually the dominant color of the tongue body and most detailed structures are contained in the red channel (Pang et al., 2005), we use the red color plane to process the tongue body segmentation.

We use the watershed algorithm (Vincent & Soille, 1991) to make an initial segmentation of the tongue image. However, the watershed algorithm is very sensitive to noise, and it often leads to severe oversegmentation. Therefore, we perform preprocessing on the tongue image to suppress noises. To this end, the GVF approach (Xu & Prince, 1998), which is an effective edge-preserving noise reduction method based on the partial differential equation (PDE), is employed. In recent years, image segmentation using PDE with a watershed transform has attracted much research interest (Weickert, 2001). The advantage of the proposed GVF-based gradient magnitude diffusion is to work with the gradient (magnitude) image, and it can remove noise and more effectively reduce the trivial details in the tongue image while preserving the main features. The PDE equation for GVF is:

$$\mu\nabla^2 u - (u - f_x)\left(f_x^2 + f_y^2\right) = 0, \mu\nabla^2 v - (v - f_x)\left(f_x^2 + f_y^2\right) = 0, \tag{6.1}$$

where ∇^2 is the Laplacian operator, (u, v) represents the gradient vector after diffusion, and its initial value is (f_x, f_y), the gradient vector of f. The Laplacian operator in (6.1) is a diffusion operator, whose function is similar to Gaussian smoothing. Therefore, GVF can remove the trivial structures (i.e., weak edges) and reduce the interference of noise so that the Snake curve can better converge toward the true boundary of the object.

In Xu and Prince (1998), the GVF was applied to gradient vector images to obtain an external force field for the snake model. In this study, we apply GVF diffusion to gradient magnitude images to construct a good watershed structure in order to reduce oversegmentation. To this end, we change (6.1) to the following form.

$$\mu\nabla^2 g - f^2(g - f) = 0, \tag{6.2}$$

where f is the gradient magnitude image, and g is the diffused result of f. Equation (6.2) can be viewed as a scalar version of the classical GVF. It has essentially the same diffusion principle as that of Eq. (6.1).

After the above preprocessing, a new gradient magnitude image can be obtained, in which the trivial structures are substantially reduced and the watershed structure is well generated. Figure 6.2 shows an example. Figure 6.2a is the tongue gradient image in which Fig. 6.2a, b shows the segmentation result by applying the watershed algorithm to it. The severe oversegmentation in the segmentation output, which makes the following region merging process very difficult can be seen. However, by using GVF processing to remove noise and trivial structures, the oversegmentation can be significantly reduced. Figure 6.2c shows the GVF processed result of and Fig. 6.2d is the watershed segmentation result of it. It can be seen that many trivial structures in the gradient magnitude image are removed, and thus the oversegmentation is greatly. In addition, the whole tongue body contour is well preserved.

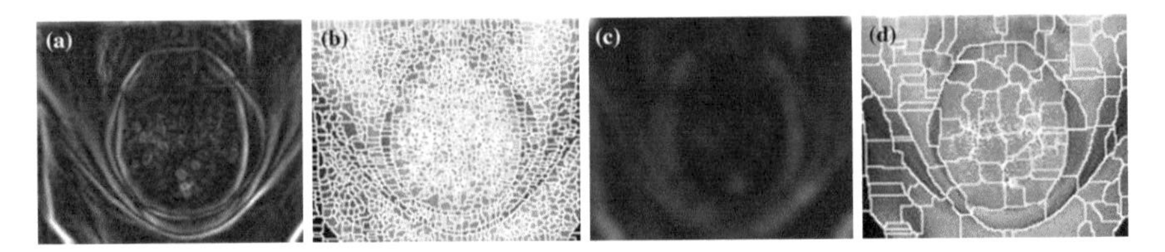

Fig. 6.2 An example of tongue image segmentation using watershed algorithm. **a** The gradient image of the image in Fig. 6.1; **b** the watershed segmentation result of (**a**); **c** the GVF processing result of (**a**); **d** the watershed segmentation of (**c**). Reprinted from Ning et al. (2012), with permission of Springer

6.3 Extraction of Tongue Area

By applying the watershed algorithm to the diffused tongue image, the tongue image is segmented into many small regions. Now the problem is how to merge the segmented regions so that the tongue body can be separated from the background. Some region merging methods have been proposed based on watershed segmentation. For example, in (Hernandez, Barner, & Yuan, 2005), a region merging method was proposed to make use of the homogeneity in joints with edge integrity to enhance the segmentations results. Due to the specialty of tongue images, however, the above region merging method is not applicable to extracting the tongue body from the tongue images.

The background objects in the captured tongue image include face, beard, lips, teeth, and cloth. In general, color is the most important feature in distinguishing the tongue body from the background objects. While some texture features such as the Local Binary Pattern (Ojala, Pietikainen, & Maenpaa, 2002; Guo, Zhang, & Zhang, 2010a, b) can be used for tongue body extraction, they are not as robust as color features. Our experiments found that employing both texture and color features in the proposed region merging algorithm cannot improve the tongue body extraction results very much but increases the computational complexity. Therefore, for simplicity, we only use color to represent the region in the following region merging development. The RGB color space is employed, while the other color spaces, such as HSV, and Lab, can also be used. To reduce the computation, we quantify the RGB space into $16 \times 16 \times 16 = 4096$ bins.

6.3.1 Similarity Metric

The basic idea of region merging-based segmentation is to merge similar regions so that the desired object can be extracted. To compare the similarity among various regions, we choose the Bhattacharyya coefficient as the metric. The Bhattacharyya coefficient between two regions P and Q is defined as follows:

$$\rho(P, Q) = \sum_{u=1}^{m} \sqrt{\text{Hist}_P^u \cdot \text{Hist}_Q^u}, \tag{6.3}$$

where Hist_P and Hist_Q are the normalized histograms of P and Q, respectively, and the superscript u represents the uth bin in Hist_P and Hist_Q.

The Bhattacharyya coefficient is a divergence-type measure that has a straightforward geometric interpretation. It is the cosine of the angle between histogram vectors P and Q. The similarity between two regions is proportional to the magnitude of their Bhattacharyya coefficient.

6.3.2 *The Extraction of the Tongue Body by Using the MRSM Algorithm*

Recently, an interactive region merging method called MSRM (Ning et al., 2010) was proposed, which is based on the maximal similarity mechanism. Its advantage is that it adapts to the image content, and the similarity threshold does not need to be set in advance. But MSRM requires the user to indicate the object marker and background marker.

With the prior knowledge that the tongue body is usually located in the center of the whole tongue image, we define a marker that is a circular region and is located in the center of the tongue image. Obviously, the marker should be a part of the tongue body. Moreover, the regions that have pixels inside the marker should belong to the tongue body. We call these regions object regions. Furthermore, the regions that have pixels located on the border of the tongue image are considered as background markers. Because the object marker and background markers can be obtained by prior knowledge, we can automatically apply the MSRM algorithm to extract the tongue body. Figure 6.3 is an example of extracting the tongue body by the MSRM algorithm.

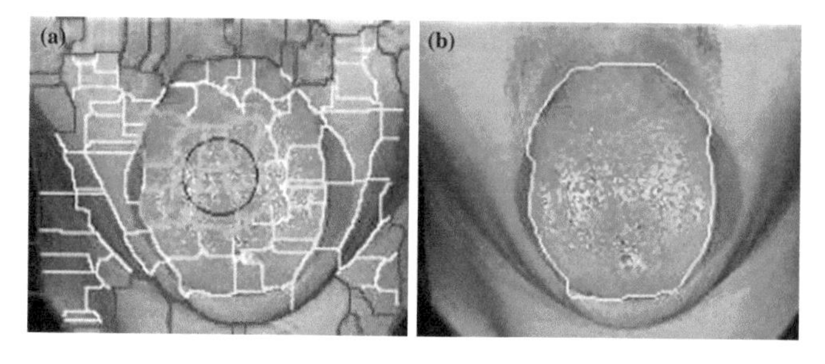

Fig. 6.3 Extracting the tongue body by using the MSRM algorithm. **a** The markers obtained by prior knowledge. **b** The extracted tongue contour by using the MSRM algorithm. Reprinted from Ning et al. (2012), with permission of Springer

By using the MSRM algorithm, the tongue body can be well segmented, and the extracted tongue contour is very close to the true tongue body boundary. However, the tongue contour in Fig. 6.3b is obtained by using the snake algorithm. Obviously, the refined tongue contour is smoother than the result obtained by region merging.

6.4 Experimental Results and Discussions

We randomly selected 200 tongue images from our database to test and evaluate the algorithms. Extensive experiments have been made to evaluate the proposed algorithm in comparison with the BEDC method in (Pang et al., 2005).

6.4.1 Experimental Results

The first example is illustrated in Fig. 6.4. In Fig. 6.4a, the bi-elliptical curve obtained by a deformable template is very close to the true tongue contour, and the extracted tongue contour (Fig. 6.4b) by using BEDC is good but still has noticeable errors in the left and right sides of boundary. Figure 6.4c shows the initial watershed segmentation, and Fig. 6.4d is the final segmentation result by the proposed method. It can be seen that the GVF preprocessing effectively suppresses the influence from background objects such as lips and teeth.

Figure 6.5 shows another example, where the tongue body is very long and the bi-elliptical model is not able to well approximate its shape to find a good initial curve (Fig. 6.5a) so that the segmentation result by BEDC fails (Fig. 6.5b). In the proposed method, the shape of the tongue contour does not need to be defined in advance. Starting from the initial watershed segmentation (Fig. 6.5c), it can completely merge the regions belonging to background objects (lips, cloth, and dark shadow.) into a large region and then accurately extract the shape of the tongue body (Fig. 6.5d).

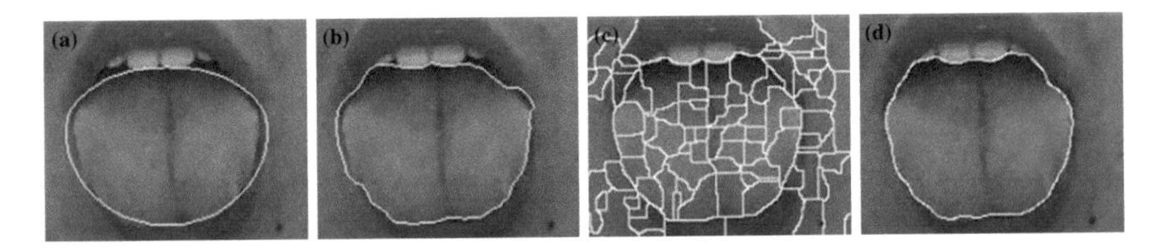

Fig. 6.4 Comparisons between the BEDC scheme and the proposed method. **a** Bi-elliptical curve, **b** tongue contour extracted by BEDC, **c** initial by watershed segmentation, **d** tongue contour extracted by the proposed method. Reprinted from Ning et al. (2012), with permission of Springer

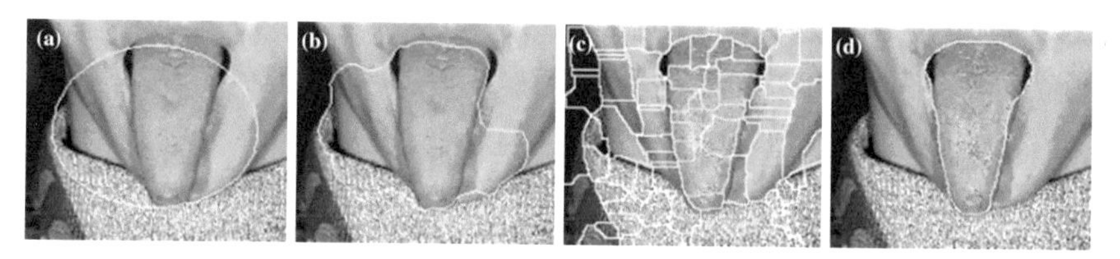

Fig. 6.5 Comparisons between the BEDC scheme and the proposed method. **a** Bi-elliptical curve, **b** tongue contour extracted by BEDC, **c** initial by watershed segmentation, **d** tongue contour extracted by the proposed method

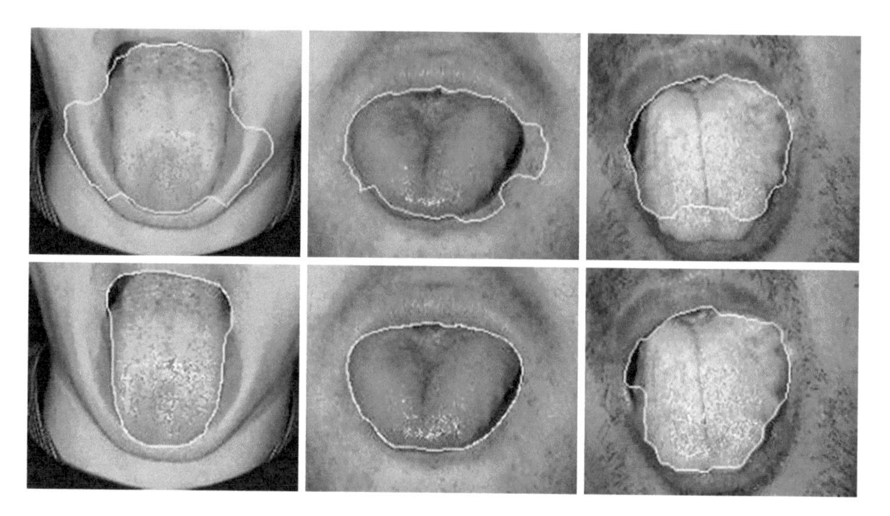

Fig. 6.6 Experimental results on some representative tongue images. The first row shows the segmentation results by BEDC, and the second row shows the three columns that present three tongue images with appendicitis, pancreatitis, and nephritis, respectively, as the results of the proposed method. Reprinted from Ning et al. (2012), with permission of Springer

More experimental results on different types of tongue images are shown in Fig. 6.6. The diseases such as appendicitis (first column), pancreatitis (second column), and nephritis (third column) cause the tongue body to present different pathological characteristics, i.e., various colors and texture features. The first row presents the segmentation results by BEDC, and the second row shows the results by the proposed method. It can be seen that the proposed method can overcome the various interferences of strong edges (e.g., cloth, lips, beards, and neck) and pathological features and obtain much better result than the BEDC method.

6.4.2 *Qualitative Evaluation*

We qualitatively evaluated the proposed method by classifying the segmentation results into three classes: "good", "poor," and "reasonable". We asked three TCM

Table 6.1 Segmentation evaluation by TCM practitioners on the two methods

Method	"Good" marks		"Reasonable" marks		"Poor" marks	
	Number	GR (%)	Number	GR (%)	Number	GR (%)
BEDC	238	39.7	251	41.8	111	18.5
The proposed method	367	61.2	185	30.8	48	8

Reprinted from Ning et al. (2012), with permission of Springer

practitioners in the 211 Hospital, Harbin, China, to independently classify the segmentation results into the three classes. If you think the tongue body is well segmented, then mark it as "good"; if you think there is much segmentation error, which may lead to wrong diagnosis, then they mark it as "poor"; if you think the segmentation is not very good but may not lead to wrong diagnosis, then mark it as "reasonable".

Table 6.1 shows the qualitative evaluation results by the three TCM practitioners on the segmentation results by the two algorithms. The proposed method obtains 61.2% "good" marks, 30.8% "reasonable" marks and 8% "poor" marks, while the BEDC method obtains 39.7% "good" marks, 41.8% "reasonable" marks, and 18.5% "poor" marks. The proposed method had much more "good" marks and much less "poor" marks than the BEDC algorithm. Clearly, it performs much better than BEDC in tongue image segmentation.

6.4.3 *Quantitative Evaluation*

Qualitative evaluation is subjective and it depends on the experience of the observers. Therefore, we then used the receiver operating characteristic (ROC) analysis (Metz, 1978; Loizou, Pattichis, Pantziaris, & Nicolaides, 2007) to assess quantitatively the proposed segmentation method by using the true-positive fraction (TPF), false-positive fraction (FPF), true-negative fraction (TNF), and false-negative fraction (FNF). Ratios of overlapping areas were assessed by applying the similarity kappa index KI (Fleiss, Cohen, & Everitt, 1969) and the overlap index (OI) (Rosenfield & Fitzpatrick-Lins, 1986).

Table 6.2 lists the ROC analysis results by using the TPF, FPF, FNF, TNF, KI, and OI indices for the two tongue body segmentation methods on 50 tongue images. From Table 6.2, it can be seen that BEDC has higher TPF of 95.36%, higher FPF of 13.78%, lower KI of 84.78%, and lower OI of 74.57%. This is because the segmentation result of BEDC is usually bigger than the true tongue body, including not only the tongue body but also part of cheek, lips, and teeth (e.g., Fig. 6.5b), which causes the BEDC to have a high TPF but low TNF.

Table 6.2 ROC analysis with TNF, TPF, FNF, FPF, KI and OI on 50 tongue images

Method	TPF (%)	FPF (%)	FNF (%)	TNF (%)	KI (%)	OI (%)
BEDC	95.36	13.78	4.64	86.22	84.78	74.57
The proposed method	92.83	2.46	7.17	97.54	93.52	88.19

Reprinted from Ning et al. (2012), with permission of Springer

However, the proposed method achieved TPF and FPF indices of 92.83 and 2.46% respectively, and the associated KI and OI indices were much higher than those of BEDC by about 10%.

6.4.4 Running Time of the Proposed Method

The proposed tongue segmentation method was implemented using Visual C++ 6.0 on a PC with P4 2.6 GHz CPU and 1,024 MB RAM. In our system, the time to segment a tongue image mainly depends on the number of regions initially segmented with the watershed algorithm.

We illustrate computational cost of the proposed method by an example. In Fig. 6.7, two different initial segmentations (Fig. 6.7a, b) for the same tongue image have different parameter settings in the modified GVF method. The numbers of the two segmented regions (Fig. 6.7a, b) are 80 and 48, respectively, and the segment time is 2.8 and 2.3 s. The final segmentation results of Fig. 6.7a, b are shown in Fig. 6.7c. The larger the number of initially segmented regions there are, the more merge time the MSRM algorithm requires.

By our experimental statistics, the time to segment a tongue image is about 2–4 s, which is fast enough for the applications of computer aided TCM tongue diagnosis.

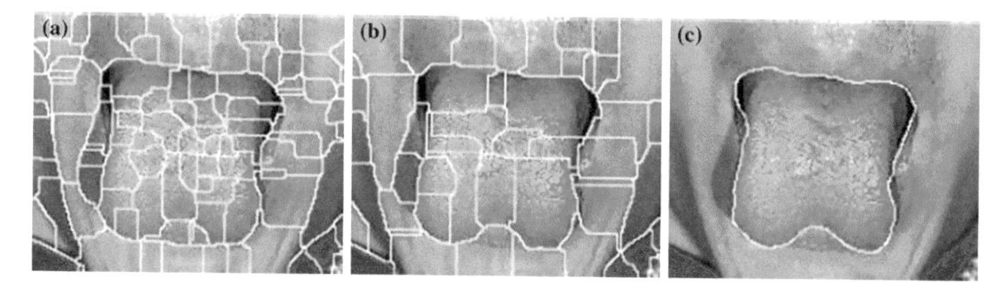

Fig. 6.7 The proposed method applied to two different initial segmentations. **a** Initial segmentation with parameter $\mu = 0.15$ and iteration numbers = 20. **b** Initial segmentation with parameter $\mu = 0.15$ and iteration numbers = 40. **c** The segmentation result by the proposed method for (**a**) and (**b**). Reprinted from Ning et al. (2012), with permission of Springer

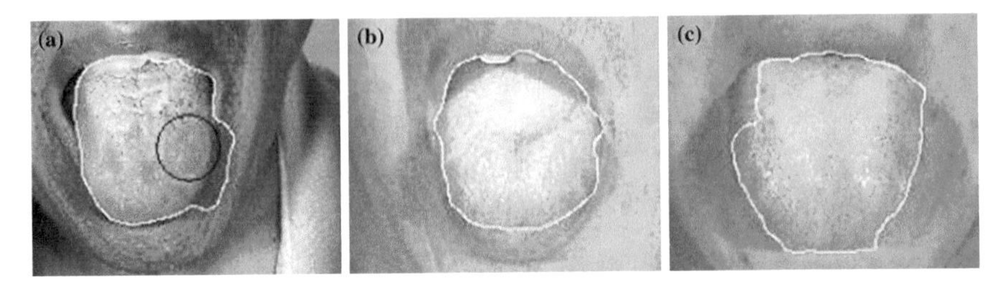

Fig. 6.8 **a** Segmentation result caused by the tongue body being very close to the borders of the tongue images. **b** Segmentation result with teeth, and **c** segmentation result caused by a week edge. Reprinted from Ning et al. (2012), with permission of Springer

6.4.5 *Limitations of the Proposed Method*

In some cases, the proposed method will fail to fully segment the tongue contour. Such limitations are summarized as follows.

(1) If the tongue body is located very close to the borders of the tongue image, the proposed method may fail because the location of the tongue marker may be inaccurate. Figure 6.8a shows an example.
(2) The segmentation result sometimes involves the tooth regions of the patient. Figure 6.8b shows an example.
(3) When the edge of the tongue body is weak or its color is very similar to the face color, inaccurate segmentation may happen. Figure 6.8c shows an example.

6.5 Summary

We proposed a fully automatic tongue segmentation method for traditional Chinese tongue diagnosis. First, the tongue gradient image was preprocessed by the modified GVF, and the watershed segmentation was used to obtain the initial segmentation. Since GVF can well preserve main edge structures while removing trivial structures, the oversegmentation of the watershed segmentation was significantly reduced. This constructs a good basis for the following region merging process. Second, the MSRM algorithm was used to extract the tongue body by segmenting the background, i.e., merging the background regions around the tongue body. Finally, the snake algorithm was used to refine the region merging result by setting the extracted tongue contour as the initial curve.

Different from the BEDC method, the proposed method extracts the contour of the tongue based on region merging instead of setting an initial shape of the tongue beforehand. Therefore, it reduces the interference of strong edges around the tongue body. The experimental results demonstrated that the proposed method achieves both high qualitative and quantitative evaluation measures. In particular, it simultaneously has a high TPF and low FPF indices, which provides a reliable foundation for the following TCM diagnosis process. It was also noted that the segmentation results may not be very desirable when the images have a weak tongue edge or the images include strong teeth or lip features. Such difficulties need to be overcome in future work.

References

Fleiss, J. L., Cohen, J., & Everitt, B. S. (1969). Large sample standard errors of kappa and weighted kappa. *Psychological Bulletin, 72*(5), 323.

Guo, Z., Zhang, L., & Zhang, D. (2010a). A completed modeling of local binary pattern operator for texture classification. *Image Processing. IEEE Transactions on, 19*(6), 1657–1663.

Guo, Z., Zhang, L., & Zhang, D. (2010b). Rotation invariant texture classification using LBP variance (LBPV) with global matching. *Pattern Recognition, 43*(3), 706–719.

Hernandez, S. E., Barner, K. E., & Yuan, Y. (2005). Region merging using homogeneity and edge integrity for watershed-based image segmentation. *Optical engineering, 44*(1), 17004.

Kass, M., Witkin, A., & Terzopoulos, D. (1988). Snakes: Active contour models. *International Journal of Computer Vision, 1*(4), 321–331.

Loizou, C. P., Pattichis, C. S., Pantziaris, M., & Nicolaides, A. (2007). An integrated system for the segmentation of atherosclerotic carotid plaque. *Information Technology in Biomedicine, IEEE Transactions on, 11*(6), 661–667.

Metz, C. E. (1978). *Basic principles of ROC analysis* (pp. 283–298). Amsterdam: Elsevier.

Ning, J., Zhang, D., Wu, C., et al. (2012). Automatic tongue image segmentation based on gradient vector flow and region merging. *Neural Computing and Applications, 21*(8), 1819–1826.

Ning, J., Zhang, L., Zhang, D., & Wu, C. (2010). Interactive image segmentation by maximal similarity based region merging. *Pattern Recognition, 43*(2), 445–456.

Ojala, T., Pietikainen, M., & Maenpaa, T. (2002). Multiresolution gray-scale and rotation invariant texture classification with local binary patterns. *Pattern Analysis and Machine Intelligence, IEEE Transactions on, 24*(7), 971–987.

Pang, B., Zhang, D., & Wang, K. (2005). The bi-elliptical deformable contour and its application to automated tongue segmentation in Chinese medicine. *Medical Imaging, IEEE Transactions on, 24*(8), 946–956.

Rosenfield, G. H., & Fitzpatrick-Lins, K. (1986). A coefficient of agreement as a measure of thematic classification accuracy. *Photogrammetric engineering and remote sensing, 52*(2), 223–227.

Weickert, J. (2001). Efficient image segmentation using partial differential equations and morphology. *Pattern Recognition, 34*(9), 1813–1824.

Xu, C., & Prince, J. L. (1998). Snakes, shapes, and gradient vector flow. *Image Processing, IEEE Transactions on, 7*(3), 359–369.

Vincent, L., & Soille, P. (1991). Watersheds in digital spaces: an efficient algorithm based on immersion simulations. *IEEE Transactions on Pattern Analysis & Machine Intelligence, 6*, 583–598.

Zhang, K., Zhang, L., Song, H., & Zhou, W. (2010a). Active contours with selective local or global segmentation: a new formulation and level set method. *Image and Vision computing, 28*(4), 668–676.

Zhang, K., Zhang, L., Song, H., & Zhou, W. (2010b). Active contours driven by local image fitting energy. *Pattern recognition, 43*(4), 1199–1206.

Chapter 7
Tongue Segmentation by Fusing Region-Based and Edge-Based Approaches

Abstract A tongue diagnosis system can offer significant information for health conditions. To ensure the feasibility and reliability of tongue diagnosis, a robust and accurate tongue segmentation method is a prerequisite. However, both of the common segmentation methods (edge-based or region-based) have limitations so that satisfactory results especially for medical use are often out of reach. In this chapter, we proposed a robust tongue segmentation method by fusing region-based and edge-based approaches. Before segmentation, the ROI (region of interest), which was used as input for the subsequent segmentation, was extracted in a novel way. Next, we merged adjacent regions utilizing the histogram-based color similarity criterion to get a rough tongue contour. It is essentially a region-based method and hence the results are less sensitive to cracks and fissures on the surface of the tongue. Then, we adopted a fast marching method to connect four detected reliable points together to get a close curve, which is based on edge features. The contour obtained by the region-based approach was utilized to act as a mask during the fast marching process (edge-based) and the mask added limits so that the ultimate contour would be more robust. Qualitative and quantitative comparisons showed that the proposed method is superior to the other methods for the segmentation of the tongue body in terms of robustness and accuracy.

7.1 Introduction

The each of methods proposed in previous chapters, has had its fair share of success, but there are corresponding limitations. Specifically, region-based image segmentation techniques can provide closed region boundaries and are robust to random noise due to their statistical basis. Nevertheless, the boundaries may not be very accurate, especially when it comes to the edges between lips and tongue due to their similar color. Similarly, despite the fact that edge-based methods can exactly locate part of edges, the detected boundaries are likely to be open curves. In addition, some post-procedures, such as edge tracking, should be performed to

D. Zhang et al., *Tongue Image Analysis*, DOI 10.1007/978-981-10-2167-1_7

obtain closed region boundaries. Furthermore, edge-based methods are sensitive to noise and often result in spurious edges. Thus, robustness cannot be guaranteed.

In tongue segmentation application, shortcomings of these two classes of methods will be further greatly aggravated owning to specific characteristics of the tongue. Specifically, the difficulties broadly fall into two categories. First, the difficulties of tongue segmentation arise when the image comes from a patient with tooth marks, evident fissures, or abnormal color that often accompany pathologies (see Fig. 7.1b, d). Second, more common and inherent problems exist. One usual difficulty comes from interference by the lips and face due to their resemblance with the tongue in the aspect of color (see Fig. 7.1a, c). Abnormal tongue shape in some occasions also challenges many segmentation approaches especially model-based

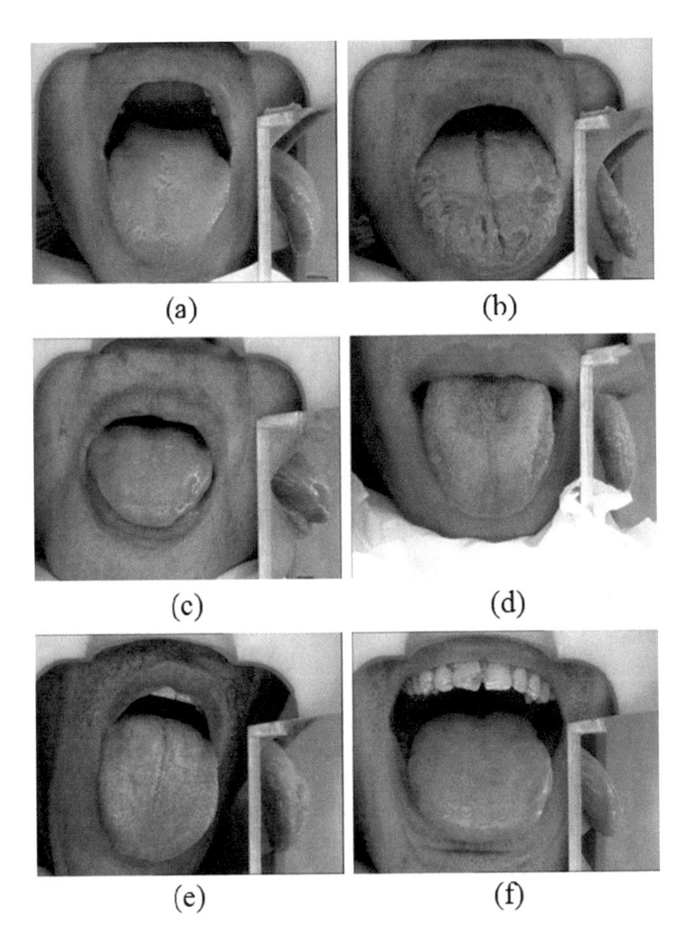

Fig. 7.1 Difficulties in tongue segmentation. **a** Tongue color is similar to face color. **b** Severe fissures on the surface of tongue. **c** Interference from lips. **d** Abnormal color on the surface of tongue. **e** Image with a complex background. **f** Image with interference from wrinkles on the lower jaw. Reprinted from Wu and Zhang (2015), with permission from Elsevier

ones. Also, images of males with beards may meet difficulty (see Fig. 7.1e) and wrinkles on the lower jaw also bring obstacles (see Fig. 7.1f). Due to those intrinsic characteristic of tongue images, a single use of the above-mentioned methods cannot achieve satisfactory results (either in terms of accuracy or robustness), whereas a combination of these two methods often performs better and the adverse influence of each method declines. Thus, we attempted to combine the region-based method with the edge-based method to get more accurate and more robust results.

The remainder of this chapter is organized as follows. Section 7.2 describes techniques used to extract the region of interest (ROI) so as to simultaneously avoid interference and reduce computational complexity. In Sect. 7.3, we give an introduction about the proposed methods, not only the adopted region-based and edge-based approaches, but also the scheme of the combination. To assess the performance, we present qualitative and quantitative comparison results in Sect. 7.4. Finally, Sect. 7.5 concludes the chapter.

7.2 Extraction of the ROI to Enhance Robustness

For any tongue segmentation routine, not only the tongue body itself but also the complex background will be involved in the computation. Generally, the background consists of the face, beard, lips, teeth, and others in the capture environments, which are collectively called non-tongue components in this book. Figure 7.2 illustrates this observation. Unexpectedly, in most of the acquired images, the non-tongue parts occupy more space than the tongue body, which will possibly interfere with segmentation accuracy and robustness. Also, the non-tongue portion will in most cases result in much higher computational complexity than the tongue body. In summary, segmentation directly from the original image will result in a large waste of time and degrade the segmentation performance. If a simple but effective preprocessing can get rid of the majority of non-tongue components while maintaining the unchanged tongue body, then this preprocessing will benefit the subsequent finer segmentation process in efficiency and accuracy. In nature, this preprocessing is to extract the region of interest (ROI). To clarify this, the ROI in

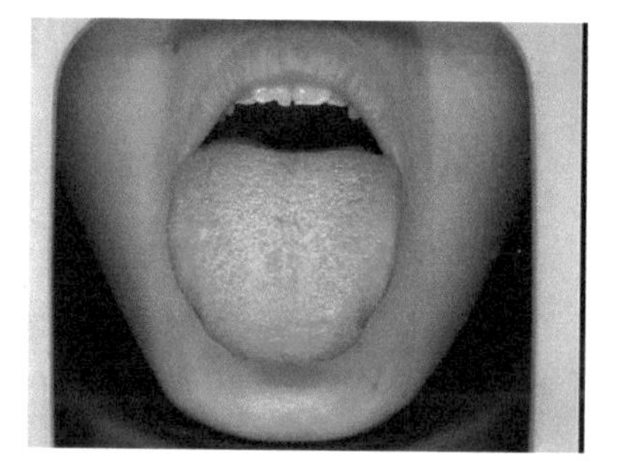

Fig. 7.2 A typical tongue image. Reprinted from Wu and Zhang (2015), with permission from Elsevier

this book refers to a rectangular area, whose main content is the tongue body. For this purpose, we proposed an efficient ROI extraction approach.

The tongue body differs from the non-tongue portion (with lips as an exception) in the aspect of color. Lips, however, are in the vicinity of the tongue body so the lips are allowed to be included in the rough ROI. Thus utilizing color information will be well suited in the extraction. To highlight the difference between the tongue and non-tongue, de-correlation and stretch algorithms of the original image (denoted as I) in the RGB format were applied. The de-correlation method was used to reduce cross-correlation among three channels and the stretch approach followed to independently enhance contrast for each of the three channels. The following Algorithm 1 gives a detailed description. To illustrate, the input I and output S of Algorithm 1 are shown in Fig. 7.3a, b.

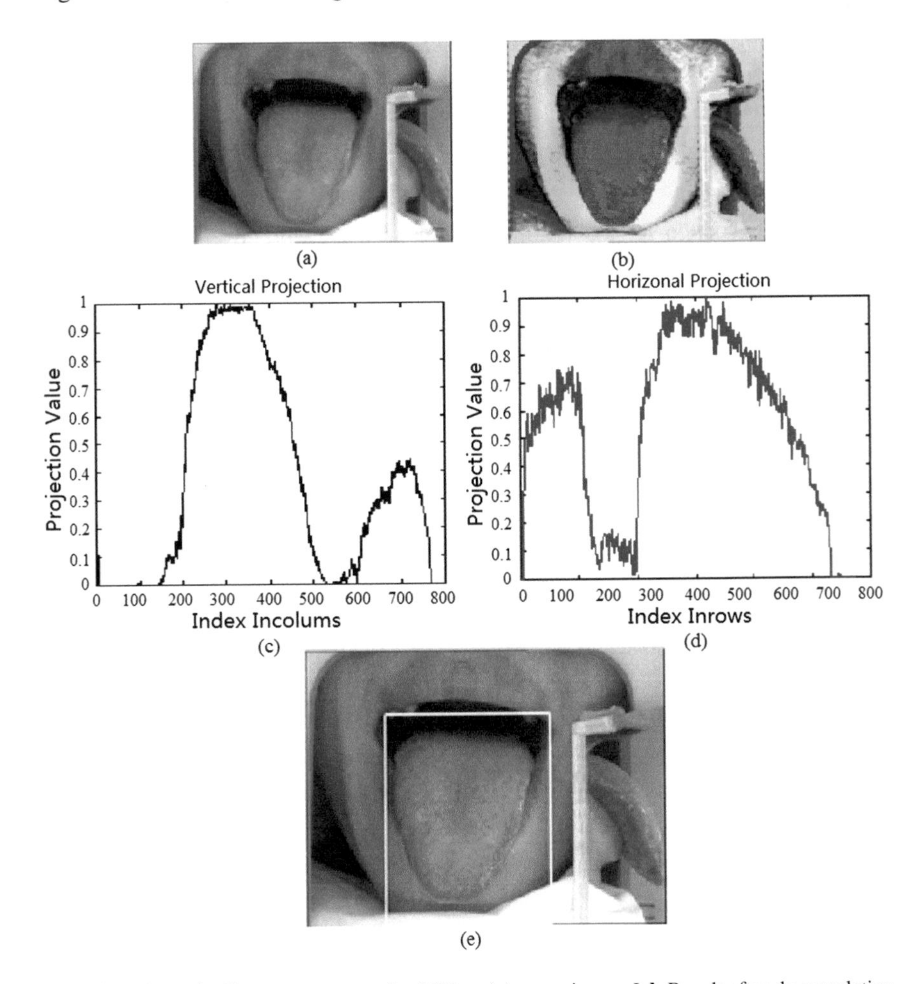

Fig. 7.3 Schematic diagram to extract the ROI. **a** A tongue image *I*. **b** Result after de-correlation stretch S. **c** Vertical projection result. **d** Horizontal projection result. **e** Sub-image inside the white rectangle is the extracted ROI. Reprinted from Wu and Zhang (2015), with permission from Elsevier

With these preparations, we then converted matrix S to HSV color space and employed the H channel image *Ih* for ROI extraction. Various tests showed that most pixels in the tongue part have a larger hue value than that in the non-tongue portion. Hence, binarization is helpful to distinguish the tongue from the background and the threshold was selected using the Otsu method. The result after binarization of *Ih* is denoted as *Ibw* and then horizontal and vertical projection on *Ibw* follow. Figure 7.3c, d show the vertical and horizontal projection plots, respectively. From the projection plot, it is evident that the horizontal projection value in the tongue zone tends to be larger than that of the non-tongue and similarly for the vertical projection. Thus, we can obtain the desired range of rows and columns with a trivial threshold operation. Then the rough boundaries gained are applied to cut image I and the ROI is available as shown by the sub-image inside the white rectangle in Fig. 7.3e.

In the gained ROI, many non-tongue components are eliminated. Hence, interference is reduced and robustness will be enhanced. Another accompanying benefit is the decrease of computational complexity in the subsequent procedure since the ROI is much smaller than the original image. With this strategy, images with a similar color of the tongue and face can also achieve satisfactory results owning to the de-correlation step (Fig. 7.4 depicts its performance). To evaluate its robustness, 150 images were applied. All of them achieved good performance. To analyze its success, both de-correlate and stretch operations are the key points since they enhance the difference between the tongue and non-tongue part. Also, both the face color and tongue color do not often deviate far from their own center color.

After this extraction, the subsequent region-based or edge-based segmentation method utilizes the extracted ROI as the input for segmentation.

Algorithm 1: De-correlation and stretch algorithm

Input: the acquired color image *I*;
Output: three-channel image *S*.

1. Suppose the height and width of the acquired color image I are m and n pixels, respectively. The image has three channels: R, G, and B. For each channel, its element is taken columnwise to form a column vector, whose length equals $(m \times n)$. Then these three column vectors are arranged in columns to form a $(m \times n) \times 3$ matrix *A*.
2. Calculation of covariance matrix Cov for A and eigen value decomposition of *Cov* will produce matrices of eigen values (*D*) and eigenvectors (*V*), so that $Cov*V = V*D$.
3. Gain transform matrix *T* using formula $T = V*D^{-1/2} * V^T$.
4. De-correlate matrix *A* using matrix *T* by right multiplication $A = A*T$.
5. Reshape *A* back to obtain a three-channel image matrix S whose size is the same to the original image I. Each column of *A* is used to make up one channel of *S*. In detail, elements for each channel of S are filled in columns (to first populate the first column) by taking pixels from the corresponding columns of *A*. In this way, the three bands for matrix S are uncorrelated with each other.
6. Enhance the contrast for each band of *S* by adjusting the histogram.

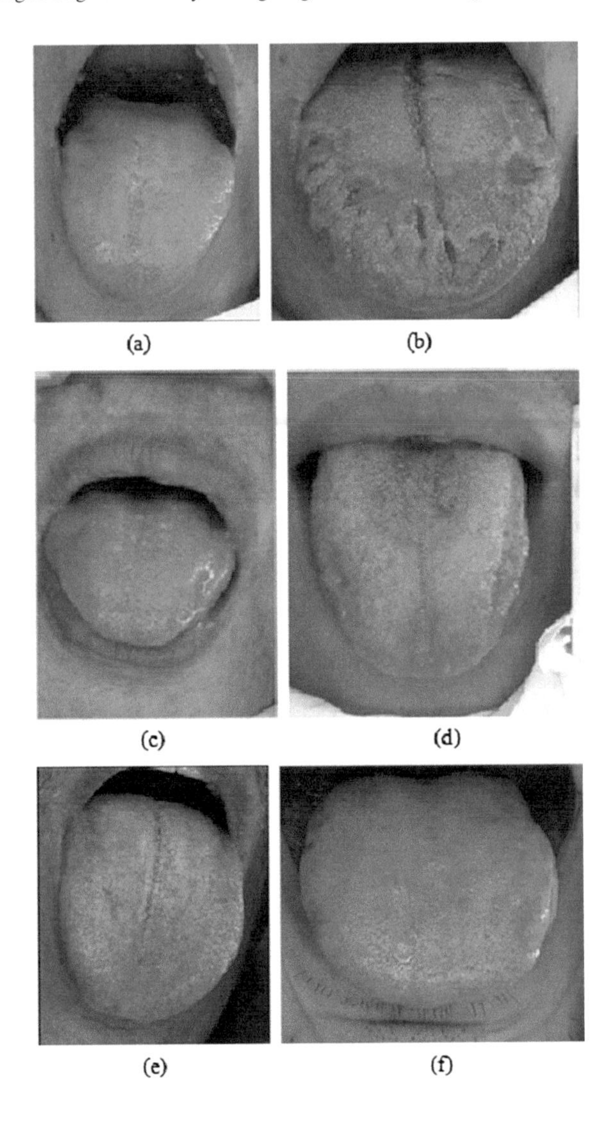

Fig. 7.4 ROI extraction results for typical images presented in Fig. 7.1. Reprinted from Wu and Zhang (2015), with permission from Elsevier

7.3 Combining Region-Based and Edge-Based Approaches

To extract the tongue body with high accuracy and strong robustness, we proposed to fuse the region-based method and edge-based method. In this section, the two methods are introduced. At the end, the fusion mechanism will be displayed as a solution.

7.3.1 Region-Based Approach: Improved MSRM

Splitting and merging are basic operations in a region-based category. For any typical region-based method, two factors are of great importance.

First, we need to regulate from where the initial regions used for splitting or merging come from. For region merging, they can be some seeds sowed manually or regions automatically obtained by employing prior knowledge. Here seed or region consists of a pixel or a cluster of neighboring pixels. On the other hands, for region splitting, the whole image is often regarded as the start. However, many region-based algorithms often include both merging and splitting, in which process, the median result gained from merging can be further assumed as the input of splitting and vice versa.

Another factor for a region-based segmentation method is to determine when the splitting (merging) should be carried out. The deciding conditions highly depend on the measure of similarity between the two regions. In other words, the similarity or homogeneity measure definition is the second factor of utmost importance. Recently, numerous measurements have been presented for various purposes and a suitable color space should be carefully chosen to adapt a specific application (for color image only) (Li, Yao, Yuan, & Zhou, 2010; Mojsilovi, Hu, & Soljanin, 2002; Deng & Manjunath, 2001). Among these variants, the color histogram distance is a simple but effective measurement for color image segmentation. The above-mentioned factors are vital for any region-based segmentation.

For tongue segmentation, the classic region-based methods are often closely related to the watershed method, which is a typical method in the region-based category. Even though over segmentation comes along with this method, many approaches have been proposed to overcome this flaw (Han & Ma, 2002; Patino, 2005; Beucher, 1994; Najman & Schmitt, 1996). In this chapter, however, we focus on the point that the watershed algorithm, which is fully automatic in its standard use, can be regarded as one way of region splitting. So the watershed algorithm provides the initial regions for subsequent region merging and annoyance over the segmentation problem can also be incidentally addressed by region merging. Ning et al. applied this approach to tongue segmentation in (Ning, Zhang, Wu, & Yue, 2012). First, the tongue image was segmented into many small regions by the watershed algorithm and these regions were then initially marked according to their positions. The markers were tongue, non-tongue, and unknown. Regions containing any pixels located at the border of the image were marked as non-tongue. Also, an area with a predefined size, which was located at the center of the image, was defined and any regions with any pixels in this predefined area were labels as tongue. The remaining unlabeled regions were stamped as unknown. In the next stage, the purpose was to tag these unknown regions as either tongue or non-tongue. The authors' strategy started with unlabeled regions adjacent to those labeled as non-tongue (near the border) and the maximal color histogram similarity measure between adjacent regions was utilized to decide whether the merging was allowed to guide the process. The merging went on iteratively until some stopping criteria were satisfied and all the unknown regions were labeled as either tongue or non-tongue. Then, those regions labeled as tongue consist of one larger region and its contour will be regarded as the tongue contour. Finally, the Snake algorithm followed to smooth the edge of tongue body. For this approach, the author abbreviated its name, which was maximal similarity based region merging, to MSRM.

This method is applicable in some occasions but many limitations still exist. First, an assumption was made to mark the tongue body for region merging: a predefined area located at the center of the whole image must be completely contained within the true tongue body. Nevertheless, this assumption disagreed with facts in many cases and thus led to a wrong initial marker. In that way, it would be impossible to accurately extract the tongue body (Fig. 7.5a shows an example). Second, the merging started from the image border (non-tongue). Nevertheless, in the whole image, the background was complex and there was a distinguished color difference in the background, resulting in a serious problem that the merging process would probably stop at the edge within the background rather than the tongue edge. Obviously, other disadvantages encompass intrinsic limitations of region-based segmentation methods. In summary, this method needs improvement.

With these considerations, an improved region-based method to overcome these limitations is proposed. First, before region merging, an adaptive labeling approach was used to mark the tongue body. Instead of using the predefined size and position, the improved algorithm adaptively obtained these parameters based on the current image. Similar to the observation in the ROI extraction step, color information in the Hue channel is the main distinguishing feature of the tongue body. After dilating the binarization result of the Hue channel gray scales image, the connected component with the largest area *Con_C* was selected as the base for computing needed parameters. To clarify it, the height and width of the smallest rectangle containing the selected region were the base to obtain the size while centroid of *Con_C* was utilized to locate the position. With these adaptively obtained parameters, the area needed to mark the tongue was defined. Apart from this improvement to automatically locate the initial tongue body marker, the initial

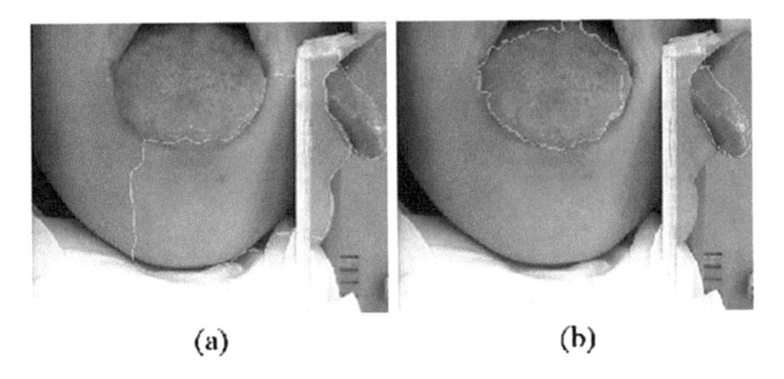

Fig. 7.5 Segmentation result when the tongue is not located at the center of the image. Reprinted from Wu and Zhang (2015), with permission from Elsevier

labels are confined to two classes, tongue and unknown, removing the non-tongue label in the original method. Also, the merging process begins inside the tongue body rather than the border (background) since there is better color consistency for the tongue body than that for the background, (Fig. 7.5b depicts the improvement). This improved method is named as improved MSRM. To sum up the improvement, an adaptive method to mark the tongue body is proposed. Unlike the original method, a more effective strategy to regulate the order to merge regions is put forward.

Under the preceding improvement, it is evident that performance will be improved compared with the original method and experiments support this prediction. The quantitatively evaluated result is shown in the section of experimental results. However, we found that the resulting boundaries are sometimes not the exact real boundaries but they tend to be in the vicinity of the real boundary. Figure 7.5b illustrates that none of the edges deviate far from the true tongue edges. This result indicates its robustness to resist the complexity of the tongue surface but fails to possess the necessary edge accuracy.

7.3.2 Optimal Edge-Based Approach: Fast Marching

While region-based approaches focus on clustering pixels using a similarity measure, edge-based segmentation approaches attempt to attach importance to dissimilarity in an image. It has attracted much attention from researchers and many algorithms have been developed under different theoretical frameworks.

Most of these methods begin by edge enhancement that is intended to heighten the image contrast in the area immediately around the edge. The conventional methods often adopt classic edge detectors, such as Canny, Roberts, and Prewitt, to compute the gradient image. However, these methods can hardly achieve satisfactory results. Some weaknesses are obvious: the results will be sensitive to noise and many trivial edges exist, leading to the fact that most of the initial results are not applicable in practice. Thus, many researchers tried to address this issue under other various frameworks. One successful attempt was made by incorporating the Gabor filter, which possesses optimal joint resolution in both spatial and frequency domains, to this area. Additionally, it has been demonstrated that simple cells in the visual cortex of mammalian brains can be modeled by Gabor functions, which ensures its indispensable role in edge enhancement. Fingerprint image enhancement has witnessed its success (Yang, Liu, Jiang, & Fan, 2003; Yin, Zhan, Tan, & Ning, 2003; Areekul, Watchareeruetai, Suppasriwasuseth, & Tantaratana, 2005; Zhu, Yin, & Zhang, 2004). In tongue segmentation, Cui et al. conducted a similar test to enhance the edge amplitude after a comprehensive analysis of the characteristics around the tongue edge and the result turned out well (Zhu et al., 2004). Its success rests with the similar waveform between the Gabor filter and the gray-level change around the tongue edge. In our method, we therefore adopted the Gabor filter for edge enhancement.

After edge enhancement, an elaborately designed post procedure is in needed to extract the desired boundary. For our specific application, the active contours approach which constitutes the majority of the existing edge-based methods as described in, (Zuo, Wang, Zhang, & Zhang, 2004; Yu, Yang, Wang, & Zhang, 2007; Han & Ma, 2002; Cui, Zuo, Zhang, & Zhang, 2013) was used. According to the difference in contour representation, active contours can be further divided into two sets: parametric active contours (snake) and geometric active contours (level set and fast marching). While snake methods employ contour points to parameterize the contour, geometric active contours instead utilize the zero level set of a higher dimensional function. Based on this intrinsic difference, the snake encodes a disadvantage that can be overcome by geometric active contours: the snake has difficulties in progressing into boundary concavities and is unable to handle topological changes, such as splitting and merging. Thus, the geometric mechanism possesses superiority to parametric ones in this sense. Nevertheless, both of these techniques suffer from a disability: their performances highly rely on the contour initialization. Unfortunately, it is never an easy task to automatically obtain an appropriate initialization and it is difficult to guarantee its robustness. Moreover, the user has to set a reasonable iteration number, which is not consistent among different images, in order to obtain an accurate boundary. This is another factor threatening robustness.

To address these problems, Cui et al. utilized the fast marching method differently (Cui et al., 2013). Unlike the traditional technique of gradually evolving an initial closed curve to obtain the tongue edge, Cui first located four reliable end points on the tongue edge by introducing threshold strategy to the image after edge enhancement and then the fast marching method was employed. The fast marching method was intended to compute the geodesic path between two points and then these geodesic paths would be adopted to successively connect these four points to form a closed curve, which was substantially the closed tongue contour.

Despite this algorithm's effectiveness for some acquired tongue images, it will fail in other cases, thus displaying disability in terms of robustness (Fig. 7.6 gives an example). With close investigation of the factors leading to failure, one in particular is prominent. It is closely related to the specific inherent characteristics of the tongue. Fissures and other complex components inside the tongue body will cause great interference when computing the geodesic paths and the paths are apt to go across the tongue body, which obviously leads to false results. Thus, this method suffers from a weak robustness but exhibits relatively high edge accuracy.

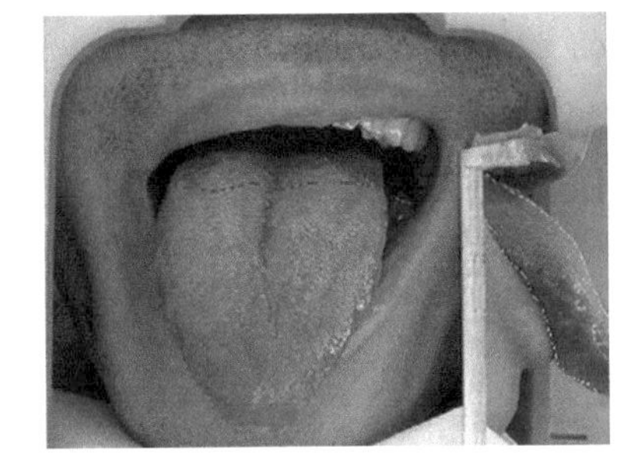

Fig. 7.6 Segmentation failure using the fast marching method. Reprinted from Wu and Zhang (2015), with permission from Elsevier

7.3.3 The Fusion Approach as a Solution

Based on the previous analysis, neither the edge-based nor region-based approach alone can form a robust segmentation algorithm. However, the combination of these two categories of methods tends to compensate for the deficiencies in the individual method. In this chapter, we integrate the methods to enhance robustness and accuracy for practical use. We start with detailed comments for each method and then the combination will be presented.

In the edge-based method, two drawbacks hinder to a certain extent its medical use. First, the annoying and time-consuming edge linking process, which is necessary for the traditional method, has been successfully addressed by computing geodesic paths in our method. The other defect, which is the high sensitivity to noise, is still an issue. However, the region-based method, serving as the counterpart of the edge-based method, has one extremely intriguing outstanding property that can alleviate this critical drawback for edge-based (sensitivity to noise) in our specific application. Since the region-based method has a statistical basis, interference from tiny complex edges inside the tongue body, which constitutes the main characteristics of the tongue, will be reduced compared with edge-based method. The region-based method has a disadvantage, which is its inability to obtain the exact boundary.

Thus, we attempted to fuse these two methods together. For the region-based method, we adopted the improved MSRM as described above whereas for the edge-based method, the fast marching method is utilized. A detailed description of the fusion is as follows.

First, a mask is generated using the result contour obtained by the improved MSRM. This mask shares the same size with the image and all pixels inside the contour will be assigned a zero value and the remaining pixels will be assigned a one. This mask is further improved by morphological erosion and dilation. Since the initial contour is obtained using the region-based method, the generated mask can often cover the region where fissure and complex components lie inside the tongue body. In addition, the edge map (result of edge enhancement) should be ready before fusion.

After these steps, the fusion begins by revising the edge map, where each element in it is replaced by the result of multiplying the corresponding elements of the edge map and acquired mask together. Thus, for the revised edge map, most of the pixels in the region of the tongue body will be assigned zero, thereby conveying the information that no tongue edge exists inside those regions, and the prominent interference inside the tongue body will be eliminated in the revised edge map. In addition, the altered edge map will be the base in the following computation of geodesic paths. First, the four needed reliable end points are extracted based on the binarization of the revised edge map instead of the original one, avoiding the interference inside the tongue body. During the calculation of geodesic paths between the end points, the revision of the edge map will implicitly add a limiting condition that the paths cannot contain any pixel inside the mask, which

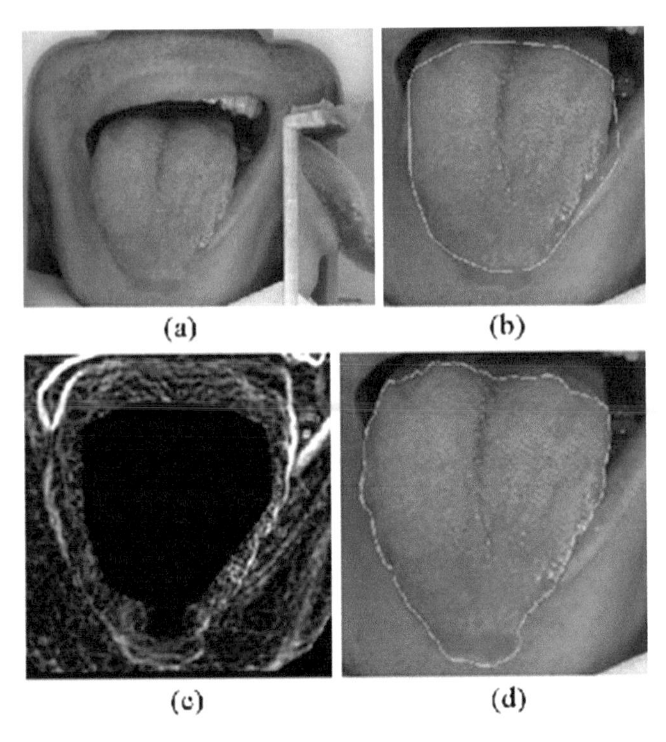

Fig. 7.7 Schematic diagram of the fusing method. **a** A tongue image. **b** Extracted ROI. **c** Revised edge map. **d** Segmentation result by combining the region-based and edge-based methods. Reprinted from Wu and Zhang (2015), with permission from Elsevier

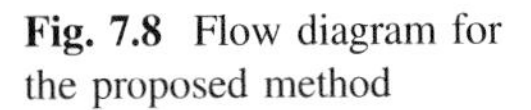

Fig. 7.8 Flow diagram for the proposed method

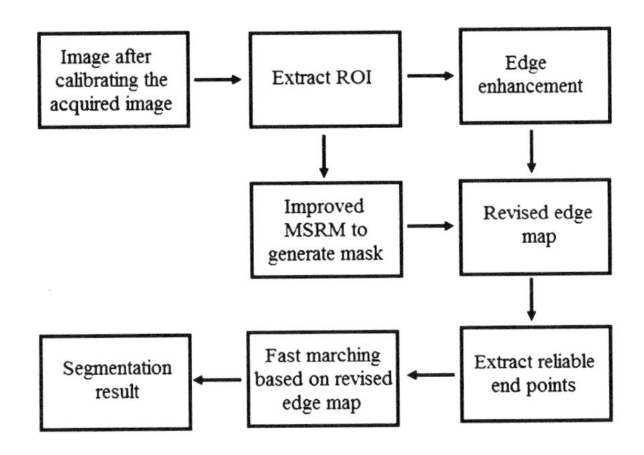

again avoids interference from tongue surface. Figure 7.7 illustrates the whole process by showing every intermediate result while Fig. 7.8 describes the whole scheme for tongue segmentation.

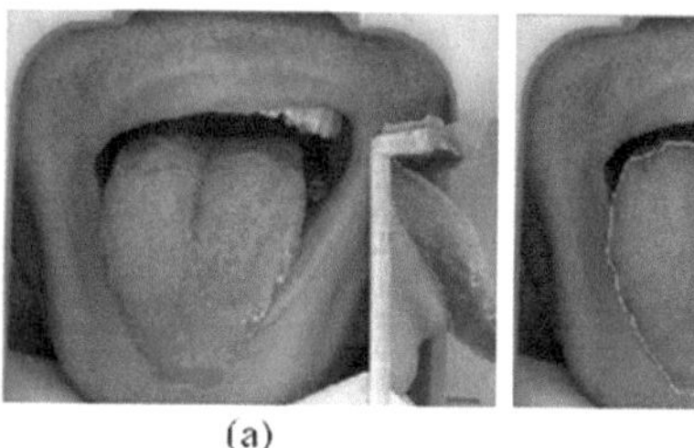
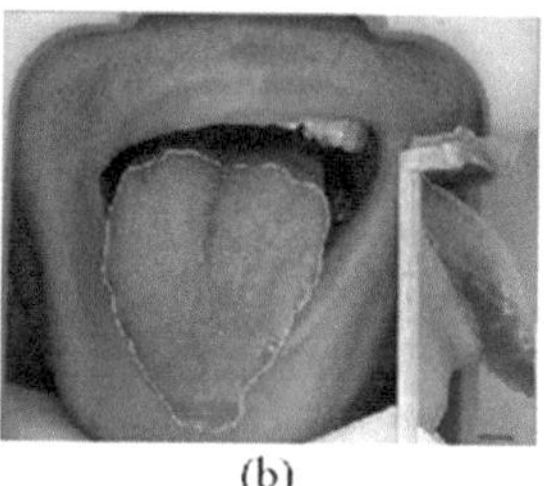

Fig. 7.9 Improved performance. **a** Segmentation result by fast marching method. **b** Segmentation result with the proposed method. Reprinted from Wu and Zhang (2015), with permission from Elsevier

The simple fusion has brought great improvement. Two instances (Fig. 7.9) are displayed to intuitively demonstrate its effectiveness.

7.4 Experiments and Comparisons

In this section, the performance of the proposed method of integrating the edge-based method and region-based method is evaluated. For a comprehensive assessment, both qualitative and quantitative evaluations were carried out. Here a brief introduction of the data set employed is given.

The data set employed consists of 150 selected images and these images were acquired using the same device but under two different cases. The difference lies in whether to take a tongue lateral view or not. For example, Fig. 7.2 only takes the front view while both front and lateral views are acquired in Fig. 7.1a.

In spite of this difference, it will not cause trouble in the tongue segmentation since this difference often disappears after ROI extraction. In addition, considering the influence of different illuminations, the captured image will be calibrated before segmentation by employing the approach presented in (Li, Zhou, & Zhang, 2004). Even though the size of the data set is not remarkably large, all of the selected images were carefully chosen to cover as many typical images as possible. Thus, the evaluation performance on this data set can be used to predict its practical property. Specifically, these images were captured from individuals with various health states: healthy, sub-healthy, and ill (diverse diseases). From the prospect of gender and age, the distribution is also relatively even. For the different clinical manifestations for various diseases, the data set also covers typical instances. Based on these considerations, it is reasonable to apply this data set to simulate the practical situation and its performance evaluation will be of great significance.

7.4.1 Qualitative Evaluation

The purpose of a tongue segmentation algorithm is to extract the tongue body from the captured image and then the segmentation result will serve as the input for future analysis for diagnosis and monitoring. Being the basis for a medical application, the segmentation algorithm has to be robust to handle all possible contingencies. Here, we focus on the acknowledged issues listed in the introduction. In (Fig. 7.10), typical results exhibiting the capability of our proposed method to cope with the acknowledged issue are presented. (a) and (b) are the segmentation results of images with tooth marks; (c) and (d) are the segmentation results of images with an evident fissure; (e) and (f) are the segmentation results of images with an abnormal color; (g) and (h) are the segmentation results of images with interference from the lips; (i) and (j) are the segmentation results of images with interference from faces; (k) and (l) are the segmentation results of images with a strange tongue shape; (m) and (n) are the segmentation results of images with a complex background; (o) and (p) are the segmentation results of images with interference from wrinkles on the lower jaw.

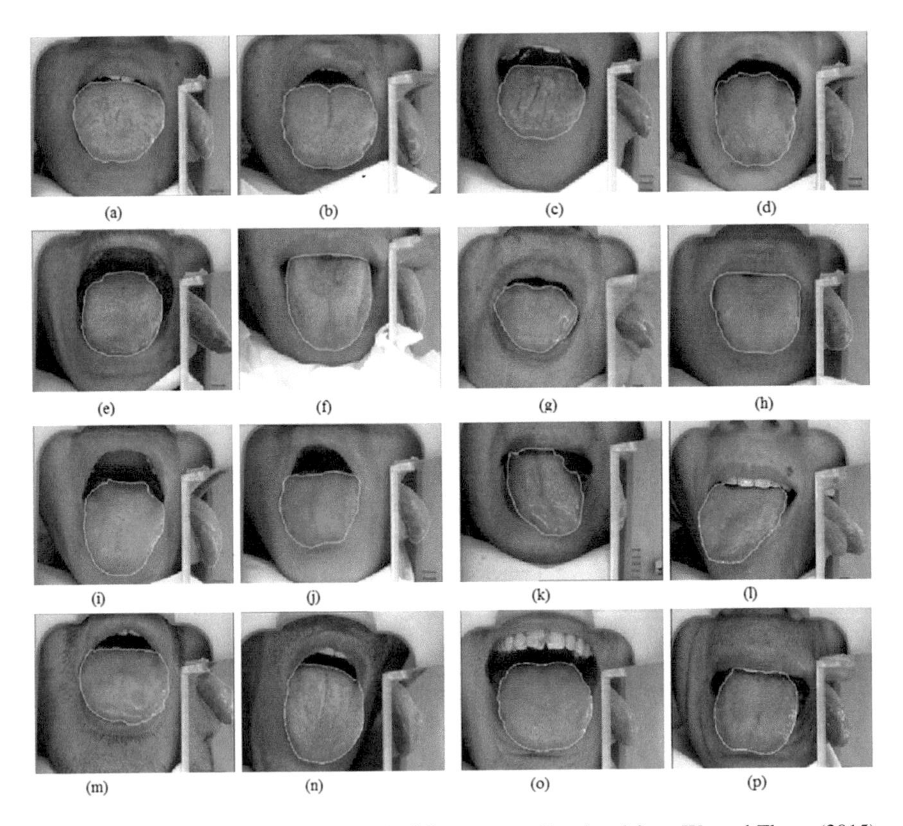

Fig. 7.10 Qualitative evaluation results in different cases. Reprinted from Wu and Zhang (2015), with permission from Elsevier

For these variants, the proposed method performs well and thus its superiority in terms of robustness is well established.

7.4.2 *Quantitative Evaluation*

In this subsection, we attempt to display the quantitative evaluation results to manifest its effectiveness. We compared the proposed methods with three other methods: the MSRM (Ning et al., 2012), Polar Snake (edge-based) (Zuo, Wang, Zhang, & Zhang, 2004), and improved MSRM (improved by utilizing the strategy described in the region-based method part).

There are many methods to evaluate the quality of segmentation methods, including comparison with manual segmentation. Unlike other medical applications, delineation of the tongue contour requires little expertise and some practice under instruction will suffice. Thus, we compared resulting segmentation contours with human delineations using the Hausdorff distance (HD) and the mean distance (MD) (Wang & Zhang, 2010) as the evaluation index to assess segmentation methods. To compute the distances between these two curves, first, each point on one curve relates to a point on the other curve so that the distance between those two points is minimum. Thus, each point on the first curve has one corresponding distance and these distances consist of a set. The Hausdorff distance then finds the maximum value of this set while the mean distance equals the average value of this set. Hence, each image in the data base will have its HD and MD after the computation. Finally, the mean value and standard deviation were computed from the database and Table 7.1 shows the comparison results.

This table demonstrates that our method has overwhelming advantages over the other three methods, from both the perspective of HD and MD. On one hand, its average values are much lower indicating its excellence in terms of accuracy. On the other hand, its standard deviations possess a similar property in comparison and thus its dominance is established concerning its robustness.

Thus from the qualitative and quantitative comparison results, we conclude that our method is superior to the other three methods, not only in sense of robustness, but also in terms of accuracy. Moreover, since the experiments were based on data collected from the real world, the feasibility of our proposed method in practice is further verified.

Table 7.1 The HD and MD distances of the MSRM, improved MSRM, Polar Snake, and proposed method

	HD	MD
MSRM	52.95 ± 33.21	11.48 ± 6.48
Polar Snake	35.38 ± 30.57	9.34 ± 7.92
Improved MSRM	34.06 ± 17.35	8.96 ± 6.05
Proposed means	15.18 ± 7.09	4.80 ± 1.4569

Reprinted from Wu and Zhang (2015) with permission from Elsevier

7.5 Summary

This chapter aims to address the issue of tongue segmentation in medical applications. Due to its special application background, accuracy and robustness are very important demands. Thus, it is proposed to combine the region-based approach with the edge-based approach to achieve better performance compared with the existing methods. In addition, to reducing the computation complexity, we optimized the use of color information to extract the ROI before segmentation.

In this chapter, we first introduced a novel but simple ROI extraction method employed in the preprocessing stage to reduce the computation time and enhance robustness by reducing the latent interference. Second, we analyzed the underlying reasons for the difficulties in tongue segmentation and summarized the characteristics of typical tongues. This is meaningful for the specific topic. Third, an improvement was made to the traditional MSRM. Also another mechanism to combine region-based and edge-based segmentation methods was presented and it can be extended to other segmentation problems, especially those with strong demands for accuracy and robustness. Fourth, experimental results based on a data set collected from the real word showed the success of the proposed method, which is meaningful in the field of tongue segmentation. Finally, it demonstrated the generally acknowledged fact that the integrated algorithm will highly improve the performance.

Although we believe this work has achieved good result in the field of tongue segmentation, this work can be further improved and extended to other fields. Despite that the proposed method has advantages in terms of accuracy and robustness, this method is a little more time-consuming especially in the region-based stage (both watershed and region merging take a relatively longer time), and time needs to be reduced to some extent by extracting the ROI before segmentation. One possible solution is put forward for future improvement. Since for the region-based method, the requirement for resolution is not strict, down sampling the image before region-based segmentation can reduce the run time and the result in this stage which should be up sampled before use in the fusion stage. In addition, the proposed method can also be extended to other medical segmentations, such as lung and brain tumor segmentation, since robustness and accuracy are essential needs in these medical applications.

References

Areekul, V., Watchareeruetai, U., Suppasriwasuseth, K., & Tantaratana, S. (2005). Separable Gabor filter realization for fast fingerprint enhancement (p. 253). IEEE.

Beucher, S. (1994). Watershed, hierarchical segmentation and waterfall algorithm. In *Mathematical morphology and its applications to image processing* (pp. 69–76). Springer.

Cui, Z., Zuo, W., Zhang, H., & Zhang, D. (2013). Automated tongue segmentation based on 2D Gabor filters and fast marching. In *Intelligence science and big data engineering* (pp. 328–335). Springer.

Deng, Y., & Manjunath, B. S. (2001). Unsupervised segmentation of color-texture regions in images and video. *IEEE Transactions on Pattern Analysis and Machine Intelligence, 23*(8), 800–810.

Han, J., & Ma, K. (2002). Fuzzy color histogram and its use in color image retrieval. *IEEE Transactions on Image Processing, 11*(8), 944–952.

Li, W., Yao, J., Yuan, L., & Zhou, Q. (2010). The segmentation of the body of tongue based on the improved level set in TCM. In *Life System Modeling and Intelligent Computing* (pp. 220–229). Springer.

Li, W., Zhou, C., & Zhang, Z (2004). The segmentation of the body of the tongue based on the improved snake algorithm in traditional Chinese medicine (pp. 5501–5505). IEEE.

Mojsilovi, A., Hu, J., & Soljanin, E. (2002). Extraction of perceptually important colors and similarity measurement for image matching, retrieval and analysis. *IEEE Transactions on Image Processing, 11*(11), 1238–1248.

Najman, L., & Schmitt, M. (1996). Geodesic saliency of watershed contours and hierarchical segmentation. *IEEE Transactions on Pattern Analysis and Machine Intelligence, 18*(12), 1163–1173.

Ning, J., Zhang, D., Wu, C., & Yue, F. (2012). Automatic tongue image segmentation based on gradient vector flow and region merging. *Neural Computing and Applications, 21*(8), 1819–1826.

Patino, L. (2005). Fuzzy relations applied to minimize over segmentation in watershed algorithms. *Pattern Recognition Letters, 26*(6), 819–828.

Wang, X., & Zhang, D. (2010). An optimized tongue image color correction scheme. *IEEE Transactions on Information Technology in Biomedicine, 14*(6), 1355–1364.

Wu, K., & Zhang, D. (2015). Robust tongue segmentation by fusing region-based and edge-based approaches. *Expert Systems with Applications An International Journal, 42*(21), 8027–8038.

Yang, J., Liu, L., Jiang, T., & Fan, Y. (2003). A modified Gabor filter design method for fingerprint image enhancement. *Pattern Recognition Letters, 24*(12), 1805–1817.

Yin, Y. L., Zhan, X. S., Tan, T. Z., & Ning, X. B. (2003). An Algorithm Based on Gabor Function for Fingerprint Enhancement and Its Application. *Journal of Software, 3,* 29.

Yu, S., Yang, J., Wang, Y., & Zhang, Y. (2007). Color active contour models based tongue segmentation in traditional Chinese medicine (pp. 1065–1068). IEEE.

Zhu, E., Yin, J., & Zhang, G (2004). Fingerprint enhancement using circular gabor filter. In *Image Analysis and Recognition* (pp. 750–758). Springer.

Zuo, W., Wang, K., Zhang, D., & Zhang, H. (2004). Combination of polar edge detection and active contour model for automated tongue segmentation (pp. 270–273). IEEE.

Chapter 8
Tongue Shape Classification by Geometric Features

Abstract Traditional Chinese Medicine diagnoses a wide range of health conditions by examining features of the tongue, including its shape. This chapter presents a classification approach for automatically recognizing and analyzing tongue shapes based on geometric features. The approach corrects tongue deflection by applying three geometric criteria and then classifies tongue shapes according to seven geometric features that are defined using various measurements of the length, area, and angle of the tongue. To establish a measurable and machine-readable relationship between expert human judgments and machine classifications of tongue shapes, we used a decision support tool, the analytic hierarchy process (AHP), to weigh the relative influences of the various length/area/angle factors used in classifying a tongue, and then applied a fuzzy fusion framework that combines seven AHP modules, one for each tongue shape, to represent the uncertainty and imprecision between these quantitative features and tongue shape classes. Experimental results show that the proposed shape correction method reduced the deflection of tongue shapes and that our shape classification approach, tested on 362 tongue samples, achieved an accuracy of 90.3%, making it more accurate than either KNN or LDA.

8.1 Introduction

A tongue body is composed of a body, tip, and root (Pae & Lowe, 1999). These parts give the tongue its shape, which is not permanent but may change. In TCM, these changes are taken to indicate particular pathologies (Li, 2011). The normal tongue is regarded as being an ellipse tongue, but TCM also has six other classes of tongue shape: square, rectangular, round, acute triangular, obtuse triangular, and hammer (see Fig. 1.2). A square tongue is as long as it is wide. A rectangular tongue is long, but equally wide at the root, body, and tip. The round tongue will look round. The hammer tongue is wider at the tip than at the root while the triangular tongue is the opposite, being wider at the root than at the tip. Triangular tongues may be either acute or obtuse triangular. Numerous clinical reports (Lin & Wang, 2002; Gong, Chen, Pu, Lian, & Chen, 2005; Li, 2011; Liu, Xu, Zhao, & Liu,

D. Zhang et al., *Tongue Image Analysis*, DOI 10.1007/978-981-10-2167-1_8

2008; Pae & Lowe, 1999; Ryan & Bradley, 2005; Wang & Liu, 1994) have associated particular tongue shapes with diseases in clinical medicine (Rotblatt & Ziment, 2002). For example, a round tongue is associated with gastritis, an obtuse triangular tongue with hyperthyroidism, and a square tongue may indicate coronary heart disease or portal sphygmo-hypertension.

To our knowledge, no previous work has sought to automatically classify and recognize tongue shapes for computerized tongue diagnosis. However, based on our experience, there are three initial difficulties in tongue shape classification. First, capturing an image of a tongue requires that the tongue be protruded. However, a protruding tongue often deflects or tends to move to one side. Such deflection can interfere with the accurate positioning of local characteristics, which will inevitably influence the final diagnostic accuracy of the tongue image. The second difficulty is that it is hard to define and represent what it is that experts regard as round, elliptical, square, etc., in particular cases, yet these subjective analyses must be summarized and rendered as a well-defined and readable machine representation. The third difficulty is the changes in the tongue shape, which do not begin and complete in 24 h, but may occur and persist over many months, reflecting the course of the disease. Such persistent variation produces diagnostic uncertainty, which is the ambiguity that belongs to one or more classes and then, only to some degree. This uncertainty should also be represented within any framework.

In this chapter, we propose a novel medical biometric approach (Zhang, 2013) that automatically classifies and recognizes tongue shapes. The proposed approach first corrects tongue deflection using automatic contour extraction and a combination of length, area, and angle criteria. Then, the features of tongue shapes are defined using seven sub-features defined from the length, area, and angle information. To convert the human judgment into classification decisions, we first apply a decision support tool called the analytic hierarchy process (AHP), wherein the relationship of each sub-feature to a shape has been characterized on a standardized numerical scale and given a weight. We then use a fuzzy fusion framework to combine seven modules of the AHP to classify each tongue image into seven classes of tongue shapes and model the relationship between diagnostic uncertainty and defined classes.

The organization of this chapter is as follows: Sect. 8.2 describes how we correct the deflection of a tongue image. Section 8.3 proposes the feature extraction of seven sub-features based on length, area, and angle information. Section 8.4 presents our method of shape classification. Section 8.5 describes our experiments. Section 8.6 offers our conclusion.

8.2 Shape Correction

In most cases, a tongue is symmetrically reflected, but a deflective tongue will not appear so in an image and must be corrected before being processed. In this section, we describe a number of techniques that are used to automatically extract the contour of a tongue and then correct the deflection using three criteria based on the length, area, and angle of the tongue.

8.2.1 Automatic Contour Extraction

Automatic contour extraction extracts the geometric contours of the tongue body, which usually includes the lips, parts of the face, or the teeth. Our approach begins by segmenting the tongue area from its surroundings using a model derived from a parameterization of the Bi-Elliptical Deformable Template (BEDT) (Pang, Zhang, & Wang, 2005), a structure that is composed of two ellipses with a common center. BEDT makes the algorithm more robust to noise, which in this case is usually caused by pathological details. BEDT produces a rough segmentation through an optimization in the ellipse parameter space by using a gradient descent method. BEDT is then sampled to form a deformable contour, known as BEDC (Pang et al., 2005). To further improve the performance of BEDC, we also replaced the traditional internal force in the BEDC with an elliptical template force which allows accurate local control. We then used BEDC to obtain a series of k points, (120 in this chapter), and defined the contour of the tongue body. Given this set of edge points, it is then possible to use the seed-filling algorithm to define every pixel in a tongue image as either inside or outside the boundary of the tongue body.

8.2.2 The Length Criterion

The length criterion is calculated as follows: let $x_{\max}$, $x_{\min}$, $y_{\max}$, and $y_{\min}$ be the maximums and minimums of contour points on the *x-axis* and *y-axis*, respectively (see Fig. 8.1). Point P_{md} (x_{md}, y_{md}) is the "middle center" of the tongue shape, where $x_{md} = (x_{\max} + x_{\min})/2$ and $y_{md} = (y_{\max} + y_{\min})/2$. We denote the set of all pixels in the region of the tongue body by $\{(x_s, y_s), s = 1,2, \ldots, S\}$, where S is the size of this set. The barycenter of the tongue shape is then P_c (x_c, y_c), where $\sum_{s=1}^{S} x_s/S$, $y_c = \sum_{s=1}^{S} y_s/S$, Fig. 8.2 shows the various measurements that are used to calculate the tongue length criterion. The vertical line $X = x_c$ is parallel to the *y*-axis and crosses point P_c (x_c, y_c). The length criterion is defined as the distance from two points with max X and min X to the vertical line $X = x_c$. This can be derived by

$$\nabla L = |x_{\max} - x_c| - |x_{\min} - x_c| \tag{8.1}$$

The length criterion is not an equally good indicator of deflection on all shapes. It is a good indicator of deflection in tongue shapes which are only approximately symmetrically reflected (triangular and hammer tongues) because the value of the length criterion changes with rotation, which means that it is able to represent the difference between a deflective and corrected (post-rotation) tongue. However,

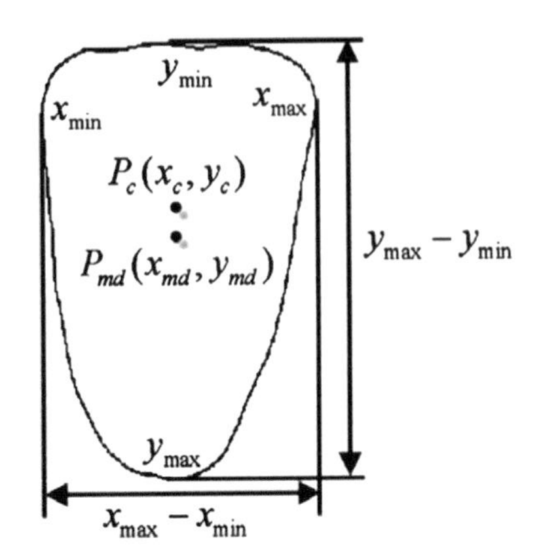

Fig. 8.1 Some basic definitions of the points and length in a tongue shape. Reprinted from Huang, Wu, Zhang et al. (2010), with permission from Elsevier

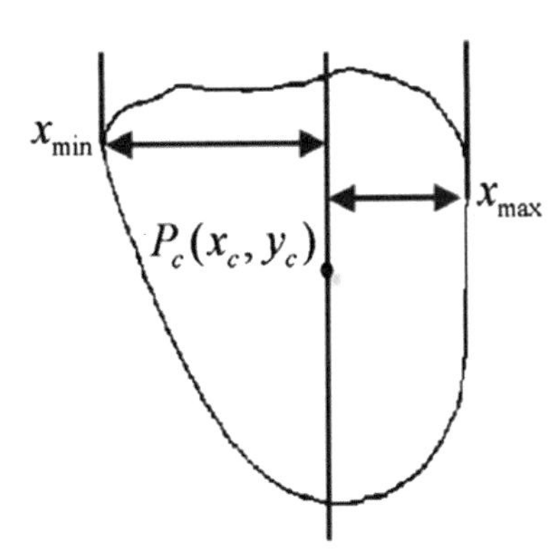

Fig. 8.2 Length criterion for shape correction. Reprinted from Huang et al. (2010), with permission from Elsevier

when a shape is approximately rotationally symmetrical (round and square tongues), the value of the length criterion remains approximately the same when rotated and any changes in the length criterion are too small to be reliable in discriminating between the deflective and corrected tongues.

8.2.3 *The Area Criterion*

Figure 8.3 shows how the area is calculated on the left and right parts of the tongue tip below the horizontal line $Y = y_c$. The difference in their areas is derived by

$$\nabla A = \left|\text{Area}_{\text{left}} - \text{Area}_{\text{right}}\right|, \tag{8.2}$$

where $\text{Area}_{\text{left}}$ and $\text{Area}_{\text{right}}$ represent the areas of the left and right parts of the tongue tip, respectively, and are obtained with a seed-filling algorithm. When the tongue is deflective, the value of the area criterion is large. When the tongue is not deflective, $\text{Area}_{\text{left}}$ and $\text{Area}_{\text{right}}$ are similar and the value of the area criterion is small.

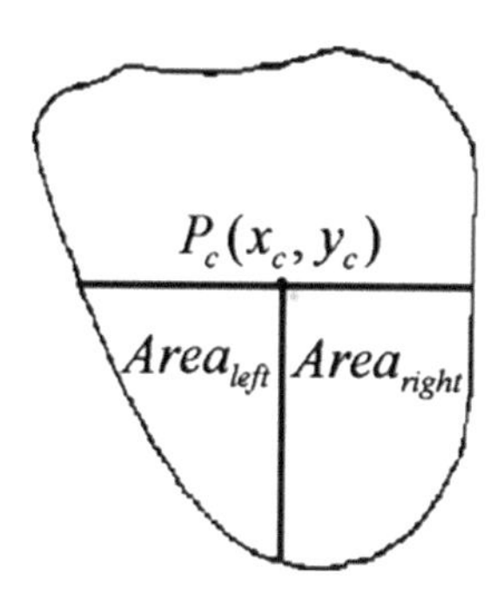

Fig. 8.3 Area criterion for shape correction. Reprinted from Huang et al. (2010), with permission from Elsevier

This criterion can be applied to any class of tongue shape except the round tongue. The value of the area criterion for the round tongue is always so small that there is no difference between the deflective and corrected tongues.

8.2.4 The Angle Criterion

The angle criterion is a measurement of the difference between two angles, which are formed by the two sides of the tongue contour that intersect with the horizontal line $Y = y_c$. From each side (left or right) of the tongue contour, we select γ contour points near the horizontal line $Y = y_c$. These points are denoted as (x_1, y_1), (x_2, y_2), …, (x_y, y_y). Using the linear regression method (Jammalamadaka, 2012), we can fit the γ points of each side into a slanted line. When $\sum_{i=1}^{\gamma}[y_i - (\beta x_i + \varepsilon)]^2$ is the minimum, the fitted line $Y = \beta X + \varepsilon$ intersects with horizontal line $Y = y_c$. It can be shown that the value of β and ε are

$$\beta = \left(\gamma \sum_{i=1}^{\gamma} x_i y_i - \sum_{i=1}^{\gamma} x_i \sum_{i=1}^{\gamma} y_i\right) \Bigg/ \left(\gamma \sum_{i=1}^{\gamma} x_i^2 - \left(\sum_{i=1}^{\gamma} x_i\right)^2\right) \tag{8.3}$$

$$\varepsilon = \left(\sum_{i=1}^{n} y_i - \beta \sum_{i=1}^{n} x_i\right) \Bigg/ \gamma. \tag{8.4}$$

Figure 8.4 shows the fitted lines and crossing angles: Line_1, Line_2, α_1, and α_2. Crossing angle α_1 is the angle between the fitted line Line_1 and the horizontal line $Y = y_c$. This angle is computed clockwise from the horizontal line to the fitted line Line_1. α_2 is the angle between the fitted line Line_2 and the horizontal line $Y = y_c$. This is computed counterclockwise from the horizontal line to the fitted line Line_2.

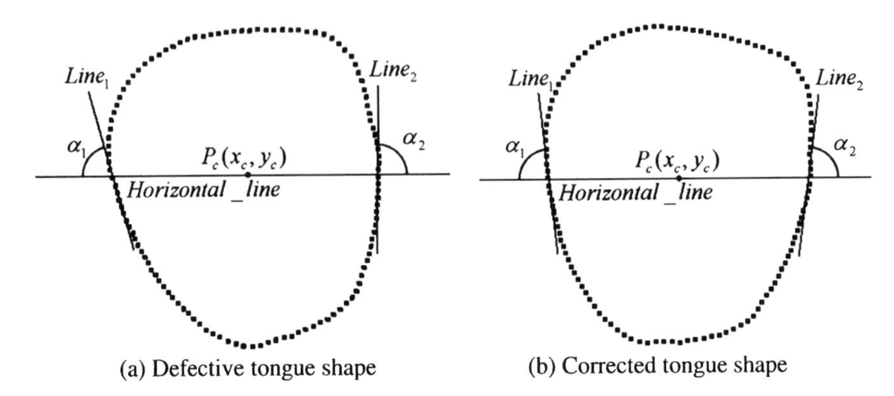

Fig. 8.4 Angle criterion for shape correction. Reprinted from Huang et al. (2010), with permission from Elsevier

The difference between these two angles can be computed by

$$\nabla\alpha = |\alpha_1 - \alpha_2| \tag{8.5}$$

When the tongue shape is deflective (see Fig. 8.4a), the value of the criterion is large. When it is not deflective, it is small (see Fig. 8.4b). This suggests that angle difference can be used to measure symmetry in all tongue shapes.

8.2.5 Correction by Combination

Tongue shape correction must also take account of the differences between the left and right parts of a tongue shape. To do this, we combine all three criteria, length, area, and angle. Each has its own limitations, while together, they are complementary. The area criterion refers to the interior area of a tongue body, the angle criterion refers to its external contour, and the length criterion refers to both internal and external information. We combine these complementary criteria when calculating the correction angle w by

$$w = \arg\min\nabla = \arg\min(a\nabla L + b\nabla A + c\nabla\alpha), \tag{8.6}$$

where ∇ is the value of the combined criterion without reference to dimensions (physical units), the physical units of ∇L, ∇A and $\nabla\alpha$ are the corresponding dimensions of length, area and angle, and a, b and c are the corresponding powers of the three criteria. We derive these powers empirically.

The quantity w is the amount of rotation that is required. A larger ∇ signifies that the tongue is increasingly more deflective. Similarly, a smaller ∇ means that the tongue is increasingly less deflective. The angle of rotation that gives us the smallest ∇ is the w. This is found by rotating the tongue shape degree-by-degree

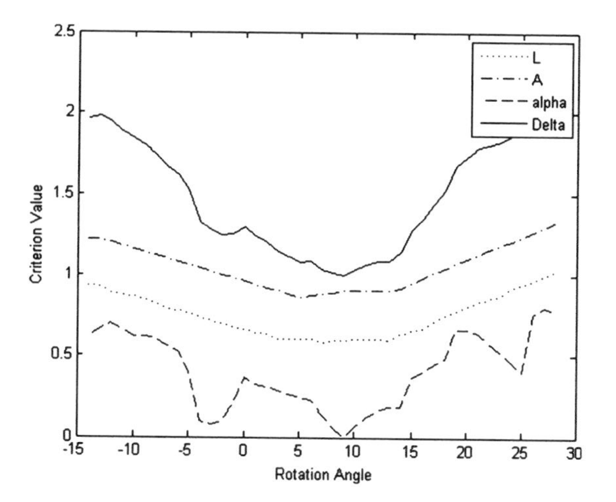

Fig. 8.5 Relationship between the criterion value and the rotation angle. Reprinted from Huang et al. (2010), with permission from Elsevier

until we are able to identify the minimum of the combined criterion. The direction of rotation can be seen in that when $w < 0$, the tongue shape is rotated clockwise and when $w \geq 0$, it is rotated counterclockwise.

Figure 8.5 shows the relationship between the criterion value and rotation angle. The solid curve is ∇ and the dotted curves: ∇L, ∇A and $\nabla \alpha$, represent the curves of the length, area, and angle criteria, respectively. The points of interest are their minimums, but the curves are not smooth since their contour points are discretely distributed and as a result, their minimums are not easy to distinguish (see Fig. 8.5). In contrast, the minimum of curve ∇ is obvious. At this point, the tongue shape is perpendicular; that is, it is not deflected. The formula for tongue shape rotation is as follows:

$$\begin{cases} x' = (x - x_c) \times \cos w - (y - y_c) \times \sin w + x_c \\ y' = (y - y_c) \times \cos w + (x - x_c) \times \sin w + y_c \end{cases}, \tag{8.7}$$

where (x, y) is the original contour point, and (x', y') is the corresponding new point.

8.3 Feature Extraction

TCM diagnosticians classify tongues according to seven shapes: elliptical, square, rectangular, round, acute triangular, obtuse triangular, and hammer. We do not use the full tongue shape in our machine-readable representation. Rather, our approach extracts three kinds of shape feature: length-based, area-based, and angle-based. The length-based and area-based shape features are all relative values of the length and area and thus are all scale invariant. The angle-based feature is also scale invariant.

8.3.1 The Length-Based Feature

The length-based feature contains three sub-features: the length–width ratio, (describing the global length ratio of the tongue shape), the off-center ratio (describing the ways that the local area affects the location of the off-center), and the radial line ratio (describing the ways that tongue shapes affect the local length).

8.3.1.1 The Length–Width Ratio

The length–width ratio can be defined as follows:

$$\mathrm{Lw} = (y_{\max} - y_{\min})/(x_{\max} - x_{\min}) \tag{8.8}$$

When the tongue shape is elliptical, rectangular, hammer, or acute triangular, Lw is larger than when it is square, round, or obtuse triangular. This sub-feature is in most cases, a good discriminator.

8.3.1.2 The off-Center Ratio

The horizontal line $Y = y_{\min}$ intersects with the tongue contour and touches two edge points on the edge contour: (x_{p1}, y) and (x_{p2}, y). We can define the y coordinate having the longest line segment as $y_{\mathrm{mw}} = \arg\max_y |x_{p1} - x_{p2}|$. The horizontal line $Y = y_{\mathrm{wn}}$ intersects with the tongue body and also touches two edge points on the edge contour. x_{mw1} and x_{mw2} are the two x coordinates corresponding to these two edge points. Point $P_{\mathrm{mw}} = (x_{\mathrm{mw}}, y_{\mathrm{mw}})$ is the off-center of the tongue shape, where $x_{\mathrm{mw}} = (x_{\mathrm{mw1}} + x_{\mathrm{mw2}})/2$.

The off-center ratio can thus be defined as follows (see Fig. 8.6):

$$\mathrm{Oc} = (y_c - y_{\mathrm{mw}})/(y_{\max} - y_{\min}) \tag{8.9}$$

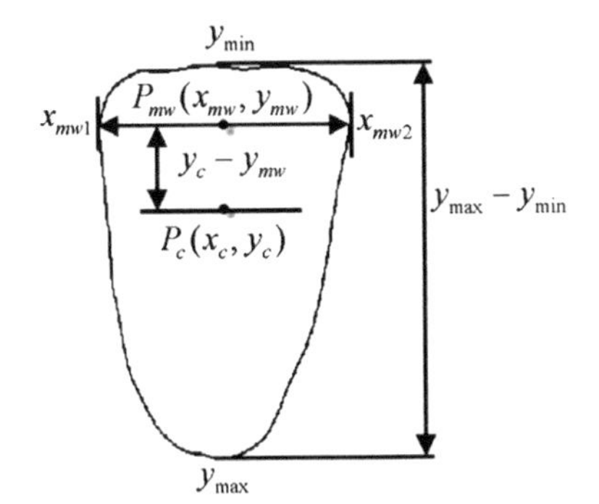

Fig. 8.6 Length-based feature B for tongue shape representation. Reprinted from Huang et al. (2010), with permission from Elsevier

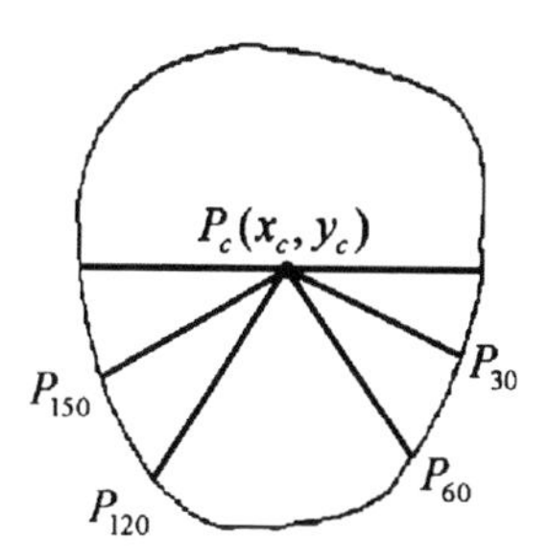

Fig. 8.7 Length-based feature C for tongue shape representation. Reprinted from Huang et al. (2010), with permission from Elsevier

When $O_c < 0$, the off-center is closer to the tip of the tongue than the barycenter and the tip is larger than the root of the tongue. In most cases, this matches the hammer tongue. When $O_c > 0$, the off-center is closer to the root than the barycenter and the tip is smaller than the root of the tongue. This shape is a better match for the obtuse or acute triangular tongue. When the tongue shape is rectangular, elliptical, square, or round, y_c is close to y_{mw}, and then $|O_c| \approx 0$.

8.3.1.3 The Radial Line Ratio

From the barycenter point $P_c(x_c, y_c)$, we can connect four radial lines to the contour at four points: P_{30}, P_{60}, P_{120}, and P_{150}. These four radial lines respectively form four angles with the horizontal line $Y = y_c$ at 30°, 60°, 120°, and 150° (see Fig. 8.7). Their respective lengths are L_{30}, L_{60}, L_{120}, and L_{150}. The radial line ratio is defined as follows:

$$\text{Rl} = (L_{30} + L_{150})/(L_{60} + L_{120}) \tag{8.10}$$

For square and round tongues, this ratio is close to 1. For obtuse triangular tongues, Rl is greater than 1, and for acute triangular tongues, Rl is less than 1.

8.3.2 *The Area-Based Feature*

The area-based feature also contains three sub-features: the total area ratio, which defines a similarity to a regular round, the triangle area ratio, which defines a similarity to a triangular, and the top–bottom area ratio, which defines a ratio between the area of the root and tip of the tongue, and is useful in discriminating between different shapes.

8.3.2.1 The Total Area Ratio

The total area ratio is used to describe the similarity of a shape that is approximately a regular round, and its corresponding area is also approximately the area of a

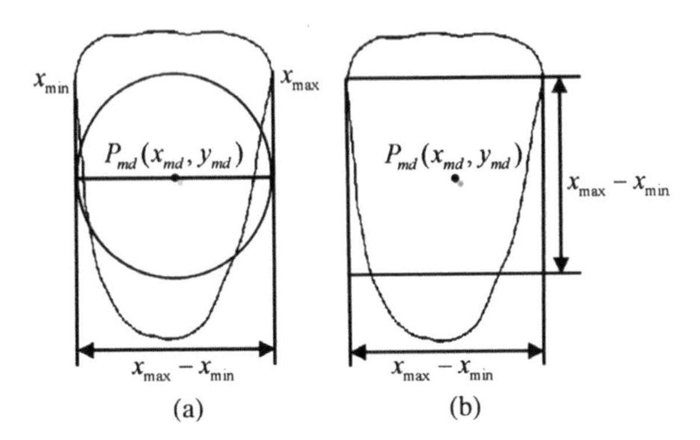

Fig. 8.8 Area-based feature D for tongue shape representation. Reprinted from Huang et al. (2010), with permission from Elsevier

regular round. To determine whether a shape is a round tongue, we first define what constitutes roundness for the given area. We then compare our definition of roundness against the target shape. The radius of this round shape is $r = (x_{max} - x_{min})/2$, so we can take the area πr^2 as a reference. We define the total area ratio as follows:

$$\text{To} = \text{Tongue\_area}/r^2 \tag{8.11}$$

where Tongue_area is the area of the entire tongue body that is obtained by applying a seed-filling algorithm. When $T_0 \approx \pi$, the tongue shape is roundish and the tongue should be classified as a round tongue (see Fig. 8.8a).

The total area ratio can also be used to describe the degree of similarity of a shape to a regular square. The area of a square is $4r^2$ (see Fig. 8.8b), so it shares an item, r^2, with the formula for the area of a circle, πr^2. This means that the shape of the tongue will be approximately square when $T_0 \approx 4$. We thus identify this shape as likely to be a square tongue.

8.3.2.2 The Triangle Area Ratio

This sub-feature is used to describe the similarity of a shape to a triangle. The areas of the obtuse and acute triangular tongues are approximately that of a regular triangle. We denote $(x_{max} - x_{min})$ as the width, and $(y_{max} - y_{min})$ as the length. Figure 8.9 shows the area of the triangle, and the triangle ratio is defined as

$$\begin{aligned} \text{Tr} &= \text{Triangle\_area}/\text{Tongue\_area} \\ &= \frac{1}{2}(y_{max} - y_{min}) \times (x_{max} - x_{min})/\text{Tongue\_area} \end{aligned} \tag{8.12}$$

As the ratio becomes increasingly closer to 1, the tongue will more closely approach a triangular shape. For rectangular and square tongues, this ratio is close to 2 and for other shapes, it is between 1 and 2.

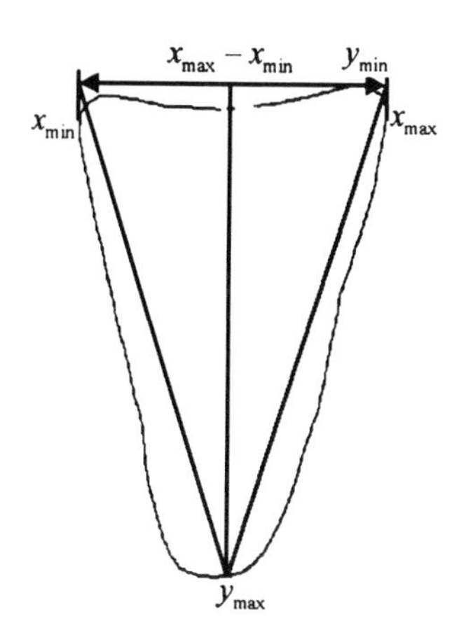

Fig. 8.9 Area-based feature E for tongue shape representation. Reprinted from Huang et al. (2010), with permission from Elsevier

8.3.2.3 The Top–Bottom Area Ratio

The top–bottom area ratio is defined as (see Fig. 8.10)

$$\text{Tb} = \text{Top\_area}/\text{bottom\_area}, \tag{8.13}$$

where Top_area and Bottom_area are the areas of the tongue root and tongue tip regions which are divided by the horizontal line $Y = y_{\text{md}}$. For hammer tongues, the Top_area is less than the Bottom_area, hence, giving the ratio $T_b < 1$. For triangular tongues, $T_b \approx 3$. For other tongue shapes, $T_b \approx 1$.

8.3.3 The Angle-Based Feature

The angle-based geometric feature has only one sub-feature. This feature is associated with two angles, a_1 and a_2, which are formed by the two sides of the tongue

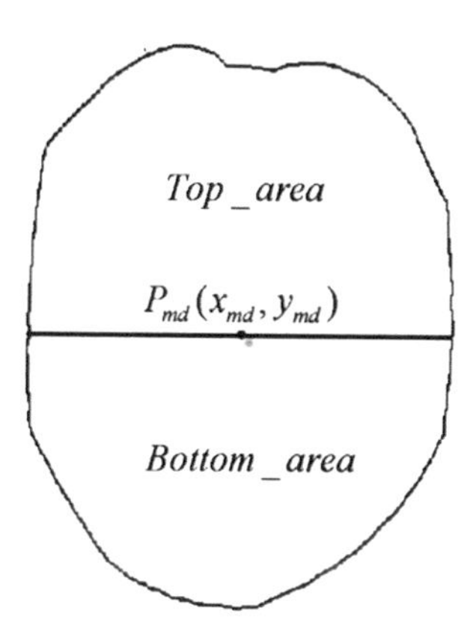

Fig. 8.10 Area-based feature F for tongue shape representation. Reprinted from Huang et al. (2010), with permission from Elsevier

shape crossing the horizontal line $Y = y_c$. We denote this sub-feature as the mean value of these two angles:

$$\alpha = \alpha_1 + \alpha_2/2 \tag{8.14}$$

This feature is used to distinguish between triangular and hammer shapes and to measure local deformation near the horizontal line $Y = y_c$. For hammer tongues, this feature is greater than 90° whereas for triangular tongues, it is less than 90°.

8.4 Shape Classification

Once the seven sub-features are calculated, they can be used to classify a tongue image so as to determine if it belongs in one of the seven shape classes. However, as some of these sub-features are correlated to more than one shape with different strengths of correlation, it is necessary to provide some reliable basis for deciding which of these features is more influential in classifying a shape and at what threshold. To help us with this, we used the analytic hierarchy process (AHP) which is a decision support tool. This method can breakdown human judgment level by level into a hierarchical structure of influential factors, and convert these more easily understood factors into comparable relative weights. Then, human judgment is converted to a measurable and readable machine representation. We can use this method to classify the current shape.

This process of shape classification is carried out in four steps. The first step is to model the classification as a hierarchy of seven self-contained AHP modules, one for each of the seven tongue shape classes. Based on the relative impact on the factor at a higher level, we next assign numerical representations (relative weights) to pairs of factors in each AHP module. The third step is to use these relative weights to calculate a global weight for each AHP module. This global weight is used to decide whether a tongue shape belongs to a given class. In the fourth and final step, a fusion framework combines these global weights to assign an image into one of the seven tongue shape classes. The following describes each of these steps in greater detail.

8.4.1 Modeling the Classification as a Hierarchy

In step 1, we model the classification as a hierarchy. As shown on the left of Fig. 8.11, our hierarchy has five levels: goal, class, feature, sub-feature, and option. This figure is the structure (not a flowchart) of classification decisions, and each element is an influential factor of the element at a higher level.

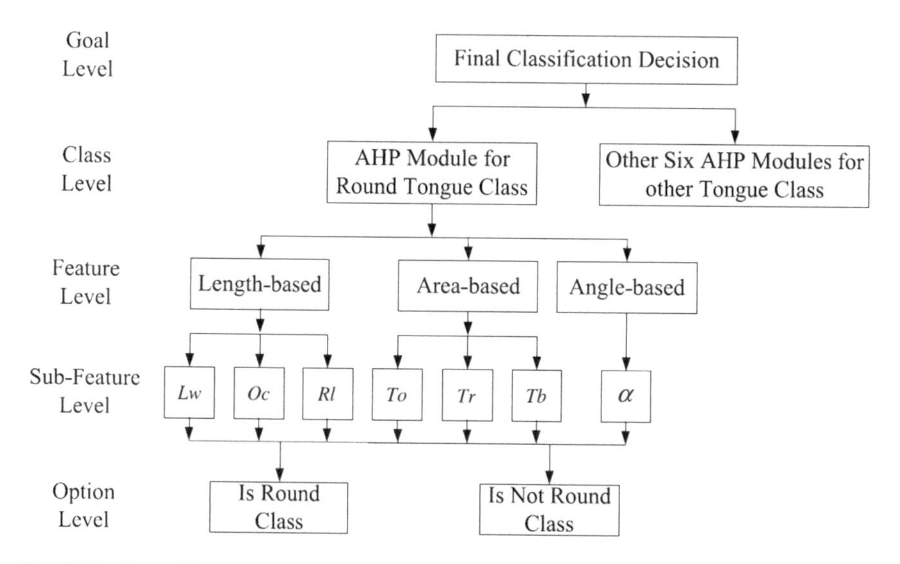

Fig. 8.11 Hierarchical structure of the fusion framework for shape classification. Reprinted from Huang et al. (2010), with permission from Elsevier

A. **Goal level**

At this level, the final decision is made as to which of the seven classes the tongue shape belongs in.

B. **Class level**

The class level is made up of seven modules, one for each class of tongue shape. For simplicity of presentation, Fig. 8.11 shows only the module of the round tongue class, which has four levels: class, feature, sub-feature, and option.

C. **Feature level**

Tongue shape is only associated with geometric information. At this level, features based on length, area, and angle as the three elements may be considered. These three elements are the influential factors which affect each element in the class level.

D. **Sub-feature level**

This level further subdivides the three features into the seven elements, or influential factors. Area-based features are subdivided into total area, triangular area, and top–bottom area ratios. The length-based feature is subdivided into length-width, off-center, and radial line ratios. Then, this level subdivides features into the seven sub-features, including an angle-based feature, as described in Sect. 8.3.

E. **Option level**

This level uses the seven sub-features to classify an image as either belonging or not belonging to one of the seven shape classes. Then, in each AHP module, this level has two options or two elements. Hence, this level has 14 elements for all seven modules.

8.4.2 Calculating Relative Weights

Relative weights are applied to decision-making at various levels of the AHP modules. In this step, we can either calculate concrete sub-features for the relative weights of the elements in the option level, or use human judgment on the relative importance of the elements in the feature and sub-feature levels. The role of human judgment is restricted to a relatively narrow area, specifically, a standardized numerical scale between 1 and 9. Then, human judgment can be used in performing evaluations which can be converted into numerical values over the entire range of the classification decision.

The relative weights in the feature and sub-feature levels are expressed as pairwise comparisons (Saaty, 1980, 1982, 1988, 1990), ratios of relative importance between pairs of factors. The weight of every factor is represented as an integer between 1 and 9 and the relative weights of factors are expressed as a ratio. For example, if the weight of the factor A is 1 and that of B is 9, the pairwise relative weight is 1/9. These values define only the weight $w = (w_1, w_2, \ldots, w_n)$. It is therefore always possible to normalize the vector w by imposing $\sum_i w_i = 1$. The ratio w_i/w_j would then be the relative weight of the ith to the jth element.

The relative weight of the option level is calculated using sub-features. These sub-features are all normalized to an interval estimate of 1–5, the thresholds of which were established empirically. We then constructed a matrix for every element a_{ij} in the hierarchy. We combined all possible pairwise relative weights into a preference matrix A as follows:

$$A = \begin{bmatrix} w1/w1 & w1/w2 & w1/w3 & \ldots & w1/wn \\ w2/w1 & & & \ldots & \\ w3/w1 & & & \ldots & \\ \vdots & & & \ldots & \\ wn/w1 & & & \ldots & wn/wn \end{bmatrix} \tag{8.15}$$

The elements of matrix A have the special property $w_i/w_j = a_{ji} = 1/a_{ji} = 1/(w_j/w_i)$ for all i and j. Each preference matrix is different at every level of a tongue shape.

8.4.3 Calculating the Global Weights

Step 3 calculates the global weight of every AHP module level by level. Of any pair, the option with a heavier global weight is the module's classification decision. The seven AHP modules for the seven classes of tongue shapes thus gave us seven global weights. These weights are determined by calculating a weight for each element at each level and then adding the relative weight obtained under each element. AHP normalizes the weight of the ith row as follows:

$$w_i = \frac{1}{n}\sum_{j=1}^{n}\frac{a_{ij}}{\sum_{k=1}^{n} a_{kl}} \tag{8.16}$$

Let $w^{(k-1)} = (w_1^{(k-1)}, w_2^{(k-2)}, \ldots, w_m^{(k-1)})^{\mathrm{T}}$ be the weight for the m elements in the $(k-1)$th level, and $p_j^{(k)} = (p_{1j}^{(k)}, p_{2j}^{(k)}, \ldots, p_{nj}^{(k)})^{\mathrm{T}}$ is the weight for the next level of n elements in the kth level, and then weight is calculated from top to bottom as

$$wi^{(k)} = \sum_{j=1}^{m} pij^{(k)} wj^{(k-1)}, \quad i = 1, 2, \ldots, n \tag{8.17}$$

The weight in the class level is the global weight of every AHP module.

It is necessary to check the consistency of the elements in each preference matrix (Saaty, 1980, 1982, 1988, 1990). A preference matrix A is said to be strictly consistent if $a_{ij} \times a_{jk} = ai_k$ for all i, j and k. However, this consistency is not forced with human judgment. We can use a simple case for illustration: "A to B" is 3 and "B to C" is 2. Then "A to C" is not always 6 in human judgment. To describe deviation or degree of consistency, we use the following formula:

$$\text{Consistency\_Index} = (\lambda_{\max} - n)/(n-1), \tag{8.18}$$

where $\lambda_{\max}$ is the largest eigenvalue, and n is the size of the preference matrix. If the Consistency_Index is less than a given threshold (this threshold changes with n) (Saaty, 1980, 1982, 1988, 1990), then the inconsistency is acceptable. Otherwise, it is necessary to reconsider the subjective judgment.

8.4.4 Fuzzy Shape Classification

Fuzzy shape classification involves classifying each tongue image into one of the seven classes of tongue shape. There are two reasons for utilizing this fuzzy method. First, although AHP converts human judgment into well-defined and measurable machine representation, each AHP module can only distinguish a class of tongue shape in the class level. Second, as we have previously noted, as it changes shape, a tongue need not belong definitively to one class or another. The fuzzy membership theory (Pedrycz & Gomide, 1998; Zadeh, 1965) is premised on the observation that many phenomena cannot be discreetly categorized as members of one class or another, but rather, share features with other phenomena so that they may be said to belong to one or more classes, and only to some degree.

Let F_{class}(class = 1, 2, …, 7) be the seven global weights extracted from the seven modules. The membership function M_{class}(class = 1, 2, …, 7) for the seven tongue shapes is found as follows:

$$M_{\text{class}} = F_{\text{class}} \Big/ \sum_{j=1}^{7} F_j \tag{8.19}$$

Each M_{class} is located in [0,1] and can be regarded as the categorical ambiguity that results from diagnostic uncertainty. A tongue is classifiable if its class membership function is greater than 0.5 and “unclassified” if its class membership functions are all less than 0.5.

8.5 Experimental Results and Performance Analysis

In this section, experiments were conducted to determine the accuracy of our shape correction and shape classification methods.

8.5.1 Accuracy of Shape Correction

To measure the accuracy of our shape correction method, we used the Hausdorff distance (HD) (Edgar, 2007) and mean distance to the closest point (MDCP) (Chalana & Kim, 1997), comparing the results against manually corrected shapes. These two measurements are advantageous in that they are not sensitive to shape changes.

Let $PA = \{pa_1, pa_2, pa_3, \ldots, pa_\lambda\}$ be the corrected shape results, and $PB = \{pb_1, pb_2, pb_3, \ldots, pb_\lambda\}$ be the manually corrected shapes, where pa_i or pb_j is a point on the corresponding shape. More formally, the HD from set PA to set PB is a maximum function defined as

$$H(PA, PB) = \max(h(PA, PB), h(PB, PA)), \tag{8.20}$$

$$\text{where} \quad h(PA, PB) = \max_{pa \in PA} \min_{pb \in PB} \|pa - pb\| \tag{8.21}$$

$$h(PB, PA) = \max_{pb \in PA} \min_{pa \in PB} \|pb - pa\|, \tag{8.22}$$

Table 8.1 Evaluation result of the correction algorithm

	Before correction	After correction
HD	93.51	23.13
MDCP	22.17	4.96

Reprinted from Huang et al. (2010), with permission from Elsevier

pa and *pb* are points of sets *PA* and *PB* respectively, and ||*|| is a metric between these points. For simplicity, we will take ||*|| as the Euclidian distance between *pa* and *pb*.

We also defined the mean of the distance to the closest point (DCP). DCP for pa_i to *PB* is defined as

$$DCP(pa_i, PB) = \min_{pb \in PB} \|pa_i - pb\| \tag{8.23}$$

We proposed the MDCP of two point sets; *PA* and *PB*, which can be defined as

$$MDCP(PA, PB) = \frac{1}{2\lambda}\left(\sum_{i}^{\lambda} DCP(pa_i, PB) + \sum_{j}^{\lambda} DCP(pb_j, PA)\right) \tag{8.24}$$

As shown in Table 8.1, the average HD and MDCP of the proposed final method are 23.13 and 4.96 pixels. The results, when not using corrected values, are 93.51 and 22.17 pixels. Hence, this method for shape correction reduces the deflection of tongue shapes.

8.5.2 Accuracy of Shape Classification

We tested the accuracy of tongue shape classification on a set of 362 pre-labeled tongue images chosen from our database. The database contains images taken from both healthy and possibly unwell volunteers. The healthy participants are students at the Harbin Institute of Technology, in the 17–23 age group. Other volunteers are in-patients from six departments at the Harbin Hospital and represent a wide range of ages, young to old. All the tongue shapes are the outputs of the segmentation algorithms proposed from Chaps. 3 to 7. Moreover, for each tongue image, five skilled TCM doctors as well as 20 students were asked to choose the best segmentation result, from the outputs of the five proposed segmentation algorithms, as the final tongue shape used in this chapter. The distribution of tongue shapes for the entire sample is as follows: rectangular; 13.3%, acute triangular; 14.4%, obtuse triangular; 14.9%, hammer; 8.3%, round; 12.7%, square; 11.6%, elliptical; 13.8%, and unclassified; 11.0% (see Table 8.2).

Manual labeling was carried out by three physicians, who are specialists in tongue diagnostics with more than 20 years of experience and members of relevant

Table 8.2 Distribution of every class for the seven tongue shapes

Class name	Number of samples	Percent (%)
Rectangular	48	13.3
Hammer	30	8.3
Acute triangular	52	14.4
Obtuse triangular	54	14.9
Round	46	12.7
Square	42	11.6
Elliptical	50	13.8
Unclassified	40	11.0
All	362	100

Reprinted from Huang et al. (2010), with permission from Elsevier

national bodies in China. They identified every sample of each class and their opinions were highly consistent. The labels given to the tongue samples were compared with the results obtained by using our approach and they formed the basis for evaluating all of the following experiments.

At the same time, we implemented a K-nearest neighbor (KNN) classifier (Xu, Zhang, Song, Yang, Jing, & Li, 2007) and a linear discriminant analysis (LDA) classifier (Xu, Yang & Jin, 2004) for comparison in order to demonstrate the superiority of our approach in tongue shape classification. The seven geometric sub-features based on length, area, and angle are considered as a seven-dimensional feature vector that was inputted into these classifiers. We also used a fivefold cross-validation to estimate the accuracy of classifiers. This cross-validation partitions all datasets into five subsets of approximately equal sizes. Each subset was used as a testing set for a classifier trained on the remaining subsets. The overall accuracy was the average of the accuracies of these fivefold classifications. As shown in Table 8.3, the overall accuracies of KNN and LDA were 78.2% and 82.9%, respectively while our approach was 90.3% accurate. The misclassification cost table assumes that all types of misclassifications are equally important. In Tables 8.4 and 8.5, we use the misclassification cost table to describe the final accuracy of every class. These results demonstrate the effectiveness of our approach and establish the potential usefulness of computerized tongue diagnosis in clinical medicine.

Table 8.3 Comparison of classification accuracy

	KNN	LDA	Our approach
Correctly classified samples	283	300	327
Classification accuracy (%)	78.2	82.9	90.3

Reprinted from Huang et al. (2010), with permission from Elsevier

Table 8.4 Classification results of the proposed method

	Rectangular	Hammer	Acute triangular	Obtuse triangular	Round	Square	Elliptical	Unclassified
Rectangular	45	0	3	0	0	0	0	0
Hammer	1	26	0	1	0	2	0	0
Acute triangular	2	0	47	3	0	0	0	0
Obtuse triangular	0	0	3	48	1	2	0	0
Round	0	1	0	1	42	1	1	0
Square	0	1	0	1	1	36	2	0
Elliptical	0	0	0	0	2	2	46	0
Unclassified	0	0	0	0	0	0	3	37

Reprinted from Huang et al. (2010), with permission from Elsevier

Table 8.5 Comparison of classification accuracy

	Correctly classified samples	Misclassified samples	Classification accuracy (%)
Rectangular	45	3	93.8
Hammer	26	4	86.7
Acute triangular	47	5	90.4
Obtuse triangular	48	6	88.9
Round	42	4	91.3
Square	36	6	85.7
Elliptical	46	4	92.0
Unclassified	37	3	92.5
All	327	35	90.3

Reprinted from Huang et al. (2010), with permission from Elsevier

8.6 Summary

As a follow-up study of the previous chapters, this chapter focuses on tongue shape, the direct output of the segmentation algorithm. We propose a classification approach for automatically recognizing and analyzing tongue shapes based on geometric features. The first step applies three geometric criteria to correct tongue deflection. Then, we develop seven geometric features using various measurements of length, area, and angle of the tongue. Moreover, a decision support tool, analytic hierarchy process, converts human judgment to machine representation. Finally, we apply a fuzzy fusion framework that combines seven AHP modules, one for each tongue shape, to represent the uncertainty and imprecision between these quantitative features and tongue shape classes. Experimental results show that this shape correction reduces the deflection of tongue shapes and our method of shape classification achieves a higher accuracy than KNN and LDA on a total of 362 tongue samples.

References

Chalana, V., & Kim, Y. (1997). A methodology for evaluation of boundary detection algorithms on medical images. *Medical Imaging, IEEE Transactions on, 16*(5), 642–652.

Edgar, G. (2007). *Measure, topology, and fractal geometry*. Springer.

Gong, Y., Chen, H., Pu, J., Lian, Y., & Chen, S. (2005). Quantitative investigation on normal pathological tongue shape and correlation analysis between hypertension and syndrome. *China Journal of Traditional Chinese Medicine and Pharmacy, 12*.

Huang, B., Wu, J., Zhang, D., et al. (2010). Tongue shape classification by geometric features. *Information Sciences, 180*(2), 312–324.

Jammalamadaka, S. R. (2012). *Introduction to linear regression analysis*. The American Statistician.

Li, N. (2011). *Tongue diagnostics*. New York: Academy Press.

Lin, Q., & Wang, M. (2002). Reorganizing analysis of genetic research materials related to tongue diagnosis in OMIM. In *Acta Universitatis Traditionis Medicalis Sinensis Pharmacologiaeque Shanghai* (02), 7–9.

Liu, M., Xu, J., Zhao, Y., & Liu, Z. (2008). The clinical research of glossoscopy of acute cerebrovascular disease. *Journal of Emergency in Traditional Chinese Medicine, 11,* 38.

Pae, E., & Lowe, A. A. (1999). Tongue shape in obstructive sleep apnea patients. *The Angle Orthodontist, 69*(2), 147–150.

Pang, B., Zhang, D., & Wang, K. (2005). The bi-elliptical deformable contour and its application to automated tongue segmentation in Chinese medicine. *Medical Imaging, IEEE Transactions on, 24*(8), 946–956.

Pedrycz, W., & Gomide, F. (1998). *An introduction to fuzzy sets: analysis and design*. MIT Press.

Rotblatt, M., & Ziment, I. (2002). *Evidence-based herbal medicine*. Philadelphia: Hanley & Belfus.

Ryan, C. M., & Bradley, T. D. (2005). Pathogenesis of obstructive sleep apnea. *Journal of Applied Physiology, 99*(6), 2440–2450.

Saaty, T. L. (1980). *The analytic hierarchy process: planning, priority setting, resources allocation*. New York: McGraw.

Saaty, T. L. (1982). *Decision making for leaders*. New York: Lifetime Learning.

Saaty, T. L. (1990). *Decision making for leaders: the analytic hierarchy process for decisions in a complex world*: RWS publications.

Satty, T. L. (1988). *Multi-criteria decision making: The analytical hierarchy process*. Pittsburgh, PA: RWS Publications.

Wang, B., & Liu, Z. (1994). Tongue shape observation on 88 patients with acute apoplexy. *Tianjin Journal of Traditional Chinese Medicine* (1), 32.

Xu, Y., Yang, J., & Jin, Z. (2004). A novel method for Fisher discriminant analysis. *Pattern Recognition, 37*(2), 381–384.

Xu, Y., Zhang, D., Song, F., Yang, J., Jing, Z., & Li, M. (2007). A method for speeding up feature extraction based on KPCA. *Neurocomputing, 70*(4), 1056–1061.

Zadeh, L. A. (1965). Fuzzy sets. *Information and control, 8*(3), 338–353.

Zhang, D. D. (2013). *Automated biometrics: Technologies and systems* (vol. 7). Springer.

Part III
Tongue Color Correction and Classification

Chapter 9
Color Correction Scheme for Tongue Images

Abstract Color images produced by digital cameras are usually device-dependent, i.e., the generated color information (usually presented in the RGB color space) is dependent on the imaging characteristics of specific cameras. This is a serious problem in computer-aided tongue image analysis because it relies on the accurate rendering of color information. In this chapter, we propose an optimized correction scheme that corrects tongue images captured in different device-dependent color spaces to the target device-independent color space. The correction algorithm in this scheme is generated by comparing several popular correction algorithms, i.e., polynomial-based regression, ridge regression, support-vector regression, and neural network mapping algorithms. We tested the performance of the proposed scheme by computing the CIE $L^*a^*b^*$ color difference (ΔE^*_{ab}) between estimated values and the target reference values. The experimental results on the colorchecker show that the color difference is less than 5 ($\Delta E^*_{\mathrm{ab}} < 5$), while the experimental results on real tongue images show that the distorted tongue images (captured in various device-dependent color spaces) become more consistent with each other. In fact, the average color difference among them is greatly reduced by more than 95%.

9.1 Introduction

In tongue analysis of traditional Chinese medicine (TCM), color and color difference often convey important diagnostic information. By the use of digital imaging and processing technology, we can briefly retrieve some physiological information of the human body condition by analyzing color features and color differences extracted from tongue images (Zhang, Pang, Li, Wang, & Zhang, 2005; Pang, Zhang, & Wang, 2005). However, there are two existing problems in such kinds of technologies when they are applied to computer-aided tongue image analysis. One problem is that the color images generated by digital cameras are usually device-dependent, i.e., these images are captured in a color space (usually an RGB-like color space) that is defined by the characteristics of a specific imaging device. As a result, the colors in images captured or rendered on one device may

D. Zhang et al., *Tongue Image Analysis*, DOI 10.1007/978-981-10-2167-1_9

differ from those captured or rendered on a different device, making it difficult to reliably and meaningfully exchange or compare images. Developed methods and obtained results on these device-dependent images may suffer from limited applicability. The other problem is, in the specific device-dependent color space, it is difficult to compute the color difference that can be useful for the tongue segmentation and diagnosis, as it is generally computed with the aid of the so-called "perceptual uniform color space," e.g., CIE $L^*a^*b^*$, which is one of the device-independent color spaces. Therefore, in order to get a consistent and standard color perception of tongue images for tongue analysis, further color correction to determine the mapping algorithm between its unknown device-dependent RGB color spaces and a particular known device-independent color space is needed.

Research on color correction methods has been extensively conducted in the color science area. Several correction algorithms were proposed for different tasks (Chang & Reid, 1996; Wandell, 1987; Finlayson, 1996; Barnard & Funt, 2002; Yamamoto et al., 2007; Vrhel & Trussell, 1999; Vrhel, Saber & Trussell, 2005; Yamamoto & James, 2006), while the polynomial-based correction method (Haeghen, Naeyaert, Lemahieu, & Philips, 2000; Luo, Hong & Rhodes, 2001) and the neural network mapping (Cheung, Westland, Connah, & Ripamonti, 2004) are most commonly used. However, most related research has focused on color correction for general imaging devices, such as digital cameras, and cathode ray tube/liquid crystal display (CRT/LCD) monitors and printers, where the color gamut covers almost the whole visible color area. Since the color gamut of human tongue images is much narrower than this, these existing algorithms cannot be directly applied to computer-aided tongue image analysis, but need to be further optimized and improved. Furthermore, although a few algorithms for color correction of tongue images have been developed, such as the polynomial-regression-based algorithm and support-vector regression (SVR)-based algorithm (Zhang, Wang, Jin, & Zhang, 2005), these algorithms were exclusively proposed for and tested in their specific imaging device. Comprehensive optimization and comparison, which are the most important parts when developing a computer-aided tongue image analysis system, have not been conducted. In view of this condition, research on the optimization of the color correction algorithms is meaningful and essential in computer-aided tongue image analysis.

In this chapter, we propose an optimized tongue color correction scheme to achieve accurate tongue image rendering. This scheme has three main steps: selection of target device-independent color space, optimization of the color correction algorithms, and evaluation of the performance. Compared with the existing approaches, the proposed scheme has several outstanding characteristics. First, to the best of our knowledge, it is the first time to propose special selection criteria among various color spaces used for tongue image correction. This is an important basic work for the accurate and efficient color correction of tongue images. Second, the proposed method is generated by a detailed comparison of the most popular color correction algorithms in the color science area, and thus the most suitable one can be applied to this specific correction task. Finally, the proposed method has been evaluated over a large tongue image database (more than 3000 samples).

Therefore, the color correction scheme, which is introduced in this chapter, is statistically more reliable.

The organization of this chapter is as follows. Section 9.2 explains why we chose the sRGB color space as the objective device-independent system color space for tongue image rendering. Section 9.3 provides the optimized tongue correction method by comparing and optimizing some color correction algorithms. In Sect. 9.4, we used the proposed method in a real situation by correcting tongue images acquired under different imaging condition and analyzed its performance. Section 9.5 provides our conclusion and discussion.

9.2 Color Space for Tongue Analysis

In this section, we describe the selection of the target device-independent color space, which plays a central role in color correction of computer-aided tongue analysis. We begin by explaining the concept of a color space (Kang, 1997; Green & MacDonald, 2011) and then present the particular requirements for color space selection in tongue image analysis. We then justify our choice of selecting the sRGB color space as the target device-independent color space and compare it with other device-independent CIE color spaces.

A color space is a mathematical model (for example, RGB and CMYK are color models) for describing the way colors can be represented as tuples, typically as three or four values of color components. A device-independent color space is one where a set of parameters will produce the same color, whatever color input or output device is used. Table 9.1 shows a variety of color spaces, which have been developed for a variety of special applications, which can be classified as either CIE- or RGB-like color spaces.

Not all color spaces are equally useful for different color correction tasks. Therefore, there are a number of requirements that must be satisfied when selecting a device-independent color space for tongue image analysis. First, according to TCM diagnostic practice, the standard illumination for tongue inspection is sunshine in an open area at 9 A.M. Therefore, we need to render the tongue image in such a color space, which has the same illumination as daylight sunshine. Currently, the standard D65 (color temperature is 6500 K) illuminant is recommended by the CIE (International Commission on Illumination) to simulate daylight sunshine.

Table 9.1 Common color spaces are either device-dependent or device independent

Group name	Color space name
Device-independent	sRGB, Adobe RGB, Apple RGB, CIE XYZ, CIE Lab, CIE LUV, etc.
Device-dependent	RGB, HSV, HSL, YIQ, YUV, YCbCr, CMYK, etc.

Thus, the color space that has a white point of 6500 K color temperature or D65 should be chose to render the tongue image. Second, the selected device-independent color space should be an RGB-like color space in order to directly display images on monitors. Third, the color space should have a constant relationship with CIE $L^*a^*b^*$ so that it is possible to calculate color differences. Finally, the color space should be commonly used, making it easy for images to be stored and exchanged.

The sRGB color space very well satisfies these criteria (Stokes, Anderson, Chandrasekar, & Motta, 2012). It is a well-defined color space and has been endorsed by many companies. It has many advantages and the most useful one in tongue image analysis is that the sRGB color space is based on phosphors, which are used in many modern CRT-based display devices. Therefore, images rendered in the sRGB color space can be exchanged among various imaging systems and directly shown on a monitor without any other further transformation while all users need to do is to change the working mode of the monitor to "sRGB." Although the rather limited gamut is a drawback of sRGB, this is not a significant limitation since vivid and saturated colors are not abundant in tongue images. Thus, we chose sRGB as the device-independent color space in our tongue image analysis.

The sRGB color space plays a central role in tongue image analysis. We first capture tongue images in various source RGB color spaces, i.e., the device-dependent color spaces. Then, the color correction algorithm is applied to these images and they are finally rendered in a target color space, i.e., the device-independent sRGB color space.

In order to compute the color difference, it is necessary to connect the sRGB color space to the CIE standard color space (Ohta & Robertson, 2006). The transformation of the sRGB color space to the CIE XYZ color space is defined as

$$\begin{pmatrix} X \\ Y \\ Z \end{pmatrix} = \Phi_{\text{sRGB}\rightarrow}\text{XYZ}\begin{pmatrix} R \\ G \\ B \end{pmatrix} = \begin{pmatrix} 0.4125 & 0.3576 & 0.1804 \\ 0.2127 & 0.7152 & 0.0722 \\ 0.0193 & 0.1192 & 0.9503 \end{pmatrix}\begin{pmatrix} R \\ G \\ B \end{pmatrix} \tag{9.1}$$

The color difference between two images is defined on the CIE $L^*a^*b^*$ color space. This color space is defined in the following, and the X_0, Y_0, Z_0 are the CIEXYZ values of the reference white point

$$\begin{cases} L^* = 116f\left(\frac{Y}{Y_0}\right) - 16 \\ a^* = 500\left[f\left(\frac{X}{X_0}\right) - f\left(\frac{Y}{Y_0}\right)\right] \\ b^* = 200\left[f\left(\frac{Y}{Y_0}\right) - f\left(\frac{Z}{Z_0}\right)\right] \end{cases} \quad f(x) = \begin{cases} x^{1/2} & (x > 0.00886) \\ 7.787x + \frac{16}{116} & (x \leq 0.00886) \end{cases} \tag{9.2}$$

Finally, the Euclidean distance between two colors (L_1^*, a_1^*, b_1^*) and (L_2^*, a_2^*, b_2^*), denoted as ΔE_{ab}^*, which is more or less proportional to their color difference as perceived by a human observer, is defined as the color chromatic aberration between images (Ohta & Robertson, 2006). The formula is

$$\Delta E = \sqrt{\left(L_1^* - L_2^*\right)^2 + \left(a_1^* - a_2^*\right)^2 + \left(b_1^* - b_2^*\right)^2}. \tag{9.3}$$

9.3 Color Correction Algorithms

In this section, we compare and optimize some common color correction algorithms: polynomial transforms, ridge regression, a SVR-based algorithm (Smola & Schölkopf, 2004; Cristianini & Shawe-Taylor, 2000; Muller, Mika, Ratsch, Tsuda, & Scholkopf, 2001), and artificial neural networks (ANNs) (Specht, 1991; Haykin & Network, 2004; Bishop, 2006). We begin in Sect. 9.3.1 by providing definitions of the three algorithms and then in the following sections compare their performance when applied to tongue images and choose the best parameters for tongue image analysis.

In this study, we chose the color reference target-based method to correct the tongue image (Green & MacDonald, 2011). Figure 9.1 shows the schematic diagram of the correction procedure. A reference target (Munsell Colorchecker (X-Rite, 2007) in our experiment) that contains a certain number of color patches was chosen to train the parameters provided by the color company. After both of the values of the colorchecker were extracted, they were inputted into different regression algorithms to train the correction parameters. Finally, we applied this color correction algorithm to the tongue images to obtain the corrected tongue images.

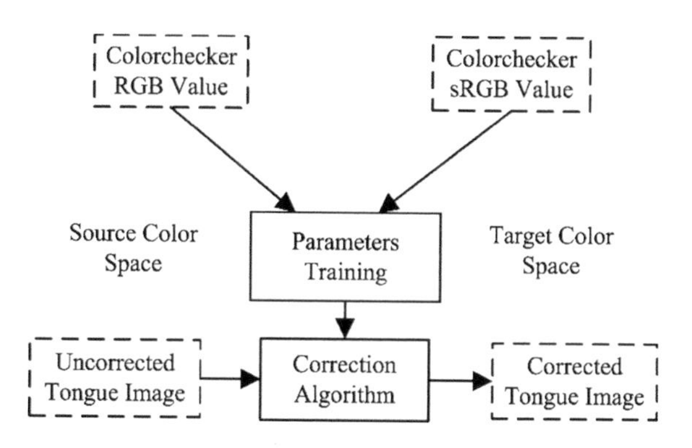

Fig. 9.1 Procedure of the color correction algorithm. © 2016 IEEE. Reprinted, with permission, from Wang and Zhang (2010)

9.3.1 Definitions of Algorithms

The first algorithm to be compared and optimized in this chapter is the polynomial transform, which is widely used in color correction and the characterization of color devices. The principle of the polynomial transform is as follows: suppose that the reference colorchecker has N color patches. For each patch, the corresponding quantized color values generated by a digital camera can be represented as a vector V:(R_i, G_i, B_i) (i = 1, 2, ..., 24) and the corresponding device-independent sRGB tristimulus values are S:(SR$_i$, SG$_i$, SB$_i$) (i = 1, 2, ..., 24). If only R, G, and B values are used for mapping from the RGB to the sRGB, the transformation is a simple linear transform. The idea of the polynomial transform is to add more terms (such as R^2, G^2, B^2) for the mapping matrix to increase the transformation accuracy, for example, if we use the combination of polynomial x: [R, G, B, 1], the transformation model can be represented as

$$\begin{cases} \mathrm{SR}_i = a_{11}R_i + a_{12}G_i + a_{13}B_i \\ \mathrm{SG}_i = a_{21}R_i + a_{22}G_i + a_{23}B_i \; (i = 1,\, 2,\, \ldots,\, 24) \\ \mathrm{SB}_i = a_{31}R_i + a_{32}G_i + a_{33}B_i \end{cases} \tag{9.4}$$

This equation can also be rewritten in matrix format as

$$S = A^T \cdot X, \tag{9.5}$$

where A is the mapping coefficient matrix and X is the matrix generated by different polynomial combinations x. Using the least-square regression method, the solution to (9.5) is as follows:

$$A = \left(X^T X\right)^{-1} X^T S \tag{9.6}$$

Thus, the mapping coefficient matrix A to correct the color tristimulus values from the device-dependent RGB color space to the sRGB color space can be derived. We can apply this transform to the tongue image. Suppose the polynomial image matrix X for the tongue image is X_{in}, then the output image matrix X_{out} is

$$X_{\mathrm{out}} = A^T \cdot X_{\mathrm{in}} \tag{9.7}$$

Different combinations of polynomial terms can be used for color correction, as in the following combinations, where there are three elements in the first row and 5, 9, and 11 elements in the second, third, and fourth rows, respectively,

$$\begin{cases} x : [R,\, G,\, B] \\ x : [R,\, G,\, B,\, \mathrm{RGB},\, 1] \\ x : [R,\, G,\, B,\, \mathrm{RG},\, \mathrm{RB},\, \mathrm{GB},\, R^2,\, G^2,\, B^2] \\ x : [R,\, G,\, B,\, \mathrm{RG},\, \mathrm{RB},\, \mathrm{GB},\, R^2,\, G^2,\, B^2,\, \mathrm{RGB},\, 1] \end{cases} \tag{9.8}$$

In our proposed color correction scheme, we tested these four combinations (9.8) and obtained an optimization one among these polynomial combinations.

Ridge regression (the second algorithm) is a linear regression technique whose goal is to circumvent the problem of predictor's collinearity (Hoerl & Kennard, 1970). In this experiment, we will test the linear combination of the ridge regression method and compare it with other correction algorithms. The parameter that needs to be optimized is the ridge parameter K.

The third algorithm compared here is SVR (Mangasarian & Musicant, 2000). Like the support-vector machine (SVM), SVR uses a nonlinear kernel to transform the training data into a high-dimensional feature space, where linear regression can be performed. Here, we chose the Gaussian radial basis function (RBF) kernel and polynomial kernel to optimize the parameters.

The fourth algorithm is ANN in which a large number of inputs are mapped onto a small number of outputs. This feature makes it suitable for regression problems. There are many different types of ANNs, but in this chapter, we mainly focus on the optimization of back propagation (BP) neural networks.

9.3.2 Evaluation of the Correction Algorithms

To evaluate the performance of the correction algorithm, we calculated the color difference among the color tristimulus values for each patch on the Munsell colorchecker before and after color correction, this color difference is calculated according to (9.3). Moreover, since some colors of color patches in the colorchecker are unlikely to appear in the tongue images, in order to achieve remarkable performance for tongue images correction, we divided the colorchecker patches into two groups: tongue-related (numbered from 1 to 13) and unrelated (other patches without number, see Fig. 9.2). Different evaluation weights are applied to them (tongue-related colors will have bigger weight than the irrelevant ones in the colorchecker).

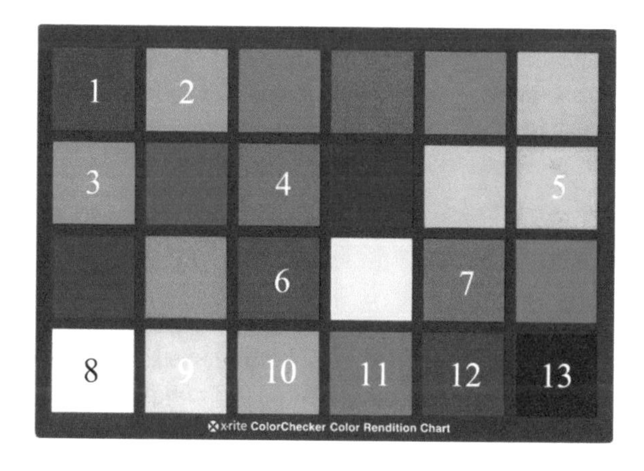

Fig. 9.2 Numbered color patches were given larger weights to evaluate the correction performance. © 2016 IEEE. Reprinted, with permission, from Wang and Zhang (2010)

There are 24 patches in the colorchecker. Supposing the patches that are most likely to be found in the tongue color space are represented as c_i (i = 1, 2, ..., M) and the other patches are represented as d_i (i = 1, 2, ..., N), we can calculate the color difference between the target value and the corrected value for each patch by (9.3). The total color difference for the whole colorchecker can be calculated as

$$F = \alpha \sum_{i=1}^{M} f_{c_i} + (1 - \alpha) \sum_{j=1}^{N} f_{d_i} \quad (M + N = 24) \tag{9.9}$$

The α is the weight value for the two groups. Generally, it will be greater than 0.5, and in our experiment, we set it to 0.7. This is done to achieve better correction performance on the tongue color space than other colors.

9.3.3 *Experiments and Results*

This section describes the optimization and comparison experiments among various correction algorithms. First, the imaging device and the dataset used in this experiment are introduced. Second, optimized parameters for each algorithm are separately analyzed. Finally, we provide the performance comparison among these algorithms.

9.3.3.1 Imaging Device

The imaging device in this research was a three-chip CCD camera with 8-bit resolution for each channel and 768 × 576 spatial resolutions. The illuminants were two standard D65 fluorescent tubes with a 6500 K color temperature and a color rendering index (CRI) larger than 90. In order to obtain uniform illumination, these two tubes were symmetrically placed around the CCD camera (above and under the camera). The illumination and viewing geometry was approximately 45/0° (Ohta & Robertson, 2006). In this viewing geometry, the sample was illuminated with one or more beams of light incident at an angle of about 45° and measurements were made along the normal. The whole imaging system was installed in a dark box that had only one small open window to capture the tongue image.

9.3.3.2 Dataset

In this experiment, we used the Munsell colorchecker 24 charts as the training sample because we can obtain the source RGB values and the corresponding target sRGB values. For the performance comparison, two kinds of test images were utilized, i.e., colorchecker images and real tongue images. We captured four sample colorchecker images at four different times after turning on the fluorescent light: 0, 3, 5 and 10 min. This produced four image groups, which we labeled as A0–A3. One of them was chosen as the training sample and the others were used for testing. For the tested tongue images, we captured two tongue images, the source tongue image and the target image under different imaging conditions to compare the performance.

9.3.3.3 Parameters Setting

Polynomial functions were used to map between a device-dependent RGB vector and a standard sRGB vector. Obviously, the order of the polynomial would strongly affect the training and testing performance. When the order was 1 and the number of polynomial elements was 3, i.e., [R, *G*, *B*], the transform was a linear transform. Increasing the polynomial number would reduce the number of training errors. However, over-fitting may occur when the number of polynomials exceeds some specified extent such as the total number of variables. This experiment tested the polynomial combinations, where there were 3, 5, 9, and 11 elements (later referred to as polynomial 3, 5, 9, and 11).

For ridge regression, we used the ridge function in the statistical toolbox of MATLAB to implement the color correction code. We obtained the optimized ridge parameter (K) by selecting the K value where the lowest regression error was reached. Figure 9.3 shows the relationship between the K value and the regression error. The best ridge parameter for ridge regression was $K = 0.432$.

For SVR, in this experiment, we utilized the library of SVM (libsvm) (Chang & Lin, 2011) to implement the SVR correction algorithm. There were three parameters in the RBF kernel, i.e., C, σ, and ε, C was the penalty factor for the regression, σ was the gamma of the RBF kernel that determined the RBF width, and E was the

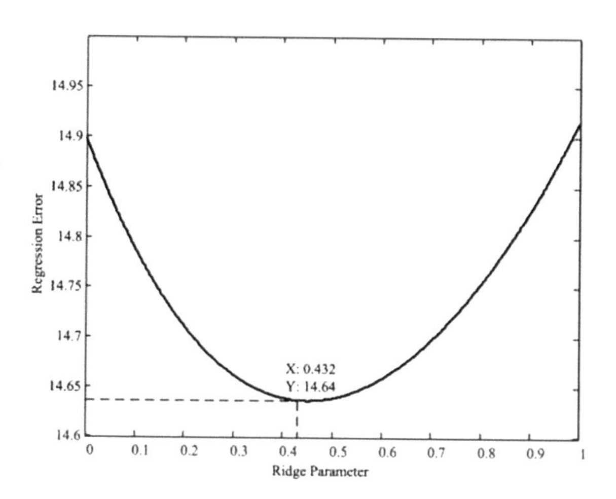

Fig. 9.3 Relationship between the ridge parameter and the regression error. © 2016 IEEE. Reprinted, with permission, from Wang and Zhang (2010)

factor of the lost function. Among these three parameters, a large value of σ made the regression similar to a linear regression. Furthermore, adjusting the values of ε can avoid over-fitting of the regression and control the amount of support vectors. In our experiment, to achieve the lowest regression error, C was set to infinity, and the other two were set to 5 and 0.025, respectively. There were two parameters in the polynomial kernel, i.e., C for the penalty factor and d for the order of the polynomial kernel. In our experiment, these two parameters were finally set at $C = 10$ and $d = 3$.

For neural network mapping, we used fully connected multilayer perceptron networks to derive a mapping between the device-dependent RGB values and the standard sRGB values. The networks contained three input units to receive the camera responses and three output units to output the corrected values. We used one hidden layer while the number of units N in the hidden layer was 10. The activation functions of the units in the hidden and output layers were the sigmoid function and linear function. The weight and offset parameters were randomly set.

9.3.3.4 Experimental Results on the Colorchecker

Table 9.2 shows the performance of the optimized correction algorithms. These experimental results were achieved on a notebook that has a hardware specification: Intel Core 2 CPU T5500, 2-GB memory, and Windows XP professional system. This table contains two kinds of information. One is the correction accuracy and the other is the time complexity of these algorithms. For the correction accuracy, the small number of the training error means a better regression performance. Moreover, the testing errors reflect the robustness of these algorithms. From the Table 9.2, regarding the accuracy, the SVR-based algorithm with the Gaussian RBF kernel was the most accurate one, with a training error of 0 and a test error of 0.68–3.03. The polynomial kernel in SVR performed much worse than the Gaussian RBF, with a test error of around 7.91. The polynomial-based methods had a training error of 4.26,

Table 9.2 Performance comparison between color correction algorithms

Algorithms	Training error	Testing error				Training time (s)	Testing time (s)
		A0	A1	A2	A3		
Polynomial	4.26	4.52	5.11	5.23	5.87	0.0006	0.00020
SVR(RBF)	0.00	0.68	1.74	2.03	3.03	0.0100	0.00090
SVR (Polynomial)	7.23	7.42	7.89	7.91	8.19	0.1153	0.00080
ANN (sigmoid)	9.70	9.92	10.27	10.88	10.90	3.3000	0.02770
ANN(linear)	7.65	7.55	7.81	7.82	8.98	2.8511	0.02570
Ridge regression	14.66	14.79	15.24	15.30	15.58	0.1107	0.00001

which was not the lowest among all these tested algorithms, but it was more robust to fluctuations in the environmental illuminant because the test error changed from 4.52 to 5.87 (test error in A0 and A3). This robust feature is very important in real cases, where the environment imaging conditions change a lot. For the time complexity, the polynomial-based method was much faster than the other algorithms, running at less than 0.001 s both in the training and testing stage. Both the linear function and sigmoid function in the ANN performed worse than polynomials. They need the longest training time among all the tested algorithms. The ridge regression performed worst having more training and testing errors than the others. This may be due to usage of the linear combination of the training sample. Moreover, the ridge regression may be inappropriate to be applied in the color correction task, because in the color correction task, there are not strong correlations among the training sample values.

There appears to be a tradeoff between these algorithms. SVR is the most accurate. Polynomial-based algorithms are the fastest but not as accurate as SVR, though still acceptable. Both algorithms produce a color difference less than 5 (4.26 for SVR and 0 for polynomials). In a real computer-aided tongue-analysis application, we might adopt a strategy of using an optimized polynomial-based algorithm for online color correction and an SVR-based algorithm for offline color correction.

9.3.3.5 Experimental Results on Tongue Images

These source and target tongue images were captured under two different sets of imaging conditions: normal imaging conditions, which used a common camera and illuminant, and standard imaging condition, which used the standard CIE lighting conditions and an industrial camera. Tongue images captured under the standard imaging condition can be regarded as the reference target image. To correct the tongue images captured under the source imaging conditions, we used the trained color correction algorithm. It was expected that after correction, the source images should be a close match for those captured under the target image condition. Figure 9.4a shows the tongue images captured under the target imaging condition (target tongue images), and Fig. 9.4b–d shows the tongue images corrected using polynomial 3, polynomial 11, and SVR-based algorithms, respectively. It can be seen that the polynomial 3 algorithm produces a better color match for the target tongue image than the other non-optimized algorithms (polynomial 11 and the SVR-based algorithms). Figures 9.5 and 9.6 show the CIEXYZ distribution of images in a chromatic diagram, which are transformed from images in Fig. 9.4. From Fig. 9.5a, it should be noticed that the distribution of the image corrected by polynomial 3 and the target image almost overlap each other (more than 95%), while there is large difference between the image corrected by polynomial 11 and the target image. Figure 9.5b, c shows the comparison of these two algorithm in *x*- and *y*-coordinates, respectively. From Fig. 9.5b, it can be found that the line of the x-corrected and x-target almost follow the same orientation of the perfect line of

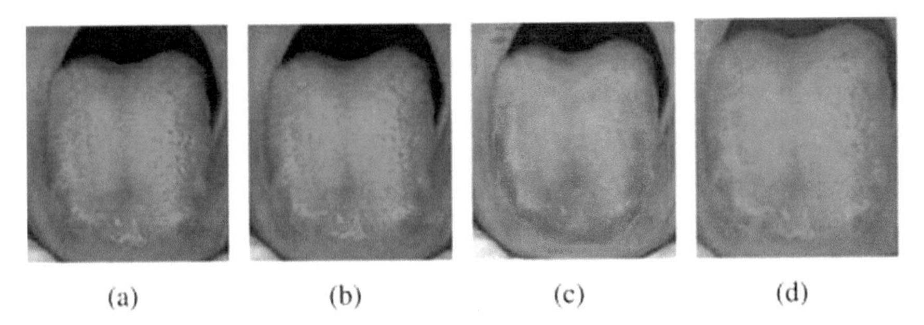

Fig. 9.4 Comparison of image perception among images corrected by different algorithms. **a** Target image. **b** Corrected image by polynomial 3. **c** Corrected image by polynomial 11. **d** Corrected image by the SVR-based algorithm. ©2016 IEEE. Reprinted, with permission, from Wang and Zhang (2010)

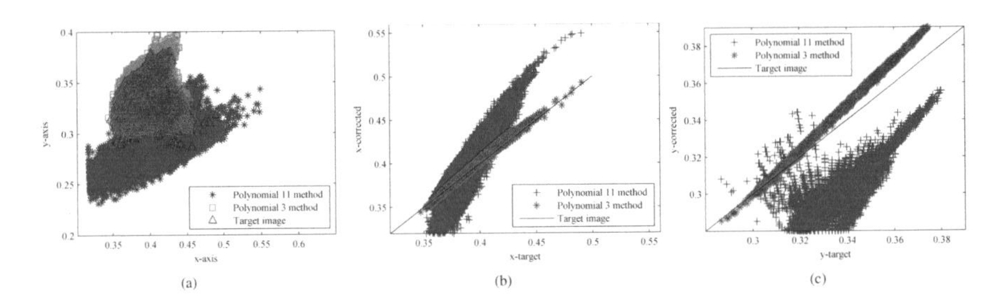

Fig. 9.5 Chromatic distribution of images corrected by using different algorithms. **a** Images corrected by polynomial 11 and polynomial 3 algorithms. **b** Image distribution in x-coordinates. **c** Image distribution in y-coordinates

x-corrected = x-target in polynomial 3, while there is large difference in polynomial 11. In Fig. 9.5c, both lines, polynomial 3 and polynomial 11, have a distance to the perfect line, but obviously, polynomial 3 is much closer than polynomial 11. Figure 9.6a shows the comparison between the image corrected by polynomial 3 and SVR-based algorithms. We can also determine that the image corrected by the algorithm based on polynomial 3 is much closer (more than 96% overlap) to the target image than the image corrected by the SVR-based algorithm. Figure 9.6b, c also shows that polynomial 3 outperforms the SVR method. On the basis of these experimental results, we selected the polynomial-3-based algorithm as our tongue image correction algorithm and optimized it for our purposes. The correction matrix derived from polynomial 3 in our experiments is given as

$$\begin{pmatrix} 1.3007 & -0.3918 & -0.1125 \\ 0.0268 & 0.8507 & -0.0155 \\ 0.0759 & -0.1889 & 0.9897 \end{pmatrix} \tag{9.10}$$

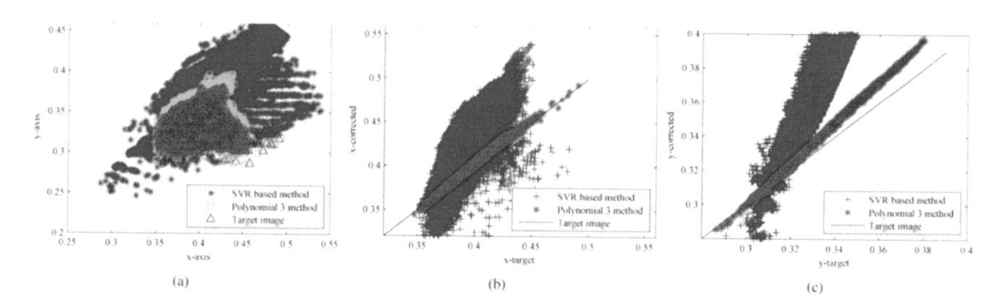

Fig. 9.6 Distribution of images corrected using different algorithms. **a** Comparison of images corrected using SVR and polynomial 3 algorithms. **b** Comparison in *x*-coordinates. **c** Comparison in *y*-coordinates. from Wang and Zhang (2010)

9.3.3.6 Discussion

There are some interesting findings in Figs. 9.5 and 9.6: the algorithm can achieve a better regression in the *x*-coordinate than in the *y*-coordinate. A possible explanation may be as follows: in the CIE chromatic diagram, starting from the central white point, if we increase the x-coordinate while keeping the *y*-coordinate constant, the color perception will become more reddish. If we increase or decrease the *y*-coordinate and keep the *x*-coordinate constant at the same time, the color perception will become more bluish or purplish. Thus, we may consider that the *x*-axis is more sensitive to the red variation, while the *y*-axis is more sensitive to the variation of blue and purple. In this research, the main task is to correct the tongue images in the computer-aided tongue image analysis system. Since the majority of tongue colors are red-related colors, and the red color information is crucial to the analysis of tongue image, our proposed color correction algorithms focused on the correction of such a small red color space in the whole space. Therefore, the correction algorithm will better correct the red colors than the non-red colors, i.e., mapping the *x*-coordinate is better than mapping the y-coordinate. Moreover, the regression error increases with a rise of y-coordinates. Thus, we may conclude from this discussion that the selection of reference target patches is crucial to the performance of the correction algorithm. This will be useful for some specific applications such as when you want to correct human tooth color, you may need to select the color patches, which have a close color perception with human tooth color.

9.4 Experimental Results and Performance Analysis

Having concluded that the polynomial-based algorithms were the most suitable ones for automated tongue image analysis and the polynomial-3-based algorithm was optimized as our proposed color correction algorithm, in this section, we will apply it to correct various tongue images, which were captured under different imaging conditions to analyze the performance and verify the validity. Since the objective of this research is to develop a color correction scheme, which can solve the problem in the computer-aided tongue image analysis, i.e., the color distortion between images captured by various imaging device, or under different lighting condition, we will first discuss the performance of the color correction algorithm on tongue images, which were captured by different types of cameras, i.e., Cannon S2, Cannon S45, and Panasonic DXC-FX01 in our experiments. Second, correction experiments on images captured under different lighting conditions, i.e., incandescent tube, shadow, and sunshine will be presented. Finally, further discussion on these two experiments will be provided.

Evaluation criteria: Regarding the problem of how to evaluate the performance of color correction on tongue images, we can directly see and assess the color perception from the tongue images. Therefore, we will show these images before and after correction to provide the comparison between them. However, since the subjective evaluation of assessing the color perception by human visualization is hard to quantify, we need to define another quantized assessment method, which can evaluate the color difference among tongue images. Currently, there is no formula to directly measure the color difference between two color images, while there is only a formula to calculate the color difference between two specific color tristimulus values (9.3). Thus, we will calculate the average color to represent each color image, and then measure the color difference between two images by computing the color difference between the two average colors. We will first transform the images from the sRGB to the CIE xyY color space to obtain the (x, y) coordinates for each pixel, and then, for each image, the mean coordinate (mean_x, mean_y) of all the pixels will be calculated and regarded as the color center of the image. After we obtain the mean value that can be utilized to represent each image, we can compute the color difference between two images by calculating the Euclidian distance of their color centers.

9.4.1 Color Correction by Different Cameras

In this experiment, we first captured the same tongue body by utilizing different cameras: Cannon S2, Cannon S45, and Panasonic DXC-FX01 under the same lighting conditions, and then corrected these images by applying the proposed color correction algorithm. Finally, we separately compared the color perceptions between the images before and after the color correction.

Figure 9.7a shows three images captured by different cameras of the same tongue body. It can be perceived that there are noticeable color differences among these images. In contrast to this, as Fig. 9.7b shows the color difference among the three images becomes smaller and the perception for these three images changes to be much closer to each other.

Figure 9.8 illustrates the distribution of the color centers for the two groups of six images before and after color correction. After correction, the distances among the tongue images become much smaller, falling from 0.1504 to 0.0081. This

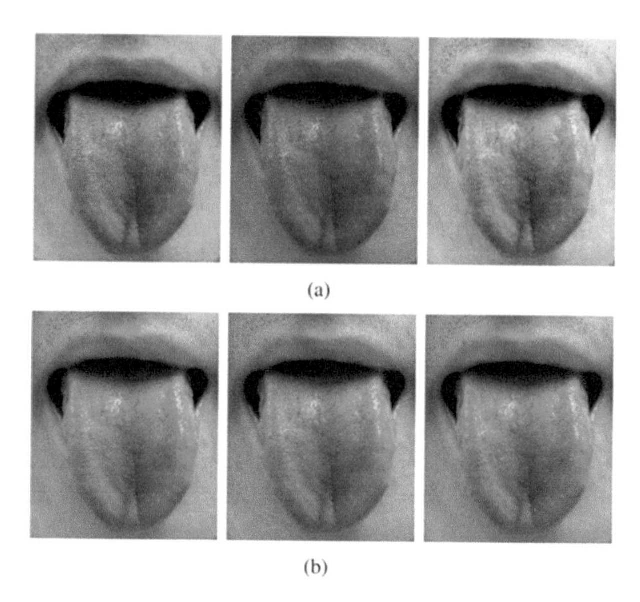

Fig. 9.7 Tongue images captured using different cameras, before and after correction. **a** The same tongue body image captured using different cameras, the color difference is obvious. **b** Images after color correction. © 2016 IEEE. Reprinted, with permission, from Wang and Zhang (2010)

illustrated that the color perception of these tongue images become similar to each other after correction. Another interesting finding generated from the figures is that these images tend to be clustered to a center. This may be explained by the assumption that the proposed color correction algorithm attempts to convert the distorted tongue images into the "ideal" tongue images, which have the same color perceptions. In this experiment, the green star in Fig. 9.8 represents such an ideal tongue image and the coordinate is (0.3923, 0.3157).

9.4.2 *Color Correction Under Different Lighting Conditions*

This experiment shows the color correction performance on the images captured by the same camera under different lighting conditions. Figure 9.9 shows six images before and after color correction. From the upper row of the original images captured under different lighting conditions, it can be seen that there are great color differences among these three images. After color correction, the images look much more similar to each other, as shown in Fig. 9.9b.

We also computed the distance of tongue images captured under different lighting conditions before and after color correction to show the improvement. Compared with tongue images captured by different cameras, the color variation between the images acquired under different lighting conditions is much bigger.

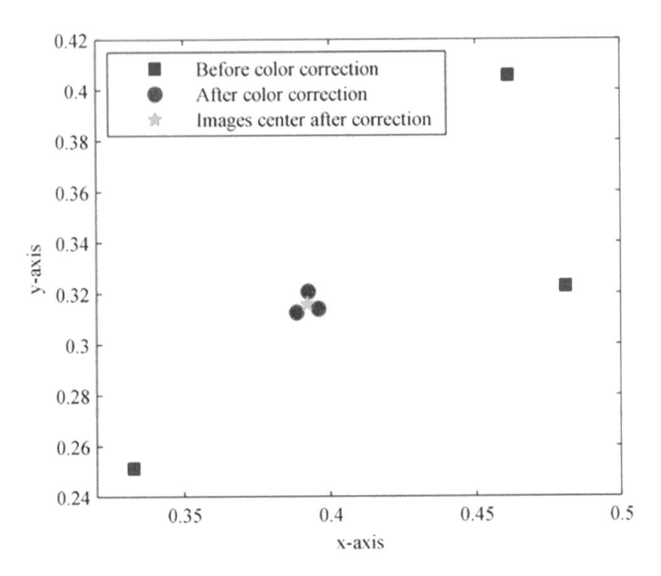

Fig. 9.8 Distribution of the color centers of the tongue images captured using different cameras before and after color correction. © 2016 IEEE. Reprinted, with permission, from Wang and Zhang (2010)

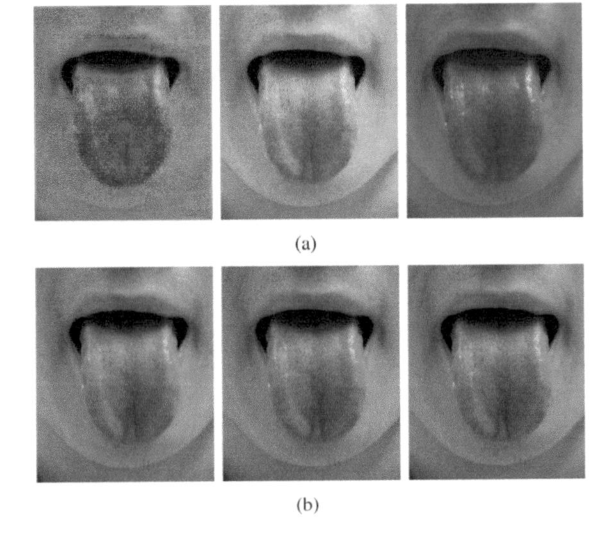

Fig. 9.9 Tongue images captured under different lighting condition, before and after correction. **a** The same tongue body captured by the same camera under different lighting conditions. **b** Images after color correction

The distance among tongue images before color correction was 0.2913, while it changed to 0.0085 after correction.

The distribution of the original and corrected images is shown in Fig. 9.10. After color correction, images became much closer to each other. Moreover, the three images tended to be clustered into a central common image, and the coordinate was (0.3939, 0.3166).

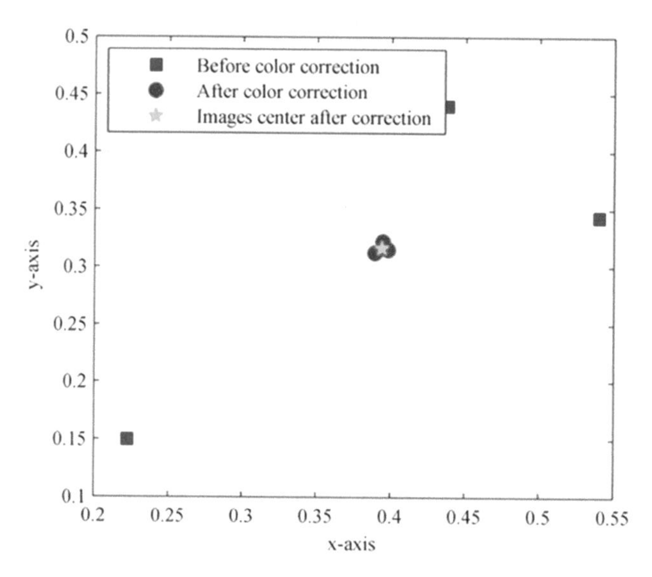

Fig. 9.10 Distribution of the color center of the tongue images captured using the same camera under different lighting conditions before and after color correction

9.4.3 *Performance Analysis*

Our experiments have shown that the proposed color correction algorithm can convert color-distorted tongue images acquired by various imaging conditions into tongue images, which appear more similar in color and which share a similar distribution on a chromatic diagram. In order to compare the performance of these two experiments, we have the following further discussions.

First, the experimental results show that whatever the great color difference between the original tongue images is, the proposed color correction algorithm can transform tongue images into similar color perception images (measured by the color distance in this research). In our experiment, the pre-correction distances between tongue images were 0.1504 and 0.2913, which fell to 0.0081 and 0.0085 after correction. Such a small color distance between images cannot even be perceived by the human eye.

Second, it can be seen that all the corrected tongue images tend to be clustered around a central point in the chromatic diagram. Table 9.3 shows the coordinates of the image centers for the two groups of corrected images. From the table, it can be found that the average distances between three tongue images and the corresponding central point dramatically dropped, i.e., from 0.0967 and 0.1734 to 0.0047 and 0.0057, respectively. Moreover, after color correction, the color difference between the corrected images was less than 0.006 in each group, which is far from that perceived by the human eye. Interestingly, even when the central points in

Table 9.3 Coordinates of image centers for two groups of images, and the average distances between tongue images and their centers, before and after correction

	Tongue images by different cameras	Tongue images under different lighting conditions
Central point coordinates	(0.3923 0.3157)	(0.3939 0.3166)
Average distance (before correction)	0.0967	0.1734
Average distance (after correction)	0.0047	0.0057
Improved ratio (average distance) (%)	95.14	96.71

these two groups of images were not the same, the distance between them was very small, less than 0.18. We may deduce that there is an ideal standard tongue image, and the tongue image after correction by the proposed algorithms can approach such an ideal image with an extremely small color difference.

9.4.4 Correction on Real Tongue Images

In order to further verify the validation of our proposed color correction on a large number of real tongue images, we provide the correction experiments in this section. Since this study is part of a research project focused on research of computerized human tongue image analysis system, we have developed a human tongue acquisition device and captured some real tongue image samples in hospital (typical samples as shown in Fig. 9.11). In this section, we will select parts of these image samples to verify the validity.

Unlike the experimental samples provided in Sect. 9.4.1, in real cases, all these real images were captured by the same imaging device, i.e., the same illuminant and same digital camera. In order to verify the validity of the correction algorithms in real tongue images, since we do not have the ground truth for each human tongue image (what does the human tongue image really looks like), we chose two samples captured from the same tongue body. Therefore, we can compare the distance between the images before and after color correction. In this experiment, these samples were captured at different times, and there may have been variations in the illumination and the response of the digital cameras between these images. Fifteen pairs of tongue images (it was not so easy to capture the image from the same patient twice) were selected to conduct the tongue image correction. In addition, the same model, the same derived parameters, proposed in this manuscript, were applied to the correction of real images.

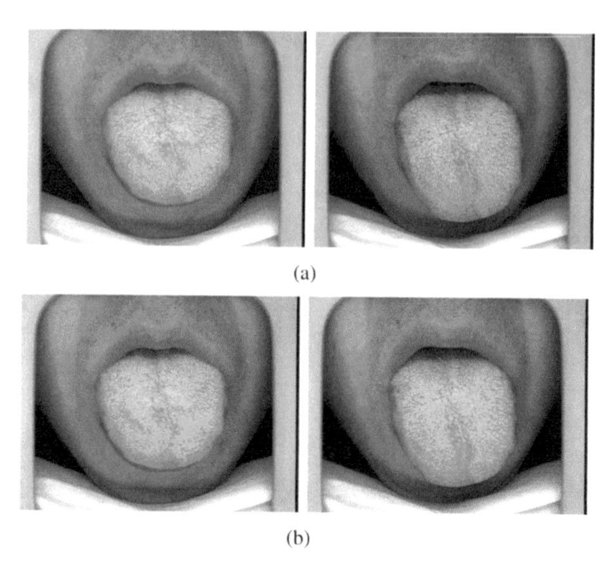

Fig. 9.11 Real tongue images corrected by the derived scheme. **a** Real tongue images before color correction. **b** Real tongue images after color correction. © 2016 IEEE. Reprinted, with permission, from Wang and Zhang (2010)

Figure 9.11 shows the color correction on a pair of tongue images. From Fig. 9.11a, it can be found that these two images have small-intensity variations (but maybe not so obvious). In Fig. 9.11b, after correction, it can be perceived that there two images become much more consistent with each other. Since it may not be easy to evaluate the performance by visualization, we have also calculated the image distance between these image pairs. Figure 9.12 shows the distance comparison between images before and after color correction. Before color correction, the color distances between images pairs ranged from 0.0096 to 0.0191, while after correction, the distances ranged from 0.0015 to 0.0045. The average distance of all the images ranged from 0.0138 to 0.0026. Although the color variations in the non-corrected images were small, our proposed scheme can still reduce the color difference between them and make them more consistent with each other.

Also, since the color correction on tongue images is crucial to the performance of tongue image analysis and diagnosis, we asked some TCM doctors to help us to evaluate the performance of the proposed color correction method. The preliminary statistical data show that after color correction, the method can achieve a better perception for the TCM doctors. Currently, this proposed algorithm has also been integrated into our tongue image acquisition system to capture the image data in real time.

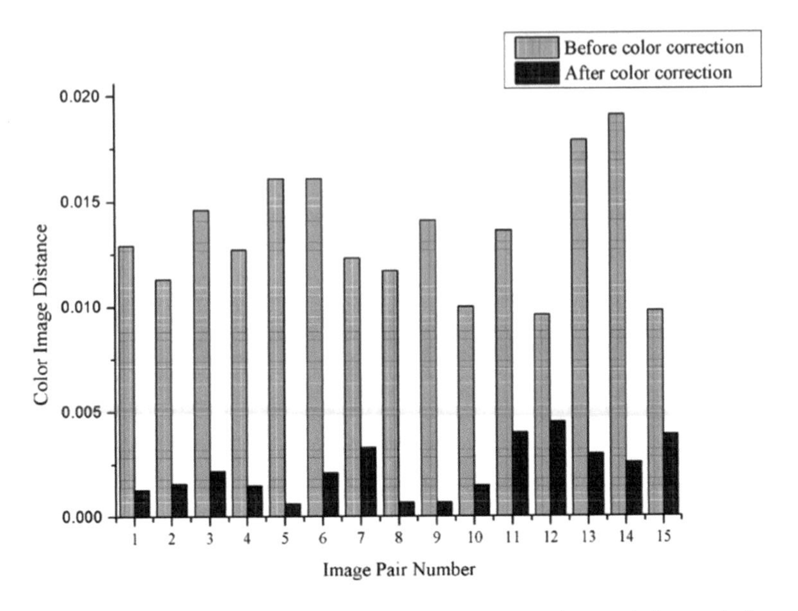

Fig. 9.12 Color image distance between 15 pair of real tongue images before and after color correction. © 2016 IEEE. Reprinted, with permission, from Wang and Zhang (2010)

9.5 Summary

This chapter presents an optimized color correction scheme for computer-aided tongue image analysis. The proposed scheme first analyzes the particular color correction requirement for selection of a device-independent target color space in tongue image analysis, and then optimizes the color correction algorithms accordingly. The proposed scheme is very effective, reducing the color difference between images captured using different cameras or under different lighting conditions to less than 0.0085, and the distances between the color centers of tongue images by more than 95% while images tend to cluster toward an "ideal" or "standard" tongue image. In addition, we have demonstrated the validity of the proposed method on real tongue images. In future research, we intend to collect a much larger, real tongue image database including a number of images of typical healthy and pathological tongues to verify the validity of our proposed scheme. In particular, we will seek to further address the ground-truth problem by using physical measurements or feedback from TCM doctors. Utilizing a colorchecker other than the Munsell colorchecker 24 as the reference target for color correction will also be studied in future research.

References

Barnard, K., & Funt, B. (2002). Camera characterization for color research. *Color Research & Application, 27*(3), 152–163.

Bishop, C. M. (2006). Pattern recognition. *Machine Learning*.

Chang, Y., & Reid, J. F. (1996). RGB calibration for color image analysis in machine vision. *IEEE Transactions on Image Processing, 5*(10), 1414–1422.

Chang, C. C., & Lin, C. J. (2011). LIBSVM: A library for support vector machines. *ACM Transactions on Intelligent Systems and Technology (TIST), 2*(3), 27.

Cheung, V., Westland, S., Connah, D., & Ripamonti, C. (2004). A comparative study of the characterisation of colour cameras by means of neural networks and polynomial transforms. *Coloration Technology, 120*(1), 19–25.

Cristianini, N., & Shawe-Taylor, J. (2000). *An introduction to support vector machines and other kernel-based learning methods*. Cambridge: Cambridge university press.

Finlayson, G. D. (1996). Color in perspective. *IEEE Transactions on Pattern Analysis and Machine Intelligence, 18*(10), 1034–1038.

Green, P., & MacDonald, L. (Eds.). (2011). *Colour engineering: Achieving device independent colour* (Vol. 30). New York: Wiley.

Haeghen, Y. V., Naeyaert, J. M. A. D., Lemahieu, I., & Philips, W. (2000). An imaging system with calibrated color image acquisition for use in dermatology. *IEEE Transactions on Medical Imaging, 19*(7), 722–730.

Haykin, S., & Network, N. (2004). A comprehensive foundation. *Neural Networks, 2*(2004).

Hoerl, A. E., & Kennard, R. W. (1970). Ridge regression: Biased estimation for nonorthogonal problems. *Technometrics, 12*(1), 55–67.

Kang, H. R. (1997). *Color technology for electronic imaging devices*. Bellingham, Washington: SPIE press.

Luo, M. R., Hong, G., & Rhodes, P. A. (2001). A study of digital camera colorimetric characterization based on polynomial modeling. *Color: Research and Applications, 26*(1), 76–84.

Muller, K. R., Mika, S., Ratsch, G., Tsuda, K., & Scholkopf, B. (2001). An introduction to kernel-based learning algorithms. *IEEE Transactions on Neural Networks, 12*(2), 181–201.

Mangasarian, O. L., & Musicant, D. R. (2000). Robust linear and support vector regression. *IEEE Transactions on Pattern Analysis and Machine Intelligence, 22*(9), 950–955.

Ohta, N., & Robertson, A. (2006). *Colorimetry: Fundamentals and applications*. New York: Wiley.

Pang, B., Zhang, D., & Wang, K. (2005). Tongue image analysis for appendicitis diagnosis. *Information Sciences, 175*(3), 160–176.

Smola, A. J., & Schölkopf, B. (2004). A tutorial on support vector regression. *Statistics and Computing, 14*(3), 199–222.

Specht, D. F. (1991). A general regression neural network. *IEEE Transactions on Neural Networks, 2*(6), 568–576.

Stokes, M., Anderson, M., Chandrasekar, S., & Motta, R. (2012). A standard default color space for the internet—sRGB, 1996. http://www.w3.org/Graphics/Color/sRGB

Vrhel, M., Saber, E., & Trussell, H. J. (2005). Color image generation and display technologies. *IEEE Signal Processing Magazine*, *22*(1).

Vrhel, M. J., & Trussell, H. J. (1999). Color device calibration: a mathematical formulation. *IEEE Transactions on Image Processing, 8*(12), 1796–1806.

Wandell, B. A. (1987). The synthesis and analysis of color images. *IEEE Transactions on Pattern Analysis and Machine Intelligence* (1), 2–13.

Wang, X., & Zhang, D. (2010). An optimized tongue image color correction scheme. *IEEE Transactions on Information Technology in Biomedicine A Publication of the IEEE Engineering in Medicine & Biology Society, 14*(6), 1355–1364.

X-Rite. (2007). Munsell Products: Colorchecker Targets. [Online]. Available: http://www.xrite.com/

Yamamoto, K., & James, U. (2006). Color Calibration for Multicamera System without Color Pattern Board. *Monash University DECSE Technical Report MECSE-4–2006.*

Yamamoto, K., Kitahara, M., Kimata, H., Yendo, T., Fujii, T., Tanimoto, M., et al. (2007). Multiview video coding using view interpolation and color correction. *IEEE Transactions on Circuits and Systems for Video Technology, 17*(11), 1436–1449.

Zhang, D., Pang, B., Li, N., Wang, K., & Zhang, H. (2005a). Computerized diagnosis from tongue appearance using quantitative feature classification. *The American Journal of Chinese Medicine, 33*(06), 859–866.

Zhang, H., Wang, K., Jin, X., & Zhang, D. (2005). SVR based color calibration for tongue image. In *2005 International Conference on Machine Learning and Cybernetics* (Vol. 8, pp. 5065–5070). New York: IEEE.

Chapter 10
Tongue Colorchecker for Precise Correction

Abstract In order to improve the correction accuracy of tongue colors by use of the Munsell colorchecker, this research aims to design a new colorchecker by aid of the tongue color space. Three essential issues leading to the development of this space-based colorchecker are investigated in this chapter. First, based on a large and comprehensive tongue database, the tongue color space is established by which all visible colors can be classified as tongue or non-tongue colors. Hence, colors of the designed tongue colorchecker are selected from tongue colors to achieve high correction performance. Second, the minimum sufficient number of colors involved in the colorchecker is attained by comparing the correction accuracy when a different number (range from 10 to 200) of colors are contained. Thereby, 24 colors are included because the obtained minimum number of colors is 20. Lastly, criteria for optimal color selection and their corresponding objective function are presented. Two color selection methods, i.e., greedy and clustering-based selection methods, are proposed to solve the objective function. Experimental results show that the clustering-based method outperforms its counterpart to generate the new tongue colorchecker. Compared to the Munsell colorchecker, this proposed space-based colorchecker can improve the correction accuracy by 48%. Further experimental results on more correction tasks also validate its effectiveness and superiority.

10.1 Introduction

As can be seen from Chap. 9, tongue images produced by digital cameras usually suffer from device-dependent color space rendering, i.e., generated color information is dependent on the imaging characteristics of specific cameras. Furthermore, there are usually noises over images due to slight variations of the illumination. Therefore, in order to correct variations caused by imaging system components and to render color images into a device-independent color space, tongue color correction is of great importance for accurate image acquisition and is ordinarily regarded as a prerequisite before further image analysis (Bala, Sharma, Monga, De Capelle, & Others, 2005; Cai, 2002; Chang & Reid, 1996; Jiang, Xu, & Chen, 2008; Vrhel &

D. Zhang et al., *Tongue Image Analysis*, DOI 10.1007/978-981-10-2167-1_10

Trussell, 1999; Wang & Zhang, 2010a, b). The color correction process normally involves deriving a transformation between the device-dependent camera RGB values and device-independent chromatic attributes by the aid of several training colors, which are often printed and arranged in a checkerboard chart, named a colorchecker (Ilie & Welch, 2005; Kang, 1997; Luo, Hong, & Rhodes, 2001; Sharma & Bala, 2002). This colorchecker, which is utilized as the reference target for training of a correction model, plays a crucial role for precise tongue color correction.

In tongue color correction, the Munsell colorchecker (McCamy, Marcus & Davidson, 1976; X-Rite, 2010), which was designed in 1976 and regarded as the de facto standard for visual evaluation of the color reproduction process in photography, television, and printing, is most commonly used. The salient advantage of this colorchecker is its representativeness and simple usage. It contains 24 scientifically selected colors, which include additive primaries and colors of typical natural objects (such as human skin, foliage, and blue sky). It thereby was utilized to correct all visible colors. Moreover, it is usually produced as a fairly small size chart which can facilitate the imaging and following correction process. However, as the Munsell colorchecker was designed to process natural color but not especially for tongue colors, most of its colors are unlikely to appear in tongue images (e.g., green and yellowish green). More theoretically, the color space (i.e., the range of colors) spanned by colors of the Munsell colorchecker is much larger than the limited color space of human tongue colors. Therefore, it is too general and less accurate to apply the Munsell colorchecker for tongue color correction. In order to improve the correction accuracy of tongue colors, which mainly include some specific colors (e.g., red color) and less so in others (e.g., green and blue color), developing a new colorchecker dedicatedly focused on tongue colors, i.e., a tongue colorchecker, is urgently needed to promote the correction performance and to improve the tongue image quality.

Several responses have been reported on this topic in the research community. In (Shen, Cai, & Zhang, 2007), Shen et al. proposed a tailor-made colorchecker for their correction task. It included 22 colors, which were made up of ten tongue colors, six primary colors, and six grayscale colors. Zhang et al. designed a larger colorchecker which included 94 colors (Zhang, Wang, Jin, & Zhang, 2005; Zhang, 2007) which included 50 tongue colors, 24 primary colors, and 20 grayscale colors. Our previous work on tongue color correction (Wang & Zhang, 2010a, b) also made an improvement on the Munsell colorchecker in which only 13 tongue colors were chosen, and the remaining colors were eliminated. These previous researches validated that the effectiveness of containing tongue colors could improve the correction performance. By adding more tongue colors and eliminating non-tongue colors than the Munsell colorchecker, one can expect to achieve better performance. However, due to the lack of establishment of a tongue color space which defines the range of tongue colors, existing researches normally subjectively chose these tongue colors based on their experience. Hence, their designs lacked a rigorous theoretical analysis and were not convincing enough. Furthermore, two more important and fundamental issues, i.e., how to determine the number of colors involved in the colorchecker and how to optimally select them, have not been thoroughly studied. Researchers chose a fixed number of colors, such as 22 in Shen's research (Shen, Cai, & Zhang, 2007) and 94 in Zhang's research (Zhang, Wang, Jin, & Zhang, 2005; Zhang, 2007), but scientific explanations on why these numbers were selected have not been given in their work. Similar situations happened on the colors selection method to design the colorchecker. Theoretically, millions of combinations of colors could be selected, but why their given colors were chosen has not been carefully studied.

This chapter aims to develop a new tongue colorchecker by solving the previous three essential problems: Where to choose colors of newly designed colorchecker? How many need to be involved? How to choose the best combination of colors? First, based on a large and comprehensive tongue image database, statistical characteristics of tongue colors were analysed and the tongue color space was established. All visible colors can be classified as tongue or non-tongue colors by the aid of this tongue color space. Hence, colors were chosen from the set of tongue colors to improve the correction accuracy. Second, the relationship between the number of colors and their corresponding correction accuracy was investigated. Different numbers of colors were utilized for correction model training, and the minimum sufficient number of colors was obtained by comparing their performance. Finally, color selection criteria to ensure an outstanding color correction performance were presented, and the objective function was proposed. To solve this function, two novel color selection methods, i.e., greedy and clustering-based methods, were proposed. Experiments were used to check which one is better for a tongue colorchecker design. Performance comparison between the proposed space-based tongue colorchecker and the Munsell colorchecker was conducted on various correction tasks to validate the effectiveness and superiority.

The remainder of the chapter is organized as follows. Section 10.2 presents the tongue color space by which tongue colors are defined. Thus, colors of the colorchecker can be selected from the set of tongue colors. In Sect. 10.3, the relationship between the number of colors and corresponding correction accuracy is obtained to decide the minimum sufficient number. Following this, color selection algorithms to generate the new colorchecker are introduced in Sect. 10.4. Section 10.5 describes the experimental results to validate the effectiveness. Finally, concluding remarks are made in Sect. 10.6.

10.2 Tongue Color Space

This section describes the tongue color space, i.e., range of tongue colors, by which all visible colors can be clearly classified as tongue and non-tongue colors: colors located inside the color space are tongue colors, and vice versa. Therefore, the colors of a newly designed colorchecker can be selected from the set of tongue colors rather than from all the visible color to improve the correction accuracy.

The method to establish the tongue color space is intuitive. First, a large image database which contains over 9000 high-quality tongue images was collected by our especially developed image acquisition device (Zhang, Wang, & Lu, 2010). The database includes images captured from subjects of different gender, age, and especially over 200 various disease types. To the best of our knowledge, this is the largest and most comprehensive database in the research community. Then, based on this database, all colors of these images were projected to two device-independent color spaces, i.e., CIELAB and CIE *xy*Y for distribution generation. This distribution can also be named as tongue color distribution (Wang & Zhang, 2011) because all colors came from tongue images. Figure 10.1 shows this distribution on the x–y plane (CIE *xy*Y) and a–b plane (CIELAB). It should be noticed that the blue points occupies a relatively small area of the whole visible color space. In order to mathematically define the range of this region, these two color distributions were modeled by a one-class support vector machine (SVM) algorithm (Manevitz & Yousef, 2002; Schölkopf, Platt, Shawe-Taylor, Smola, & Williamson, 2001). All the projected tongue colors were utilized as positive samples to train the classifier which can be regarded as the boundary of the tongue color space. The LIBSVM toolbox was employed in this study (Chang & Lin, 2011) to implement the algorithm. Figure 10.1 shows the tongue color space (red line) in two color spaces. By utilizing the boundary function of the gained tongue color space, colors can be easily classified into tongue or non-tongue colors.

After obtaining the tongue color space, it is interesting to check the relationship between the distribution of colors from the Munsell colorchecker and the tongue color space. Figure 10.2 shows the Munsell colorchecker and its corresponding sRGB coordinate in the CIE *xy*Y color space. All colors are numbered for convenience. From the figure, it can be observed that as this colorchecker is designed to process natural colors for general applications, its colors distribute evenly in the blue triangle of the sRGB color space. However, most colors are located outside of the tongue color space because they are unlikely to appear on tongue images, or

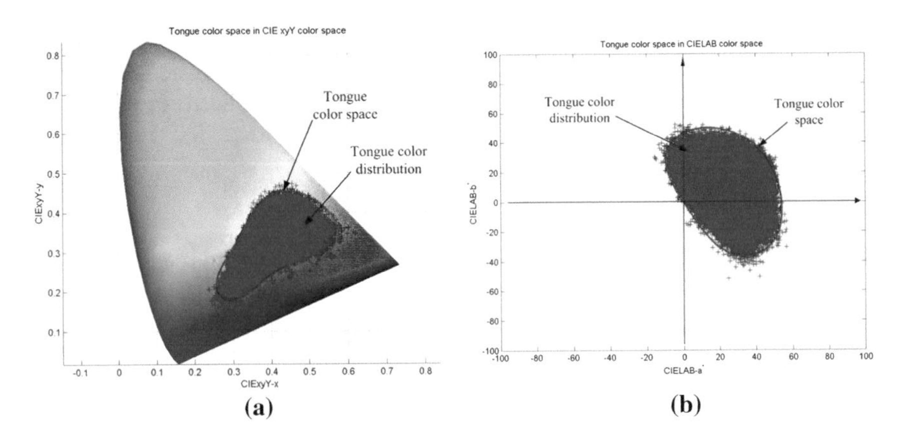

Fig. 10.1 Tongue color space in **a** CIE *xy*Y and **b** CIELAB color spaces. *Blue* points show the distribution of tongue colors. The tongue color space (*red line*) was obtained based on this distribution by a one-class SVM algorithm. © 2016 IEEE. Reprinted, with permission, from (Wang & Zhang, 2012)

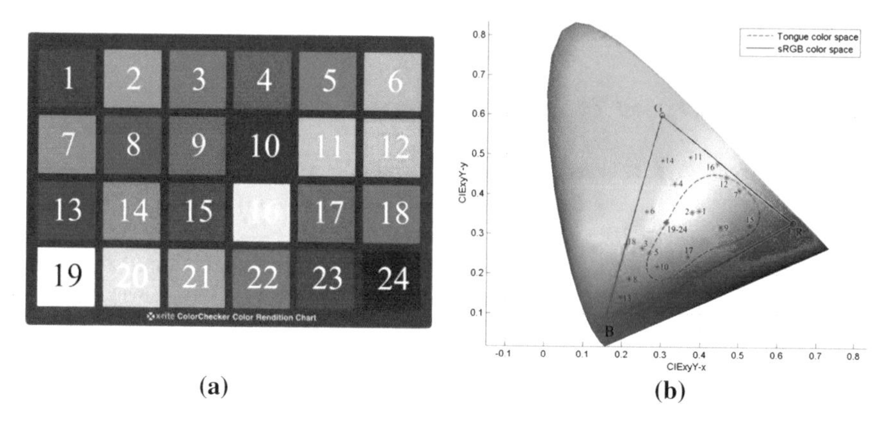

Fig. 10.2 The Munsell colorchecker and its distribution in the CIE *xy*Y color space. Obviously, most colors of this colorchecker do not distribute inside the tongue color space. © 2016 IEEE. Reprinted, with permission, from (Wang & Zhang, 2012)

they are too saturated to be involved. For example, there are not any greenish colors on tongue images, and thus nos. 11 and 14 colors are distributed outside of the tongue color space. Although tongue images have yellow and blue colors, colors in the Munsell colorchecker (nos. 6, 8, and 13) are too saturated to appear on tongue images. Therefore, in order to improve the correction accuracy, colors of the new designed tongue colorchecker were all selected from the tongue color space.

10.3 Determination of the Number of Colors

This section aims to investigate how many colors need to be involved in a tongue colorchecker. Generally, the more colors that are included in the reference colorchecker, the more accurately the trained color correction model performs. But, when more colors are included, more computational cost and time are needed. Furthermore, it can be conjectured that the increase in correction accuracy is not unlimited, and that there should be a "*minimum sufficient number*" of colors above which improvements in accuracy are negligible when the number of colors is increased. Therefore, this section studies the relationship between the number of colors in the tongue colorchecker and their corresponding color correction accuracy, in order to find such a number to achieve a balance between the correction accuracy and the computational cost in practical applications. Furthermore, stability tests on this obtained number were also conducted to check if it remains stable when various correction tasks or different correction algorithms are involved.

This part of study is somewhat an experiment-driven study, i.e., all the findings and conclusions are derived from experimental results of color correction by different numbers of colors rather theoretical analysis. Detailed information is present as follows.

10.3.1 Setting for Number Deciding Experiment

10.3.1.1 Training and Testing Dataset

In this research, we selected colors from the Munsell Book of Color (Glossy edition). This book is a set of colors which covers all the visible colors in the Munsell color system (Fig. 10.3a shows one page of this book which contains several printed colors). There are 1488 colors which are manufactured by a professional industrial company to ensure the printing quality. The distributions of these colors under illuminant D65 in CIE *xyY* and CIELAB are shown in

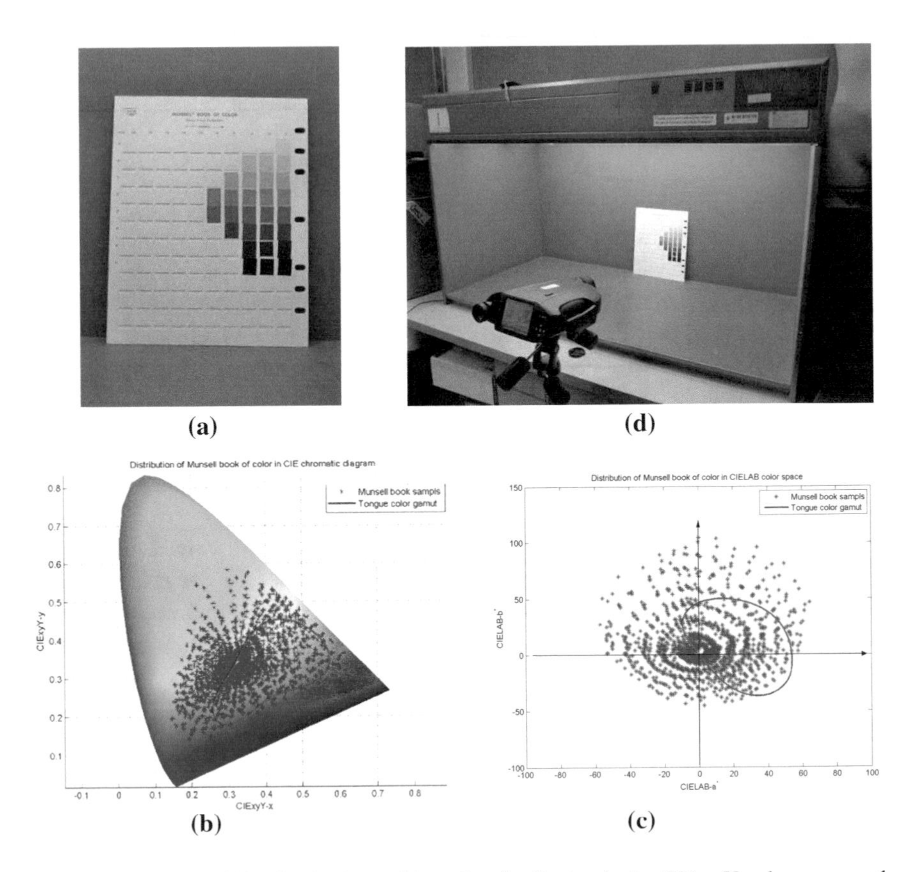

Fig. 10.3 The Munsell book of color and its color distribution in the CIE *xy*Y color space and CIELAB color space. Only colors distributed inside of the tongue color space (*red line*) were utilized for further process of the tongue colorchecker design. **a** Page of the Munsell book of color. **b** Measurement of the CIE XYZ and CIELAB value in a light box by PR-655. **c** Color distribution in the CIE chromatic diagram (xyY color space). **d** Color distribution on the *a*–*b* plane (CIELAB color space). © 2016 IEEE. Reprinted, with permission, from (Wang & Zhang, 2012)

Fig. 10.3c, d. In order to design the tongue colorchecker, only tongue colors, i.e., colors located inside the tongue color space, are considered to be used for colorchecker design. In this experiment, 688 out of the 1488 colors located inside the tongue color space could be utilized as the *selection pool*. Different numbers of colors (ranging from 10 to 200) were chosen from the selection pool and used as the *training dataset* for correction model training. All 688 tongue colors were used as the *testing dataset* to evaluate the correction accuracy. The ground truth of these 688 colors, i.e., the CIE XYZ and CIELAB of D65, was provided by the lighting box CAC 120 (VeriVide Ltd., Leicester, U.K.). Figure 10.3b shows the measurement of the ground truth.

10.3.1.2 Experimental Implementation

Figure 10.4 shows the flowchart of experiments to determine the number of colors involved in the new tongue colorchecker. *In the training phase*, different numbers of colors ranged from 10 to 200 at an interval of 2. Hence, 96 groups of colors were selected to train correction models. All these groups of colors were selected by our newly proposed clustering-based method (it will be introduced in Sect. 10.4). For the model generation algorithm which connects the imaged RGB matrix to the measured XYZ matrix, the classical polynomial regression algorithm was employed (Cheung, Westland, Connah, & Ripamonti, 2004; Johnson, 1996; Luo, Hong, & Rhodes, 2001). Since this polynomial regression by least square fitting has been adequately studied, only a brief introduction of it is provided here. The main task of

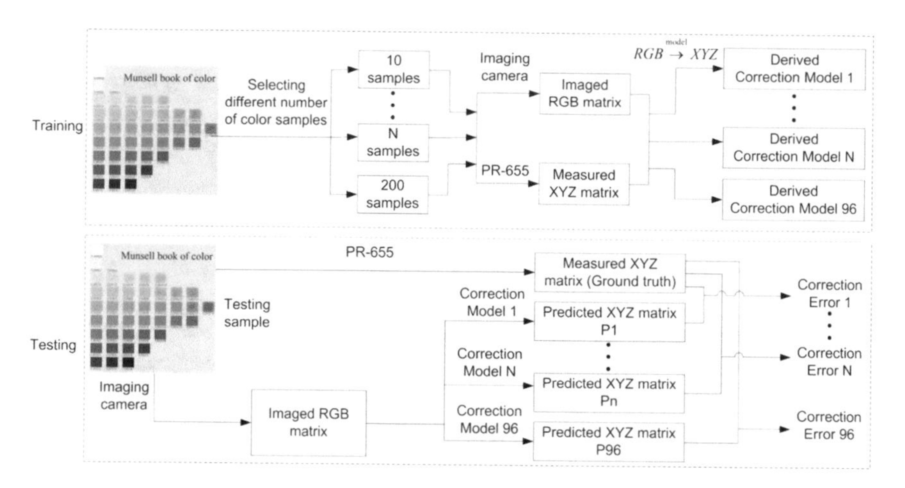

Fig. 10.4 Flowchart of color correction experiments to determine the minimum sufficient number of colors. © 2016 IEEE. Reprinted, with permission, from (Wang & Zhang, 2012)

this model generation is to obtain a transformation matrix, which can convert the RGB matrix to the XYZ matrix. Suppose the RGB matrix is $\boldsymbol{X}$, and the XYZ matrix is $\boldsymbol{S}$, we need to obtain the coefficient matrix $\boldsymbol{A}$ in the following formula:

$$\boldsymbol{S} = \boldsymbol{A}^{T} \cdot \boldsymbol{X} \tag{10.1}$$

In the polynomial regression method, both $\boldsymbol{X}$ and $\boldsymbol{S}$ are represented by polynomial terms, and by using the least square regression method, the solution to (10.1) is

$$\boldsymbol{A} = \left(\boldsymbol{X}^{T}\boldsymbol{X}\right)^{-1}\boldsymbol{X}^{T}\boldsymbol{S} \tag{10.2}$$

Although the use of different algorithms or different parameters would likely generate different correction models, we believe it may not affect the colorchecker design in which the relative performance comparisons are the key issues.

In the testing phase, the color correction performance of these derived correction models was calculated in terms of the CIELAB color difference (Sharma & Bala, 2002) by (10.3) between the measured *XYZ* values (ground truth) and the *XYZ* values predicted from the *RGB* values captured by digital cameras, and the *XYZ* values needed to be converted to LAB values beforehand. The lower the correction error, the better the correction model performs. Finally, we can compare the performance of these 96 correction models and choose the best one. One more issue that needs to be noted here is the influence of usage of different color selection methods. Although the correction results may vary with each other when different selection methods are applied, we believe that it is likely that the relative performances may remain unchanged. Our further results in the stability test also experimentally confirmed this deduction where four different selection methods were utilized for comparison of their derived "*minimum sufficient number*"

$$\Delta E_{\text{ab}}^{*} = \sqrt{\left(L_1^{*} - L_2^{*}\right)^2 + \left(a_1^{*} - a_2^{*}\right)^2 + \left(b_1^{*} - b_2^{*}\right)^2} \tag{10.3}$$

10.3.1.3 Configuration for Stability Test

In order to test the stability of the obtained *minimum sufficient number*, a series of color correction experiments under different imaging condition was conducted. All 688 colors of the selection pool were captured under four different lighting conditions by two different cameras. Table 10.1 shows the detailed information about the combination of camera type and lighting condition. Color correction on images captured under different imaging conditions can be regarded as different correction tasks. By comparing the obtained number with each correction task, the robustness and stability of such a number can be verified. Moreover, in order to verify if the color selection method affected the achieved *minimum sufficient number*, four color

Table 10.1 Four image conditions were tested to verify the stability of the derived minimum number

No.	Camera	Lighting condition
1	Casio EX-Z400	D65
2	Casio EX-Z400	Incandescent
3	Casio EX-Z400	TL84
4	Canon SX200 IS	Illuminant F

selection methods (CMMxyz, CMMxy, CMMlab, and CMMab which will be introduced in Sect. 10.4) were applied for this test.

10.3.2 Results of Number Determination

10.3.2.1 Obtained Minimum Sufficient Number

Figure 10.5 shows correction results when different numbers of training colors were employed under the no. 1 imaging condition in Table 10.1. The color selection

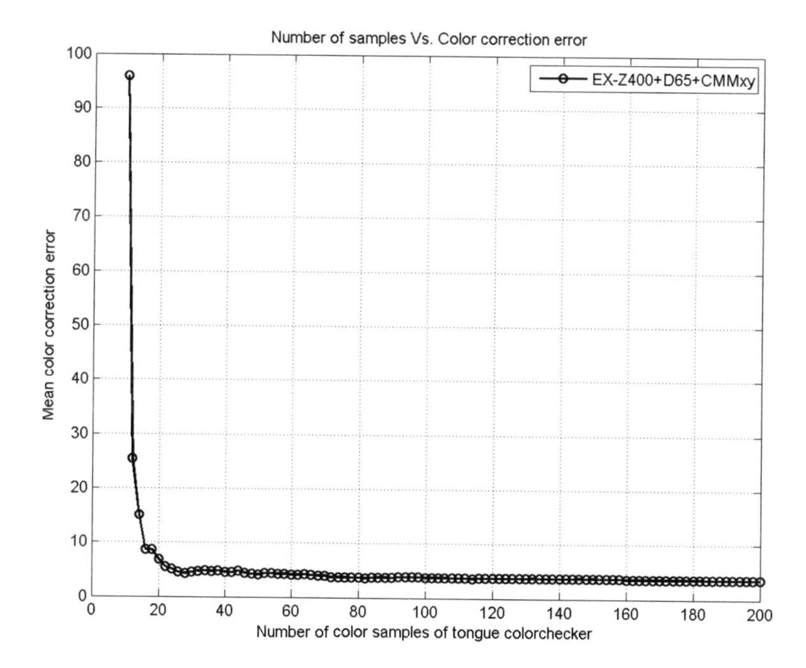

Fig. 10.5 Distribution of color correction error with respect to different numbers of training colors. © 2016 IEEE. Reprinted, with permission, from (Wang & Zhang, 2012)

method used here was the CMMlab method which will be introduced in Sect. 9.4. Since different selection methods would not affect the results of the derived number, we use this method as an example. From Fig. 10.5, it can be observed that when the number of training colors increases, the mean color correction error decreases. Furthermore, when this number is bigger than 20, the increase of correction accuracy becomes very slow though some small fluctuations may be observed. This trend is also similar to the finding of other studies (de Lasarte, Arjona, Vilaseca, & Pujol, 2010) in spectral reconstruction by using a reference target. Based on this finding, we may deduce that the minimum sufficient number is 20 (or a little bigger, such as 22). Hence, when designing the tongue colorchecker, we may select 20 or a larger number of colors to ensure the performance of the color correction.

10.3.2.2 Results of the Stability Test

We further tested the stability of the gained *minimum sufficient number* by comparing the derived number from different correction tasks. Figure 10.6 presents four accuracy curves which were obtained by correcting color images captured under the four imaging conditions (see Table 10.1) using different numbers of colors. It can

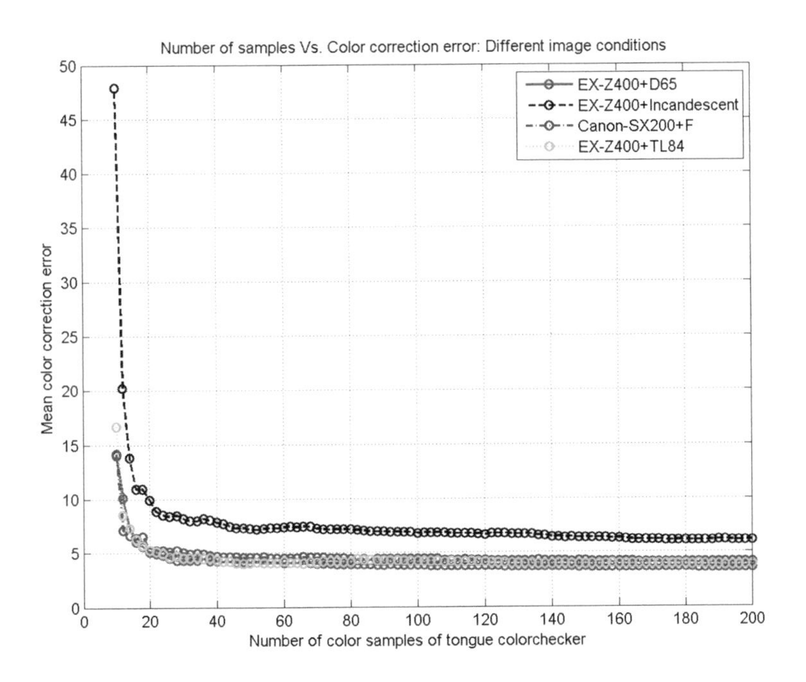

Fig. 10.6 Comparison of number selection results of four different correction tasks. © 2016 IEEE. Reprinted, with permission, from (Wang & Zhang, 2012)

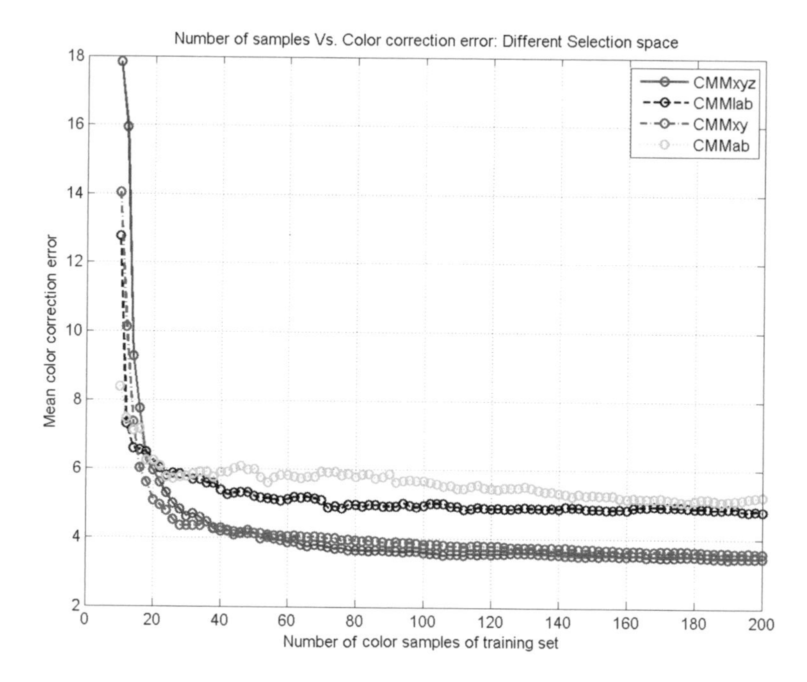

Fig. 10.7 Comparison of number selection results for four different color selection methods. © 2016 IEEE. Reprinted, with permission, from (Wang & Zhang, 2012)

be noticed that although absolute correction errors of these four correction tasks vary, such as that the minimum correction error is around 6 in no. 2 imaging condition (black line), while it is much smaller in other three conditions (around 4), the decreasing trend of these four curves is similar. The minimum number of all these four cases could be chosen as 20.

Similar to the previous study of number selection in four different color correction tasks, Fig. 10.7 describes the comparison results when different color selection methods (CMMxyz, CMMxy, CMMlab, and CMMab which will be introduced in Sect. 10.4) were employed. Though various absolute correction accuracies may be observed, the relative trend remained unchanged in terms of different selection methods. Hence, the minimum number of 20 is still valid.

Similar to the previous study of number selection in four different color correction tasks, Fig. 10.7 describes the comparison results when different color selection methods (CMMxyz, CMMxy, CMMlab, and CMMab which will be introduced in Sect. 10.4) were employed. Though various absolute correction accuracies may be observed, the relative trend remained unchanged in terms of different selection methods. Hence, the minimum number of 20 is still valid.

In brief, this section investigated the color correction accuracy in terms of different numbers of training colors to form a new colorchecker. Experimental results show that the *minimum sufficient number* is 20 or a little larger. This number remained stable when different correction tasks or different color selection methods were tested. In this study, in order to compare the newly designed tongue colorchecker with the Munsell colorchecker, and also for the sake of practical application, 24 colors were involved.

10.4 Optimal Colors Selection

This section aims to propose novel methods to select a set of colors (24 in this study) from the selection pool which has 688 colors. We first introduce the criteria and objective function for optimized color selection, and then present color selection algorithms to solve the optimization problem.

10.4.1 Objective Function

The first challenge for color selection is to establish selection criteria and thereby to derive the objective function. To the best of our knowledge, there have not been any reported studies on this topic illustrating what kind of colors should be chosen which can lead to high correction accuracy. Therefore, the most intuitive and effective way is to learn the underlying principle from the design of the most commonly used Munsell colorchecker. From Fig. 10.2; two criteria can be observed from the distribution of these colors. First, they are *complete* enough to cover the whole sRGB color space. Several colors are distributed near the boundary region of the sRGB color space (blue triangle) to occupy the whole color space. Therefore, the Munsell colorchecker can be utilized to process all visible colors. Second, these colors are *distinguishable* enough to make them as different as possible from each other. Hence, we may deduce that large diversity and small redundancy may improve the correction performance. This selection principle, i.e., to select the most different colors so as to enlarge the diversity among them, has also been verified by several similar researches on colors selection in spectral reflectance reconstruction (Cheung & Westland, 2006; Kosztyán & Schanda, 2009; Shen, Zhang, Xin, & Shao, 2008). From this literature, it was noticed that the key strategy to ensure high reconstruction accuracy was also to select colors as different or diverse as possible from each other. Interestingly, the first requirement of color selection in which colors need to be complete enough is somewhat subordinate to the second criterion. If colors are separated enough with each other, some of them will be "pushed" to the boundary and occupy the whole color space. Therefore, based on previous analysis, to select colors *as distinguishable as possible* from each other is the main objective to ensure a promising correction performance.

Let R and S denote the selection pool (688 colors) and selected subset of colors (24 colors), and $d(s)$ denotes the diversity measurement of subset S, the objective function is as follows:

$$f(s) = \arg\min_{s \in R} d(s) \tag{10.4}$$

For the diversity measurement $d(s)$, two methods are considered, i.e., the sum of distance among samples in subset S (SumD) and the minimum distance among samples in subset S (MinD). The first distance SumD is very intuitive and can easily be understood. Since the difference between two colors can be measured by the distance between them, the total difference of a subset which includes 24 samples can be measured by the sum of the distance among them. Figure 10.8a shows an example of the SumD measurement when four samples are included in the subset. For the measurement of MinD, this idea was actually stimulated by a famous management theory named *Bucket theory*. The principle of this theory is briefly that the water containing ability of a barrel is not determined by the longest piece of wood but by the shortest piece of wood. Therefore, we also deduce that the diversity of a subset is not determined by the longest or sum of the distance among all samples but by the minimum distance among them. Figure 10.8b shows an example of the MinD measurement. The distance between two colors is measured by the norm of their corresponding color values as $d\ (X_i, X_j) = \|X_i - X_j\|_p$, $p = 2$ or ∞, when p equals 2, it is the Euclidean distance, and when p equals ∞, it is the Chebyshev distance.

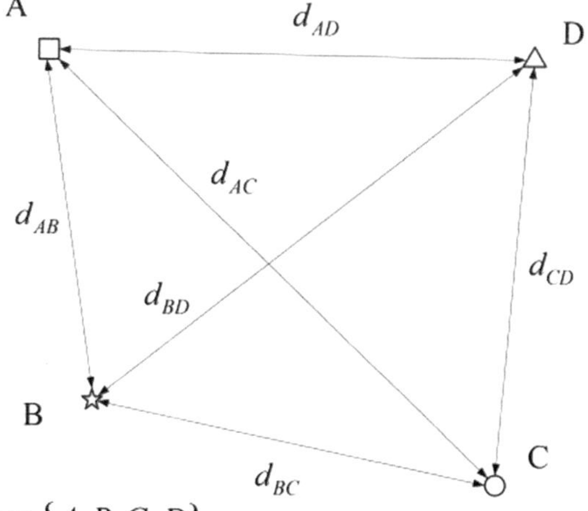

Fig. 10.8 Example for diversity measurement of a subset which contains four samples. *a* Sum of the distance of the subset (SumD). *b* Minimum distance of the subset (MinD). © 2016 IEEE. Reprinted, with permission, from (Wang & Zhang, 2012)

Based on the proposed diversity measurement, the objective function of (10.4) can be further developed as

$$f(s:p,m)=\begin{cases}\arg\max\limits_{\substack{s\in R\\ x_{i,j}\in s}}\sum\limits_{i,j}\left\|x_i-x_j\right\|_p, m=\mathrm{SumD}, \quad P=2\,or\,\infty\\ \arg\max\limits_{\substack{s\in R\\ x_{i,j}\in s}}\min\sum\limits_{i,j}\left\|x_i-x_j\right\|_p, m=\mathrm{MinD}, \quad P=2\,or\,\infty\end{cases} \tag{10.5}$$

10.4.2 Selection Algorithms

The optimization of (10.5) is an NP-hard problem for which it is difficult to obtain the optimum solution. Here, we propose two algorithms to solve the optimization problem for color selection of a tongue colorchecker. One is the greedy method (Cormen, 2009), named greedy maximizing sum distance (GMS) and greedy maximizing minimum distance (GMM). The other one is the clustering-based method, named clustering-based maximizing sum distance and clustering-based maximizing minimum distance (CMM).

10.4.2.1 The Greedy Method

Shown in Algorithm 1, the basic idea for the greedy selection method is to start with an initial selected first sample and subsequent samples are selected in turn from the selection pool such that the newly selected colors are as different as possible from the samples already selected according to the greedy rule (diversity measurement). The greedy selection method is simple and can be easily implemented, and also it may obtain the suboptimum of even optimum solutions. However, the drawbacks of this method are that it needs to select the initial samples beforehand which may cause unstable selection output, and its time and space complexity are a little bit high especially when a large selection pool is involved. According to different diversity measurements (see Sect. 10.4.1), there are two algorithms of this kind of greedy selection method, i.e., GMS and GMM.

For the first sample selection, we can choose random samples from the selection pool or choose the maximum saturation samples (far from the gray axis). However, experimental results show that although some fluctuations is observed, the relative performance of this greedy method does not heavily change when different first samples are selected.

Algorithm 1 Greedy selection method (GMM and GMS).

Input: **R** is selection pool; **N** is the number of samples of the selection pool; X_0 is the initially selected first sample; ***n*** is number of samples that need to be selected (**n** = 24); ***m*** is the greedy rule (*SumD* or *MinD*); ***p*** is the type of distance (2 or ∞).

Output: Subset of selected color samples **X**.

1) Start from the initial selected first sample X_0,

2) **for** i =1 to (**n**-1) **do**

selected color samples $\mathbf{X} = \{X_0, X_1, \ldots, X_{i-1}\}$

for j =1 to (N-i-l) **do**

for each color sample Y_j in the remaining color selection pool (**R-X**), according to the greedy rule m, calculate the diversity of subset $\boldsymbol{D}_j = \boldsymbol{d}_{\{X, Y_j\}} = \boldsymbol{d}\{X_0, X_1, \ldots, X_{i-1}, Y_j\}$

end for

selected the *kth* sample Y_k which maximizes $D_j(j \in (1, \text{N-i-1}))$,

and let $X_t = Y_k$.

Renew $\mathbf{X} = \{X_0, X_1, \ldots, X_{i-1}\}$

end for

return X

10.4.2.2 The Clustering-Based Method

In order to overcome the drawback of greedy selection methods, i.e., first color selection and computational time or space consuming, another clustering- based selection method is proposed. The basic idea of this method is to replace the 24 class centers which were initially iteratively derived from a cluster algorithm [such as fuzzy *C*-means (Bezdek, Ehrlich, & Full, 1984) or *k*-means (Lloyd, 1982)] by the within-class color samples according to the optimization rule (diversity measurement). For all color samples belonging to one class, if there exists one color which has a larger distance to the remaining (24-1) centers than the center of this class does, the center color will be replaced by this color. In this case, the total maximum distance among all these 24 centers would be gradually increased. However, this total distance would not be increased forever, and when it reaches the maximum distance, we consider that we have obtained the optimum solution for this optimization problem. Detailed information of this algorithm is shown in Algorithm 2.

Compared with the greedy method, the advantage of the clustering-based method is that the convergence rate is very fast and it can obtain the optimum solution. A possible reason is that it is generated based on the initial clustering result which already clusters samples based on their inner distance to ensure centers are far from each other.

Algorithm 2 Clustering-based selection method (CMM and CMS).

Input: $\boldsymbol{R}$ is selection pool; $\boldsymbol{n}$ is number of colors that need to be selected *{n=24}*; T is the diversity measurement of selected colors according to different methods *(SumD* or *MinD))*. ΔT is the variance of the $\boldsymbol{T}$ during the iteration which equals to $\Delta T_i = (T_{i+1}\text{-}T_i)$, i = 1, 2, …,100, ε is the tolerance threshold of ΔT.

Output: Subset of selected colors $\boldsymbol{C}$.

1) Cluster $\boldsymbol{R}$ into $\boldsymbol{n}$ classes, the set of cluster centers is $\boldsymbol{C} = \{C_1, C_2, \ldots, C_n\}$.

2) $\boldsymbol{T}$ is initially calculated ($\boldsymbol{T_0}$) based on the set of cluster centers $\boldsymbol{C}$. ε is set to a small positive number (1%).

3) **for** i =1 to 100 **do**

  for j = 1 to $\boldsymbol{n}$ **do**

    Calculate the distance between samples belong to the *jth* cluster class and remaining (***n-1***) selected color centers, and select the maximum distance D_j according to the optimization rule. Suppose the *kth* sample Y_k of the *jth* class achieves maximum distance.

    Calculate the distance between the *jth* color center C_j with other *(n-1)* selected color samples according to the optimization rule, which can be represented by F_j

    if $D_j > F_j$ **then** $C_j = Y_k$ **end if**

  end for

  $\Delta T_i = (T_{i+1}\text{-}T_i)$, if $\Delta T_j < \varepsilon$ **then break end if**

end for

return C.

10.4.2.3 Selection the Color Space

In addition to proposing the greedy and clustering-based selection methods to find the optimum solution to the objective function in (10.5), one more issue that needs to be considered is which color space is used for color selection. We have developed the tongue color space in CIELAB and CIE *xy*Y color space. These two color spaces are 3-D color spaces which are widely used as target device-independent spaces for color correction. Hence, the selection process can be conducted based on these two 3-D color spaces of CIELAB and CIEXYZ. Moreover, another two 2-D color spaces, the *x–y* space of CIE *xy*Y and *a–b* space of CIELAB, are also considered for color selection. The intention is to select colors only based on the chromatic information but without the luminance information. The selection of samples in the 2-D chromatic space may stimulate samples to be more evenly distributed and to be much more different from each other than when the selection is conducted in 3-D color space.

In sum, four factors should be considered when implementing this new colorchecker: the selection method (greedy or clustering based), diversity measurement (SumD or MinD), color spaces (CIEXYZ, CIELAB, *x–j*, *a–b*), and distance measure (*Euclidean* and *Chebyshev*). These four parameters will be optimized to choose the best combination in the following section.

10.5 Experimental Results and Performance Analysis

The section provides the design of a new colorchecker by selecting the best combination of parameters. Furthermore, this newly designed tongue colorchecker is compared with the Munsell colorchecker in terms of correction accuracy on tongue colors. Section 10.5.1 describes the configuration of the experiment. The best combinations of parameters are derived based on the experimental results in Sect. 10.5.2 to realize the design of a tongue colorchecker. Finally, Sect. 10.5.2.3 provides the performance comparison with the Munsell colorchecker.

10.5.1 Experimental Configuration

10.5.1.1 Training and Testing Dataset

Similar to the number selection experiment in Sect. 10.3.1, 24 colors were selected by different selection methods from the selection pool and utilized as the training dataset for generation of a correction model. All 688 colors in the selection pool were used as the testing dataset. CIEXYZ values of 688 tongue colors were measured by the PR-655 under standard illuminant D65 which could be used as mapping targets in the training phase and the ground truth in the testing phase.

10.5.1.2 Flowchart of the Experiment

Figure 10.9 shows the flowchart of this experiment. *In the training phase*, different parameters were applied for color selection. As described in Sect. 10.4, there are 32 combinations of parameters, i.e., four color spaces (CIEXYZ, CIELAB, x–y, and a–b), two selection methods (greedy and clustering based), two diversity measurements (SumD and MinD), and two distances (*Euclidean* and *Chebyshev*). Thus, 32 groups of colors were selected for correction model training. The polynomial regression algorithm was employed to generate 32 different correction models. In addition, in order to achieve the best result (the benchmark result) for comparison, all colors in the selection pool were employed to generate the benchmark correction model. For comparison, the Munsell colorchecker was also applied for model training.

In the testing phase, first the best combination of parameters for color selection was obtained by comparing the accuracy of the 32 correction models, and thereby the tongue colorchecker was designed by these optimal parameters. This parameter optimization procedure was presented in Sect. 10.5.2. Second, in Sect. 10.5.2.3, this newly designed colorchecker was compared with the Munsell colorchecker to validate the effectiveness and superiority.

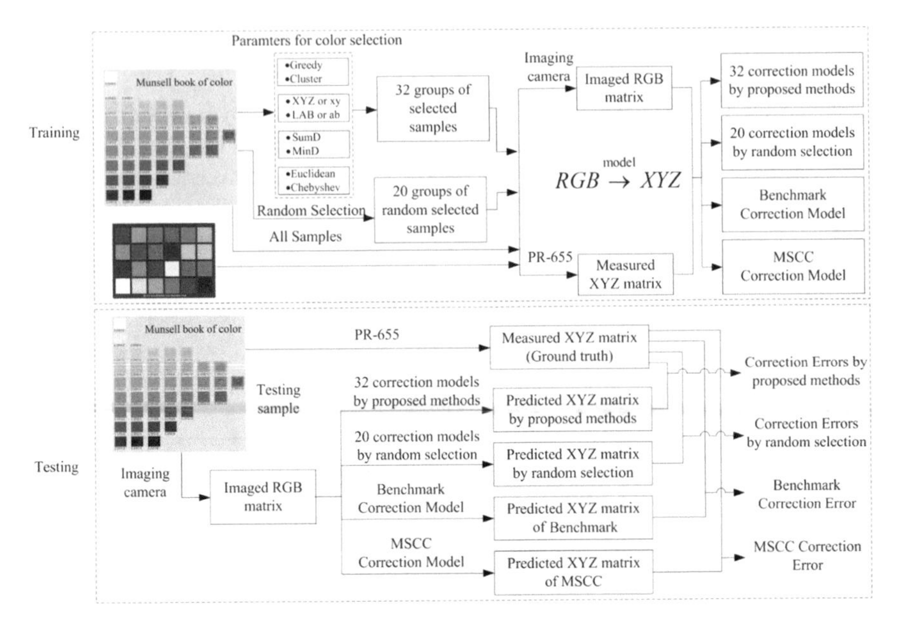

Fig. 10.9 Flowchart of performance analysis experiments. In the training phase, colors were selected according to 32 different combinations of parameters. Also, the selected colorchecker chart was compared to the Munsell colorchecker in terms of color correction performance.

10.5.2 Parameter Optimization

Four kinds of parameters were introduced earlier, and there are 32 combinations because there are only two or four choices for each parameter. In this part, one parameter was optimized by comparing the performance of different choices of this parameter when the other three parameters were the same. For example, when we selected which selection method is better, we compared the performance of the greedy and clustering- based method on the other 16 combinations of parameters.

10.5.2.1 Color Space

Figure 10.10 provides the performance comparison results. For each color space, eight groups of colors were selected according to other eight parameter sets and shown on the horizontal axis. From the figure, it can be observed that among these four subfigures which represent different correction tasks, there is not a color space which performs the best among all cases. Most times, correction accuracies of these four color spaces are close to each other except the left two most points in each curve. The possible reason for why correction accuracy of these two left points largely varies is because the greedy selection method and maximizing sum of distance were employed in these two cases. These two parameters (greedy selection and maximizing sum of distance) were found to be the two worst parameter combinations which will achieve bad and unstable correction performance (detailed results are shown in the following section). Hence, we believe that the unstable correction performance under such bad parameter combinations may affect the evaluation results to decide which color space performs the best, and we will only utilize the experimental results by the other six combinations of parameters (from 3 to 8 on the horizontal axis). Obviously, when not considering the left two results, correction accuracies are almost the same among these four color spaces. In general, all these four color space can be chosen to design the colorchecker.

However, there are still several concerns that need to be discussed. First, these four color spaces can be divided into two groups: 2-D and 3-D color space. Which one is better when conducting color selection? From the experimental results which are shown in Fig. 10.10, it is hard to decide which one is better. However, in order to select colors without any loss of information, we should select the 3-D color space. In this task of a tongue colorchecker design, the results show that the difference in using a 2-D (ab or xy) and a 3-D (LAB or *XYZ*) color space is not significant. It may be explained that all color samples were selected from tongue colors whose lightness value changes within a small range. Hence, selected colors in the 2-D color space may also have the biggest diversity in the 3-D color space. Given that a 3-D color space should be employed, the second issue is whether we

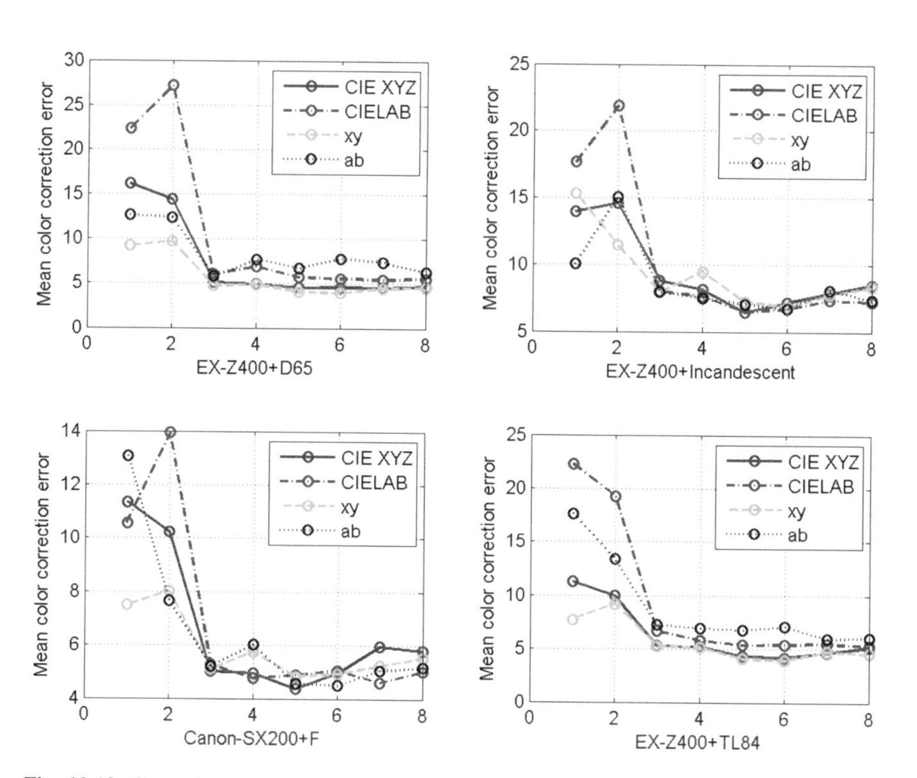

Fig. 10.10 Correction comparison based on colors selected from different color spaces. © 2016 IEEE. Reprinted, with permission, from (Wang & Zhang, 2012)

need to choose the CIE LAB or *XYZ* color space. Although these two color spaces perform almost the same in this task, we finally chose the CIE LAB color space because it is an approximately visually uniform color space and selecting colors from it may allow selected colors samples to be better distributed.

In sum, according to the result and previous discussion, each of these four color space could be applied for this color selection task, and we selected the 3-D CIELAB color space to design the tongue colorchecker.

10.5.2.2 Selection Method

Similar to color space selection, Fig. 10.11 shows the performance comparison results between the greedy and clustering-based methods. It is obvious that in most cases, the clustering-based method performs much *better* than the greedy method because the red line is below the blue one most of the time. Moreover, results show that the clustering-based method performs more *stable* than the greedy method. One possible reason is because the clustering-based method can achieve the optimum solution and the greedy selection method cannot. Based on the result, we chose the clustering-based method for color selection of a tongue colorchecker design.

Another interesting finding is that in some special cases (nos. 3, 4, 7, 8, 11, 12, 15, and 16), the performance of these two methods is close to each other (the blue

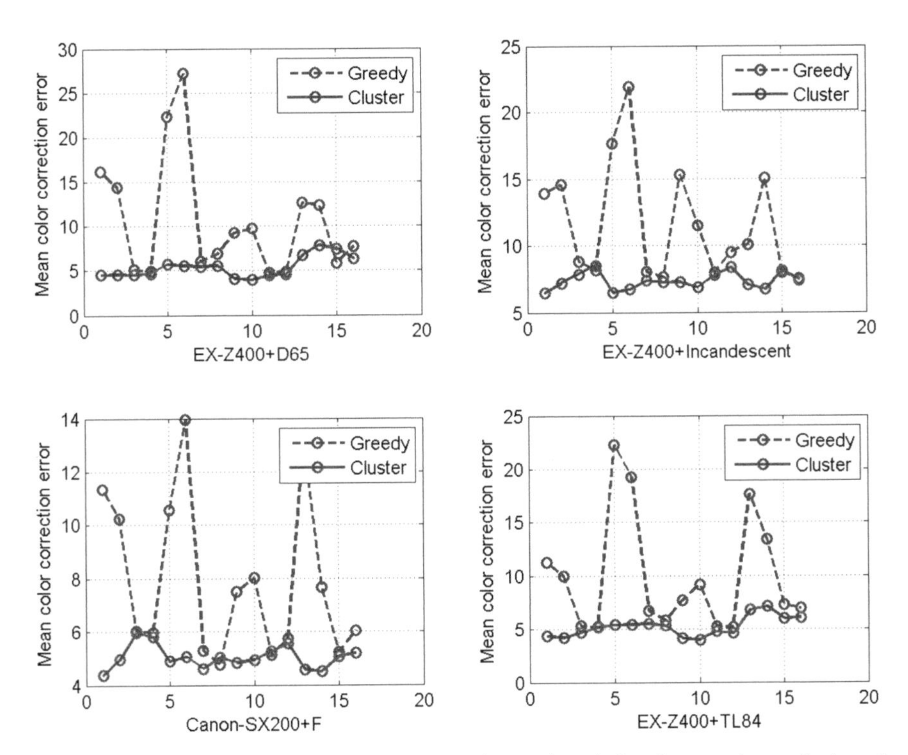

Fig. 10.11 Correction comparison based on colors selected by the greedy method and clustering-based methods. © 2016 IEEE. Reprinted, with permission, from (Wang & Zhang, 2012)

and red points are close to each other). The common thing shared among these parameter combinations is the employment of the diversity measurement of MinD. Hence, this result also validates the effectiveness of it.

10.5.2.3 Diversity Measurement

For the diversity measurement of SumD and MinD, Fig. 10.12 shows the comparison results. Obviously, the red line is always below the blue line, i.e., correction error of MinD is much lower than SumD. Therefore, the MinD performs much more effectively and stably than the SumD. Actually from the principle of the diversity measurement in Fig. 10.8, we may deduce that the MinD may outperform the SumD. The principle of maximizing the MinD could be simply understood as "to maximize the distance between me and my *nearest* neighbor," thus, it can ensure that selected samples are as diverse as possible while maximizing the SumD cannot achieve this objective. Figure 10.13 shows a selected example by the same selection method according to these two diversity measurements. Obviously, samples in (c) are distributed more evenly than samples in (b). Based on the previous analysis, we chose the MinD measurement in the objective function for the color selection of a tongue colorchecker.

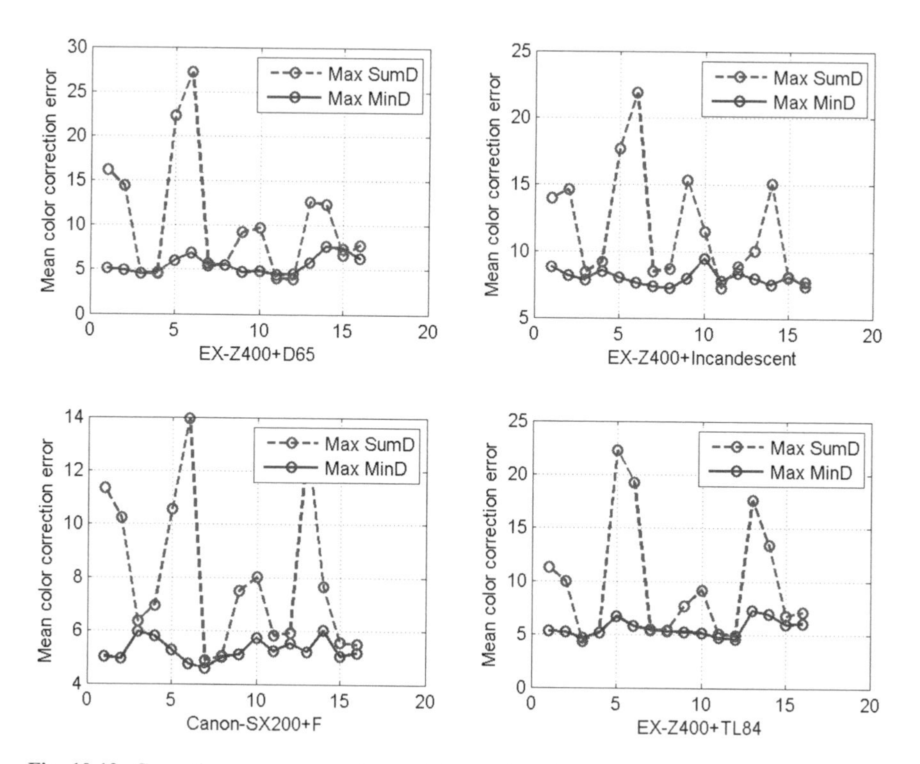

Fig. 10.12 Correction comparison of two different diversity measurements: SumD and MinD. © 2016 IEEE. Reprinted, with permission, from (Wang & Zhang, 2012)

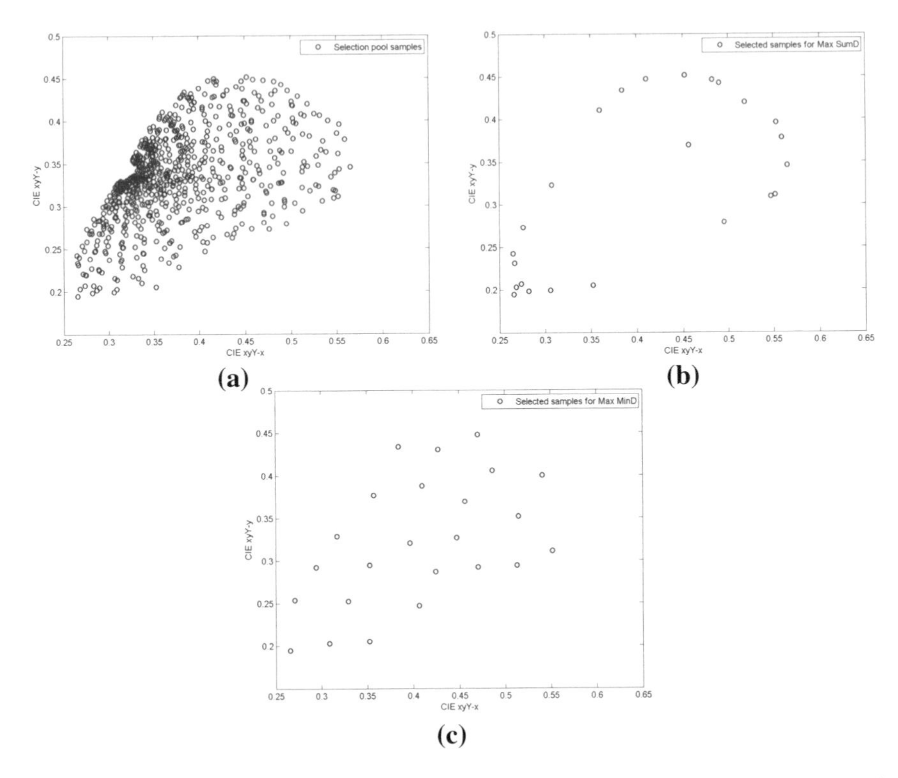

Fig. 10.13 Distribution of selected samples by different diversity measurement of SumD and MinD. Distributions of **a** selection pool samples, **b** samples by SumD, and **c** samples by MinD. It shows that samples in (**c**) are much more separated with each other than in (**b**). © 2016 IEEE. Reprinted, with permission, from (Wang & Zhang, 2012)

10.5.2.4 Distance Measure

Last, regarding which kind of distances needs to be selected in this experiment, Fig. 10.14 shows the comparison results. Between these two candidate distances, i.e., *Euclidean* and *Chebyshev* distance, it seems that these two distances perform almost the same though some variations can be observed. Therefore, either of the Euclidean or Chebyshev distance can be chosen. In our design of a tongue colorchecker, we chose *Euclidean* distance.

In sum, there are four kinds of parameters for color selection. Based on the results of previous parameters optimization, we finally proposed our new tongue colorchecker by the clustering-based selection method to maximize the MinD in the CIELAB color space (clustering-based maximizing the MinD in the CIELAB color space, or the CMMlab in short). Figure 10.15 shows the designed tongue colorchecker and its corresponding color distribution on the CIE x–y plane. Compared to the distribution of the Munsell colorchecker in Fig. 10.2, unlike colors in the

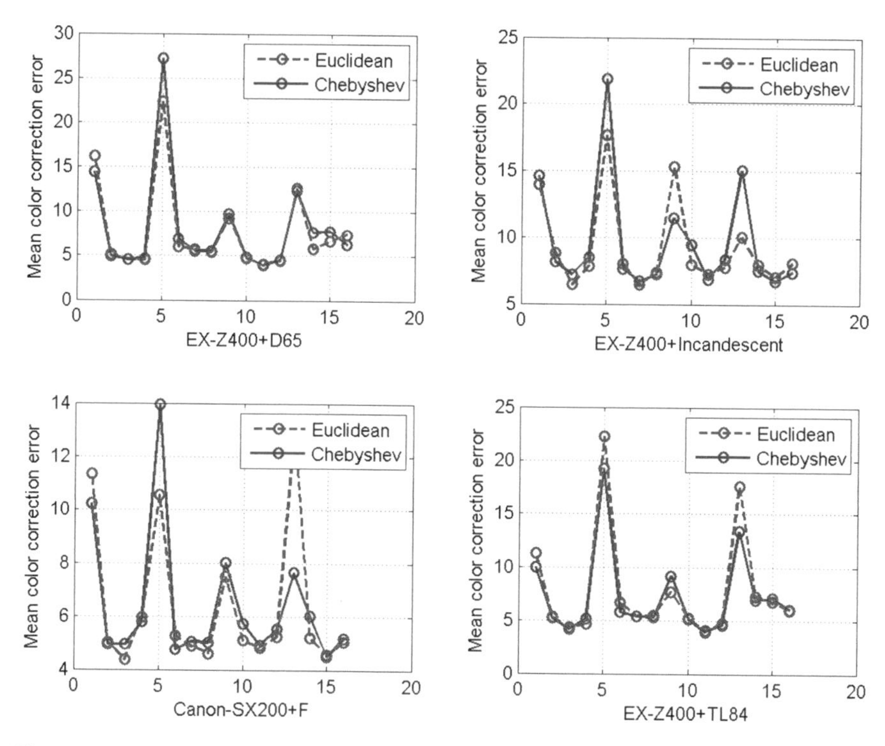

Fig. 10.14 Correction comparison of two different distances: the Euclidean distance and the Chebyshev distance. © 2016 IEEE. Reprinted, with permission, from (Wang & Zhang, 2012)

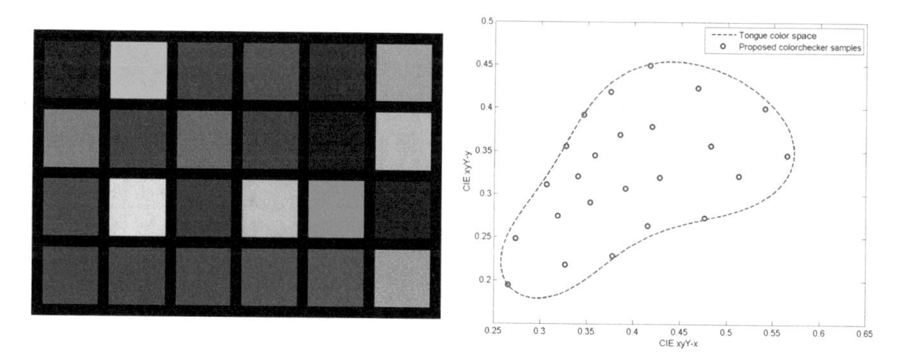

Fig. 10.15 Proposed tongue colorchecker and its corresponding color distribution on the CIE x–y plane. © 2016 IEEE. Reprinted, with permission, from (Wang & Zhang, 2012)

Munsell colorchecker are evenly scattered in the larger sRGB color space, while colors from the newly designed tongue colorchecker are only distributed inside the tongue color space. Moreover, these colors are evenly distributed thereby ensuring a promising correction performance of this tongue colorchecker.

10.5.2.5 Performance Comparison

This section compares the correction performance of the proposed colorchecker with the Munsell colorchecker and the benchmark result to validate the effectiveness and superiority. Tables 10.2, 10.3, 10.4 and 10.5 show the comparison of correction accuracy for four different correction tasks. In this study, four statistical

Table 10.2 Performance comparison between the proposed colorchecker and the Munsell colorchecker (CASIO EX-Z400+D65)

CIELAB color difference				
Methods	Mean	Median	Max	Min
Benchmark	3.6861	3.0434	30.6345	0.4427
Proposed space-based colorchecker	5.3729	4.0838	57.7473	0.4679
Munsell colorchecker	10.3528	7.7212	75.0332	0.8295

Table 10.3 Performance comparison between the proposed colorchecker and the Munsell colorchecker (CASIO EX-Z400+INCANDESCENT)

CIELAB color difference				
Methods	Mean	Median	Max	Min
Benchmark	8.0801	5.3713	89.4872	0.7248
Proposed space-based colorchecker	11.5785	7.2640	84.5281	0.7515
Munsell colorchecker	14.9662	11.7510	138.7499	0.8569

Table 10.4 Performance comparison between the proposed colorchecker and the Munsell colorchecker (CASIO EX-Z400+TL84)

CIELAB color difference				
Methods	Mean	Median	Max	Min
Benchmark	4.6885	3.7358	26.2212	0.3749
Proposed space-based colorchecker	5.6664	4.8462	26.9428	0.5700
Munsell colorchecker	11.6763	10.0367	55.4211	1.0914

Table 10.5 Performance comparison between the proposed colorchecker and the Munsell colorchecker (CANON SX200 IS+ILLUMINSNTF)

CIELAB color difference				
Methods	Mean	Median	Max	Min
Benchmark	3.7998	3.2097	32.2991	0.3022
Proposed space-based colorchecker	5.0729	4.0772	30.9739	0.3118
Munsell colorchecker	11.6644	8.4890	62.8263	0.3421

indexes: mean, median, max, and min errors were employed to describe the correction performance.

From these four tables, it can first be observed that the best correction results (benchmark) are different in terms of different correction tasks. The no. 1 imaging condition achieves the lowest correction error of 3.68, while no. 2 obtains the highest correction error of 8.08. This finding illustrates that the best correction accuracy is dependent on a specific correction task. Hence, we may deduce that the no. 2 imaging condition has more variation or color-rendering problems than the other three imaging conditions because it obtains the worst benchmark result. In addition to the benchmark results, correction errors by the proposed colorchecker also follow the same trend, where no. 1 imaging condition obtains the best result, nos. 3 and 4 performs in the middle and no. 2 achieves the worst results.

As the correction error follows a similar trend among these four correction tasks, we may take one of them as an example for deeper analysis. In Table 10.2, the benchmark result is around 3.68, and correction error on the Munsell colorchecker is 10.35 which is much worse than the best result. Compared to the Munsell colorchecker, our proposed tongue colorchecker obtains a mean correction error of 5.37 which improves the correction performance by almost 48%. Therefore, this comparison validates that the effectiveness and superiority of our proposed colorchecker for tongue color correction. Similar findings can be observed in the other three tables thus enforcing the conclusion that the newly designed tongue colorchecker performs much better than the Munsell colorchecker.

Figure 10.16 provides the overall comparison between the proposed colorchecker and the Munsell colorchecker. Obviously, among these four tasks, the proposed space-based colorchecker performs much better than the Munsell colorchecker, which

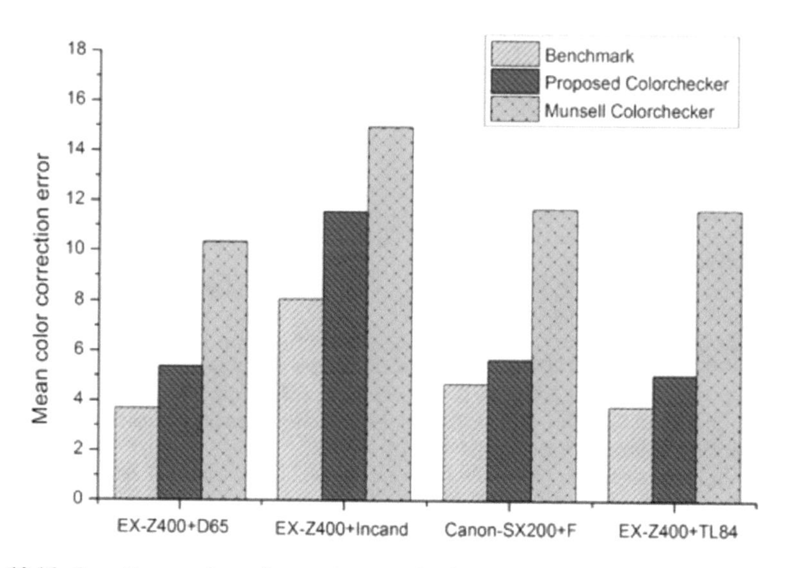

Fig. 10.16 Overall comparison of correction error for the proposed space-based colorchecker and the Munsell colorchecker. © 2016 IEEE. Reprinted, with permission, from (Wang & Zhang, 2012)

means that it corrects tongue colors more precisely than the Munsell colorchecker. Moreover, in some cases, this designed one performs even closely to the benchmark results when only 24 colors are involved. This results show that the proposed colorchecker achieves fairly accurate correction for a small number of colors.

10.6 Summary

This chapter presents a thorough and comprehensive study of the issue of a colorchecker design for precision tongue color correction. A new space-based tongue colorchecker was developed by deep analysis of three essential issues. Tongue color space was proposed to define the range of tongue colors, while 20 was found to be the *minimum sufficient number* for the colorchecker design. General selection criteria were presented to ensure promising correction performance. Two color selection methods were proposed to solve the objective function derived from these criteria. After parameter optimization, the clustering-based maximizing minimum distance in the CIELAB color space (CMMlab) was found to be the most effective one. The mean correction error of the proposed tongue colorchecker is around 5.37. Compared to the performance of the Munsell colorchecker whose mean correction error is around 10.35, the newly proposed one can improve the performance by around 48%.

Besides previous conclusive results, such as the *minimum sufficient number* is 20 and the CMMlab method performs the best, and the whole schematic framework for a colorchecker design could also be regarded as a valuable contribution to the community. Furthermore, the color selection criteria proposed in this study could be generally applied to other kinds of colorchecker designs either in other research fields, such as food color science, human dermatology, and dentistry.

References

Bala, R., Sharma, G., Monga, V., De Capelle, V., & Others. (2005). Two-dimensional transforms for device color correction and calibration. *IEEE Transactions on Image Processing, 14*(8), 1172–1186.

Bezdek, J. C., Ehrlich, R., & Full, W. (1984). FCM: The fuzzy c-means clustering algorithm. *Computers & Geosciences, 10*(2), 191–203.

Cai, Y. (2002). *A novel imaging system for tongue inspection* (pp. 159–164): IEEE; 1999.

Chang, C. C., & Lin, C. J. (2011). LIBSVM: A library for support vector machines. *ACM Transactions on Intelligent Systems and Technology (TIST), 2*(3), 27.

Chang, Y., & Reid, J. F. (1996). RGB calibration for color image analysis in machine vision. *IEEE Transactions on Image Processing, 5*(10), 1414–1422.

Cheung, V., & Westland, S. (2006). Methods for optimal color selection. *Journal of Imaging Science and Technology, 50*(5), 481–488.

Cheung, V., Westland, S., Connah, D., & Ripamonti, C. (2004). A comparative study of the characterisation of colour cameras by means of neural networks and polynomial transforms. *Coloration Technology, 120*(1), 19–25.

Cormen, T. H. (2009). *Introduction to algorithms*. Cambridge, Massachusetts: MIT Press.
de Lasarte, M., Arjona, M., Vilaseca, M., & Pujol, J. (2010). Influence of the number of samples of the training set on accuracy of color measurement and spectral reconstruction. *Journal of Imaging Science and Technology, 54*(3), 30501.
Ilie, A., & Welch, G. (2005). *Ensuring color consistency across multiple cameras* (pp. 1268–1275). New York: IEEE.
Jiang, L., Xu, W., & Chen, J. (2008). *Digital imaging system for physiological analysis by tongue colour inspection* (pp. 1833–1836). New York: IEEE.
Johnson, T. (1996). Methods for characterizing colour scanners and digital cameras. *Displays, 16*(4), 183–191.
Kang, H. R. (1997). *Color technology for electronic imaging devices*. Bellingham, Washington: SPIE press.
Kosztyán, Z. T., & Schanda, J. A. N. (2009). Adaptive statistical methods for optimal color selection and spectral characterization of color scanners and cameras. *Journal of Imaging Science and Technology, 53*(1), 10501.
Lloyd, S. P. (1982). Least squares quantization in PCM. *IEEE Transactions on Information Theory, 28*(2), 129–137.
Luo, M. R., Hong, G., & Rhodes, P. A. (2001). A study of digital camera colorimetric characterization based on polynomial modeling. *Color: Research and applications, 26*(1), 76–84.
Manevitz, L. M., & Yousef, M. (2002). One-class SVMs for document classification. *Journal of machine Learning research, 2,* 139–154.
McCamy, C. S., Marcus, H., & Davidson, J. G. (1976). A color-rendition chart. *Journal of Applied Photographic Engineering, 2*(3), 95–99.
Schölkopf, B., Platt, J. C., Shawe-Taylor, J., Smola, A. J., & Williamson, R. C. (2001). Estimating the support of a high-dimensional distribution. *Neural Computation, 13*(7), 1443–1471.
Sharma, G., & Bala, R. (Eds.). (2002). *Digital color imaging handbook*. Boca Raton, Florida: CRC Press.
Shen, L., Cai, Y., & Zhang, X. (2007). *Tongue image acquisition and analysis*. Beijing: Beijing University of Technology Press.
Shen, H., Zhang, H., Xin, J. H., & Shao, S. (2008). Optimal selection of representative colors for spectral reflectance reconstruction in a multispectral imaging system. *Applied Optics, 47*(13), 2494–2502.
Vrhel, M. J., & Trussell, H. J. (1999). Color device calibration: a mathematical formulation. *IEEE Transactions on Image Processing, 8*(12), 1796–1806.
Wang, X., & Zhang, D. (2010a). An optimized tongue image color correction scheme. *IEEE Transactions on Information Technology in Biomedicine, 14*(6), 1355–1364.
Wang, X., & Zhang, D. (2010b). A comparative study of color correction algorithms for tongue image inspection. In *Medical Biometrics* (pp. 392–402). New York: Springer.
Wang, X., & Zhang, D. (2011). Statistical tongue color distribution and its application. *Health, 2856,* 2566.
Wang, X., & Zhang, D. (2012). A New tongue colorchecker design by space representation for precise correction. *IEEE Journal of Biomedical and Health Informatics, 17*(2), 381–391.
X-Rite. (2010). Munsell colorchecker classic. [Online]. Available: http://xritephoto.com/ph_product_overview.aspx?id=1192&catid=28
Zhang, H. (2007). *Tongue image acquisition and analyzing technology*. Harbin: Harbin Institute of Technology.
Zhang, H., Wang, K., Jin, X., & Zhang, D. (2005). *SVR based color calibration for tongue image* (pp. 5065–5070). New York: IEEE.
Zhang, D., Wang, X., & Lu, G. (2010). An integrated portable standardized human tongue image acquisition system. *Chinese Patent, ZL A, 101972138.*

Chapter 11
Tongue Color Analysis for Medical Application

Abstract A novel tongue color analysis system for medical applications is introduced in this chapter. Using the tongue color gamut, tongue foreground pixels are first extracted and assigned to one of 12 colors representing this gamut. The ratio of each color for the entire image is calculated and forms a tongue color feature vector. Experimenting on a large dataset consisting of 143 Healthy and 902 Disease (13 groups of more than 10 samples and one miscellaneous group), a given tongue sample can be classified into one of these two classes with an average accuracy of 91.99%. Further testing showed that Disease samples can be split into three clusters, and within each cluster most if not all the illnesses are distinguished from one another. In total, 11 illnesses have a classification rate greater than 70%. This demonstrates a relationship between the state of the human body and its tongue color.

11.1 Introduction

The human tongue contains numerous features that can be used to diagnose disease, with color features being the most important (Chiu, 1996, 2000; DudaHart & Stork, 2012; Kirschbaum, 2000). Traditionally, medical practitioners would examine these color features based on years of experience (Li et al., 2008; Li & Yuen, 2002; Li et al., 1994; Maciocia, 1987; Ohta & Robertson, 2006; Pang, Zhang & Wang, 2005a, b). However, ambiguity and subjectivity always accompanied their diagnostic result. As a matter of fact, tongue color can be objectively analyzed through its color features, which also offers a new way to diagnose disease, one that minimizes the physical harm inflicted to patients (compared with other medical examinations).

A literature review on this topic revealed only a few papers where color features from the tongue are the main component used to diagnose disease. Su, Xu, Wang, & Xu (2011) used tongue color along with qualitative and quantitative analysis to examine 207 patients suffering from lung cancer. The patients were split into four syndrome groups according to Chinese Medicine, and the CIELAB color model was

D. Zhang et al., *Tongue Image Analysis*, DOI 10.1007/978-981-10-2167-1_11

used for quantitative classification. They reported a significant statistical difference between the four groups when it came to each tongue's CIELAB value. The correct classification rate of each group was 69.4, 54.4, 72.2, and 54.4%, respectively. A color metric was utilized (Wang, Zhang, Li, & Pang, 2001) in order to diagnose appendicitis using tongue images. Tongue samples (789) were captured from 399 patients (two samples from each person), consisting of common illnesses such as diabetes, pancreatitis, and hypertension, along with 114 images from tongues affected by appendicitis. The samples were captured using a specially designed device consisting of a 3-CCD digital camera, two D65 lights, and calibrated with a white color plate. Four color spaces (RGB, CIEXYY, CIELUV, and CIELAB) were evaluated to find the best combination. In their work, they reported a correct classification of appendicitis to be 66.67%. Pancreatitis (29 samples) and appendicitis (53 samples) tongue images again appeared in Wang & Zhang (2010), albeit this time with 56 normal samples. These images were captured with a device designed by their research center consisting of a lens, CCD sensor board, two D65 lights, and a video frame grabber. Assessing the same four spaces as Wang, Zhang, Li, & Pang (2001), the experimental results showed that normal and pancreatitis as well as appendicitis and pancreatitis can be linearly separated using color features.

In Su, Xu, Wang, & Xu (2011), the dataset was quite small and only one disease was analyzed. The patients were also diagnosed using Chinese Medicine. As for Wang, Zhang, Li, & Pang, (2001), its dataset was substantially larger but only appendicitis was classified. The samples in Wang & Zhang (2010) included two illnesses as well as normal, but their sizes were too small to have any statistical significance. Both works in Su, Xu, Wang, & Xu, (2011), Wang & Zhang (2010) did not use any image correction to ensure uniform feature extraction and analysis under different operating conditions. Also, Su, Xu, Wang, & Xu (2011), Wang & Zhang (2010), Wang, Zhang, Li, & Pang (2001) used some variation of the CIE color space to embody the tongue colors, which may not be very accurate. Therefore, there is a lack of any work on an in depth systematic tongue color analysis system for medical applications, one that accurately captures the images and represents its colors using a tongue color gamut (Wang & Zhang, 2011). In this chapter, such an application is described to address these problems. Tongue images were first captured using a specifically designed device with image correction. Afterward, the images were segmented (Zhang, 2013) with the background removed and tongue foreground remaining. Color features from each pixel were then extracted and assigned to 1 of 12 colors symbolizing the tongue color gamut (Wang & Zhang, 2011). This produced the tongue color feature vector. Experimental results were carried out on a large scale dataset consisting of 143 Healthy and 902 Disease samples (diagnosed using Western Medicine) taken from Guangdong Provincial Hospital of Traditional Chinese Medicine, Guangdong, China. The Disease class was composed of 13 specific illnesses (with at least 10 samples in each group) and one sizeable miscellaneous group (made up of various illnesses). Classification was performed between the illnesses in addition to Healthy versus Disease.

The rest of this chapter is organized as follows. An introduction to the tongue image acquisition device and dataset used is given in Sect. 11.2. Section 11.3

summarizes the tongue color gamut and explains how color features are extracted by using it. In Sect. 11.4, classification between the two classes of Healthy and Disease is performed. Following this, illnesses in the Disease class are classified. Finally, concluding remarks are made in Sect. 11.5.

11.2 Tongue Image Acquisition Device and Dataset

The tongue database is composed of 1045 images (one image per person) split into 143 Healthy and 902 Disease captured at Guangdong Provincial Hospital of Traditional Chinese Medicine, Guangdong, China. The patients' consent was obtained according to the Declaration of Helsinki and the Ethical Committee of the Institution in which the work was performed approved it. The capture device used was a three-chip CCD camera with 8-bit resolution and two-D65 fluorescent tubes placed symmetrically around the camera in order to produce a uniform illumination. The images captured were color corrected (Zhang, Pang, Li, Wang, & Zhang, 2005) to eliminate any noise caused by variations of illumination and device dependency. This allowed consistent feature extraction and classification in the following steps. Figure 2.12a shows the capture device. Healthy samples were verified through a blood test and other experiments. If indicators from the tests fell within a certain range they were deemed fit. In the Disease class, samples were collected from inpatients with illnesses determined by their admission note and diagnosed using Western Medical practices. Inpatients suffering from the same illness were grouped together into a single class. In total, there were 13 ailment groups (with at least 10 samples) and one miscellaneous group containing various illnesses. A summary of the Disease class breakdown is given in Table 11.1. Please note any future reference to a specific illness in Table 11.1 will be made using its Disease ID.

Table 11.1 Disease class statistics listing the ID, name, and number of samples

Disease ID	Disease name	No. of samples
1	Chronic kidney disease	141
2	Diabetes	69
3	Nephritis	10
4	Hypertension	66
5	Verrucous gastritis	25
6	Pneumonia	10
7	Nephritic syndrome	10
8	Chronic cerebral circulation insufficiency	14
9	Upper respiratory tract infection	12
10	Erosive gastritis	10
11	Coronary heart disease	13
12	Chronic bronchitis	11
13	Mixed hemorrhoid	11
14	Miscellaneous	500

11.3 Tongue Color Gamut and Color Features Extraction

The following section describes how color features are extracted from tongue images. The tongue color gamut is first summarized in Sect. 11.3.1. In Sect. 11.3.2, every foreground tongue pixel is compared to 12 colors representing the tongue color gamut and assigned its nearest color. This forms the color features.

11.3.1 Tongue Color Gamut

The tongue color gamut (Wang & Zhang, 2011) represents all possible colors that appear on the tongue surface and exists within the red boundary shown in Fig. 11.1 (CIE*xy* chromaticity diagram). Further investigation revealed that 98% of the points lie inside the black boundary. To represent the tongue color gamut using 12 colors, the RGB color space was employed and plotted in Fig. 11.2. On the RG line point Y (Yellow) was marked. Between R and B, point P (Purple) was marked and C (Cyan) was marked between G and B. The center of the RGB color space was calculated and designated as W (White), the first of the 12 colors (see Fig. 11.2). Then, for each R (Red), B (Blue), Y, P, and C point, a straight line was drawn to W. Each time these lines intersected the tongue color gamut, a new color was added to represent the 12 colors. This accounts for R, Y, C, B, and P. LR (Light red), LP (Light purple), and LB (Light blue) were midpoints between lines from the black boundary to W, while DR (Deep red) was selected as no previous point occupies

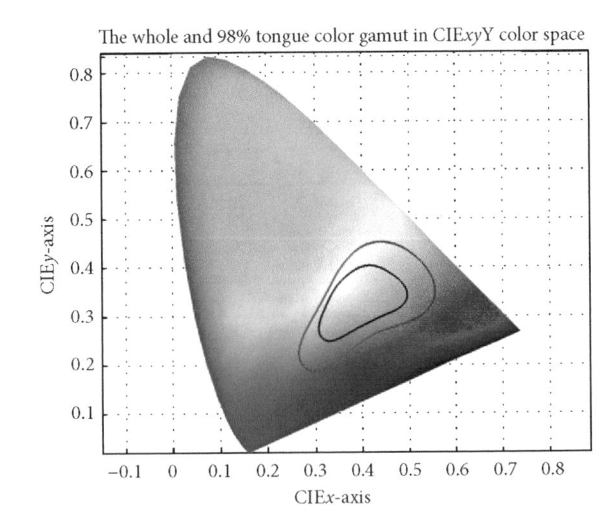

Fig. 11.1 A color gamut in the CIE*xy*Y color space depicting the tongue color gamut inside the red boundary. Furthermore, 98% of the tongue color gamut can be located within the black boundary

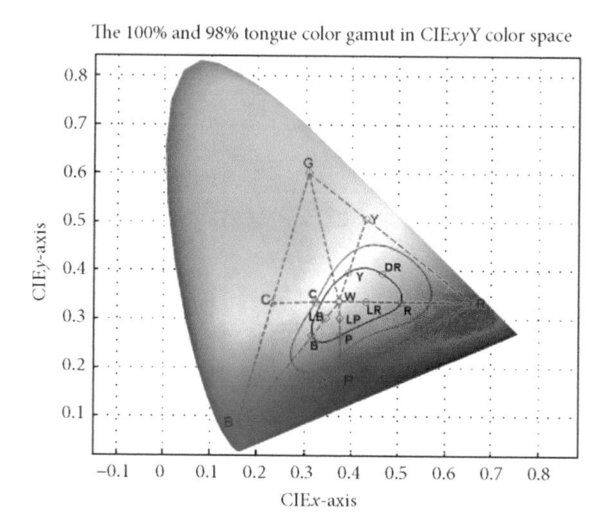

Fig. 11.2 The tongue color gamut can be represented using several points by drawing lines from the RGB color space

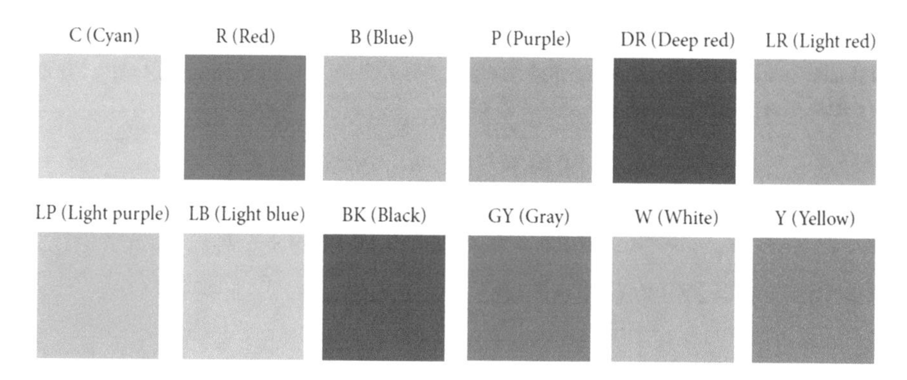

Fig. 11.3 12 colors representing the tongue color gamut with its label on top

that area. More details about the tongue color gamut can be found in (Wang & Zhang, 2011). GY (Gray) and BK (Black) are not shown in Fig. 11.2 since both belong to gray scale.

The 12 colors representing the tongue color gamut were extracted from Fig. 11.2 and shown in Fig. 11.3 as a color square with its label on top. Correspondingly, its RGB and CIELAB values are given in Table 11.2.

Table 11.2 RGB and CIELAB values of the 12 colors

Color	[RGB]	[LAB]
C (Cyan)	[188 188 185]	[76.0693 −0.5580 1.3615]
R (Red)	[189 99 91]	[52.2540 34.8412 21.3002]
B (Blue)	[183 165 180]	[69.4695 9.5423 −5.4951]
P (Purple)	[226 142 214]	[69.4695 42.4732 −23.8880]
DR (Deep red)	[136 72 49]	[37.8424 24.5503 25.396]
LR (Light red)	[227 150 147]	[69.4695 28.4947 13.3940]
LP (Light purple)	[225 173 207]	[76.0693 24.3246 −9.7749]
LB (Light blue)	[204 183 186]	[76.0693 7.8917 0.9885]
BK (Black)	[107 86 56]	[37.8424 3.9632 20.5874]
GY (Gray)	[163 146 143]	[61.6542 5.7160 3.7317]
W (White)	[200 167 160]	[70.976310.9843 8.2952]
Y (Yellow)	[166 129 93]	[56.3164 9.5539 24.4546]

11.3.2 Tongue Color Features

Given a tongue image, segmentation was first applied to locate all foreground tongue pixels (Zhang, 2013). Having located each pixel, its corresponding RGB value was extracted and converted to CIELAB (Zhang, Wang, Jin, & Zhang, 2005) by first converting RBG to CIEXYZ using

$$\begin{bmatrix} X \\ Y \\ Z \end{bmatrix} = \begin{bmatrix} 0.4124 & 0.3576 & 0.1805 \\ 0.2126 & 0.7152 & 0.0722 \\ 0.0193 & 0.1192 & 0.9505 \end{bmatrix} \begin{bmatrix} R \\ G \\ B \end{bmatrix} \tag{11.1}$$

followed by CIEXYZ to CIELAB via

$$\begin{aligned} L^* &= 116\left(\frac{Y}{Y_0}\right) - 16, \\ a^* &= 500\left[f\left(\frac{X}{X_0}\right) - f\left(\frac{Y}{Y_0}\right)\right], \\ b^* &= 200\left[f\left(\frac{Y}{Y_0}\right) - f\left(\frac{Z}{Z_0}\right)\right], \end{aligned} \tag{11.2}$$

Where $f(x) = \begin{cases} x^{1/3} & (x > 0.008856) \\ 7.787x + \frac{16}{116} & (x \leq 0.008856) \end{cases}$.

In (11.2), X_0, Y_0, and Z_0 are the CIEXYZ tristimulus values of the reference white point. The LAB values were then compared to 12 colors from the tongue color gamut (see Table 11.2) and assigned the color which was closest to it (measured using the Euclidean distance). After calculating all tongue foreground pixels, the total of each color was summed and divided by the number of pixels. This ratio of the 12 colors formed the tongue color feature vector $\boldsymbol{v}$, where $\boldsymbol{v} = [c_1, c_2, c_3, c_4, c_5, c_6, c_7, c_8, c_9, c_{10}, c_{11}, c_{12}]$ and c_i represents the sequence of colors in Table 11.2. As an example, the color features of two tongues are shown in visual form (refer to Figs. 11.4 and 11.5) along with their extracted tongue color feature vectors, where the original image is decomposed into one of the 12 colors. Figure 11.4 is from a Healthy sample and Fig. 11.5 is from a Disease sample. In the Healthy sample, the majority of pixels are LR and for the Disease sample it is GY.

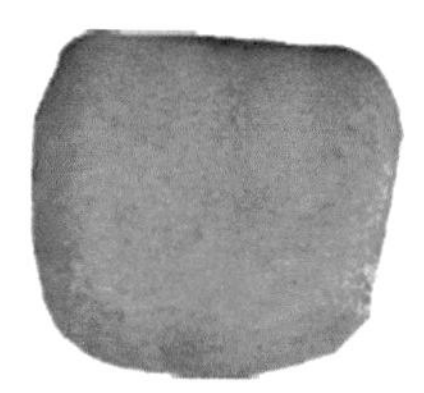

v = (0.001 17.067 0 0 6.004 54.722 0.029 0.205 5.551 4.766 3.711 7.899)

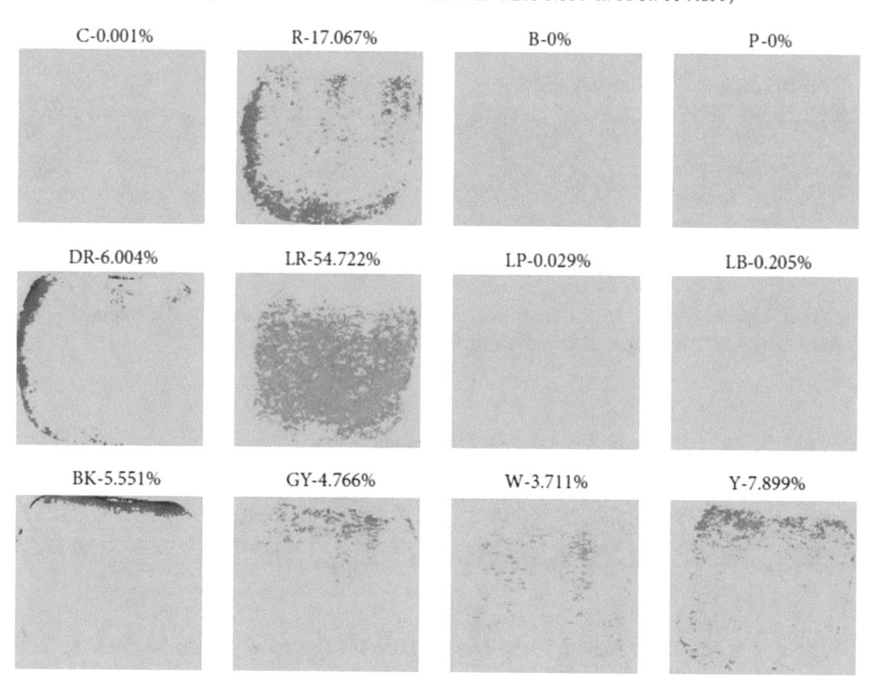

Fig. 11.4 Healthy tongue sample, its tongue color feature vector and corresponding 12-color makeup with most of the pixels classified as LR

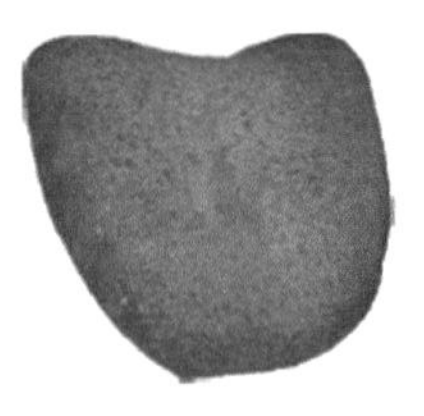

v = (0.053 0.002 0.085 0 2.092 0 0.001 0.053 35.648 61.108 0.097 0.853)

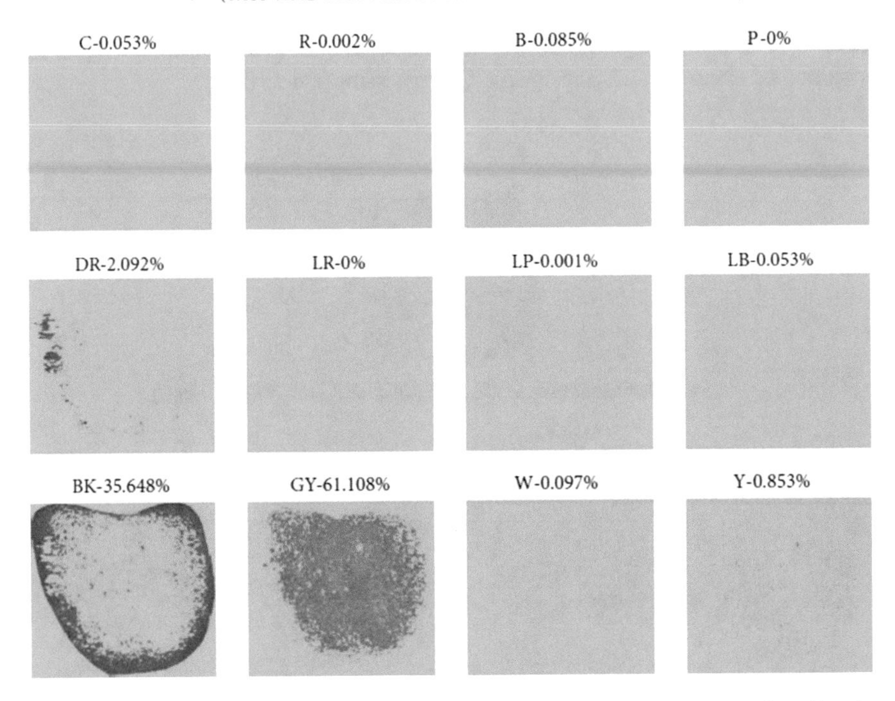

Fig. 11.5 Disease tongue sample, its tongue color feature vector and corresponding 12-color makeup with most of the pixels classified as GY

Table 11.3 Mean of the color features for Healthy and Disease

	R	DR	LR	BK	GY	W	Y
Healthy	20.9284	5.6679	33.8483	8.2356	14.5583	7.9166	8.0485
Disease	28.2901	15.5951	11.0277	15.4325	16.2247	2.4990	10.6382

The mean colors of Healthy and Disease are displayed in Table 11.3 along with three typical samples from each class shown in Fig. 11.6. Disease tongues have a higher ratio in R, DR, BK, GY, and Y according to Table 11.3. On the other hand, LR and W are greater in Healthy tongues. Only 7 colors are listed out of the 12 as the remaining 5 have ratios of less than 1%.

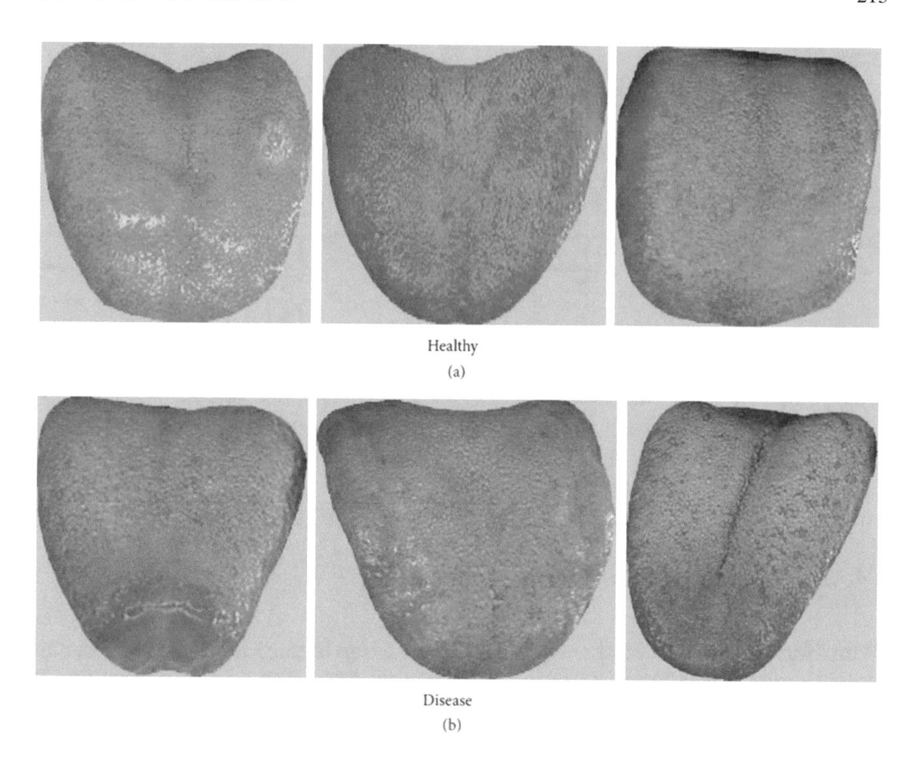

Fig. 11.6 Three typical Healthy (**a**) and Disease (**b**) samples

11.4 Results and Discussion

In this section, classification using color features is described. Classification between Healthy versus Disease is first given in Sect. 11.4.1, while illnesses in Disease are classified in Sect. 11.4.2.

11.4.1 Healthy Versus Disease Classification

Table 11.4 shows the classification rate between Healthy versus Disease on the test data. Half the images were randomly selected from either class to represent the training set and the remaining samples assigned to the test set. The training data in each class are the mean tongue color features of Healthy and Disease. To reduce the number of tongue color features, feature selection with sequential forward search was implemented. Both *k*-NN (Zhang, Liang, Wang, Fan, & Li, 2005) and SVM (Zhang, Liang, Wang, Fan, & Li, 2005) using a quadratic kernel were tested producing the same result as can be seen in Table 11.4. This means for *k*-NN and SVM the tongue color feature vector of the training set consisting of Healthy and Disease

Table 11.4 Classification result between Healthy versus Disease using *k*-NN and SVM

Classification method	Average accuracy (%)
k-NN	91.99
SVM	91.99

Table 11.5 Distribution of the illnesses within the clusters

Cluster number	Disease group
1	1 13
2	5 7 8 9 10 12
3	2 3 4 6 11

was placed in an *n*-dimensional space. Each tongue color feature vector representing the test set was mapped to this space and classified depending on its classification rule (*k*-NN or SVM).

11.4.2 Typical Disease Analysis

With Healthy versus Disease separated the next step is to examine whether certain illnesses within the Disease class can be distinguished from one another. All 13 illnesses were grouped into three clusters by the fuzzy c-means(FCM) (Zhang, Liang, Wang, Fan, & Li, 2005), with Table 11.5 illustrating to which cluster each illness belongs. The mean tongue color features of each cluster are shown in Table 11.6. R, DR, and LR are greater in Cluster 3. Cluster 2 has higher concentrations of GY, BK, and W, while Y is more significant in Cluster 1.

Table 11.7 shows the classification rate of the three clusters calculated in groups of two. In each case, the two clusters in question are clearly separable as seen in this table and Figs. 11.7, 11.8, and 11.9. Three typical samples from each cluster are depicted in Fig. 11.10. From a visual perspective the tongue color features in each cluster are quite different compared to the rest.

Table 11.6 Mean tongue color features of the three clusters

Cluster number	R	DR	LR	BK	GY	W	Y
1	21.56	13.972	12.265	12.535	9.524	3.703	26.191
2	17.116	11.980	9.437	15.574	34.733	4.111	6.539
3	40.736	15.396	15.872	8.232	10.770	1.668	7.051

Table 11.7 Classification result between the three clusters compared in groups of two

Cluster comparison	Average accuracy (%)
Cluster 1 versus Cluster 2	100
Cluster 1 versus Cluster 3	97.75
Cluster 2 versus Cluster 3	99.63

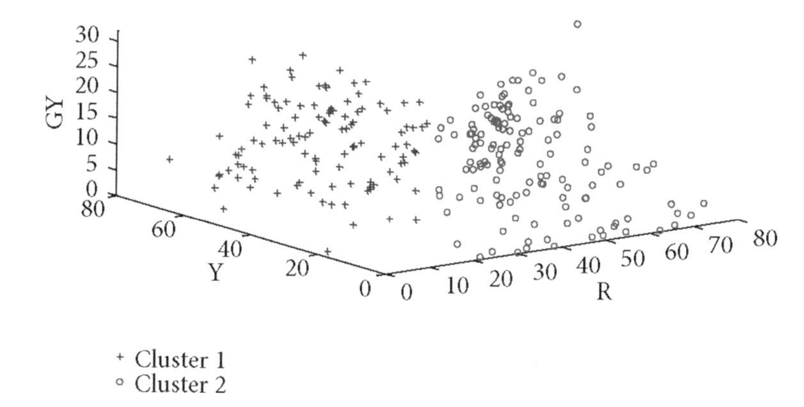

Fig. 11.7 Plot of Cluster 1 versus Cluster 2

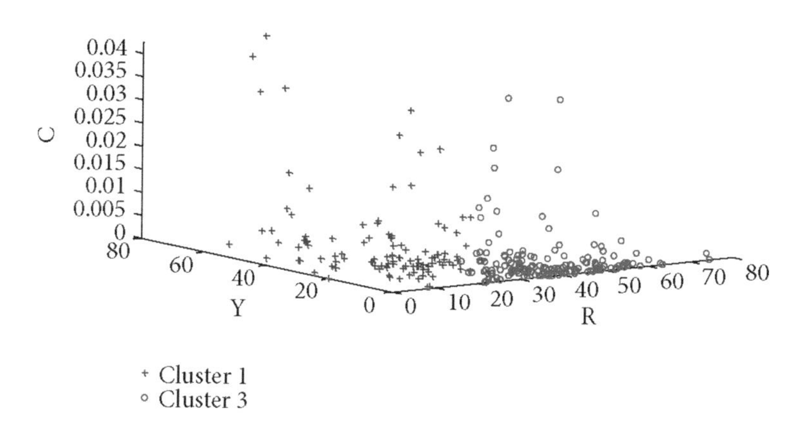

Fig. 11.8 Plot of Cluster 1 versus Cluster 3

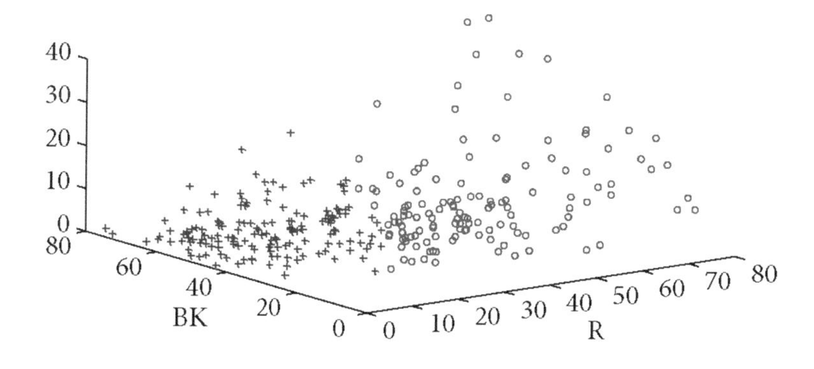

Fig. 11.9 Plot of Cluster 3 versus Cluster 2

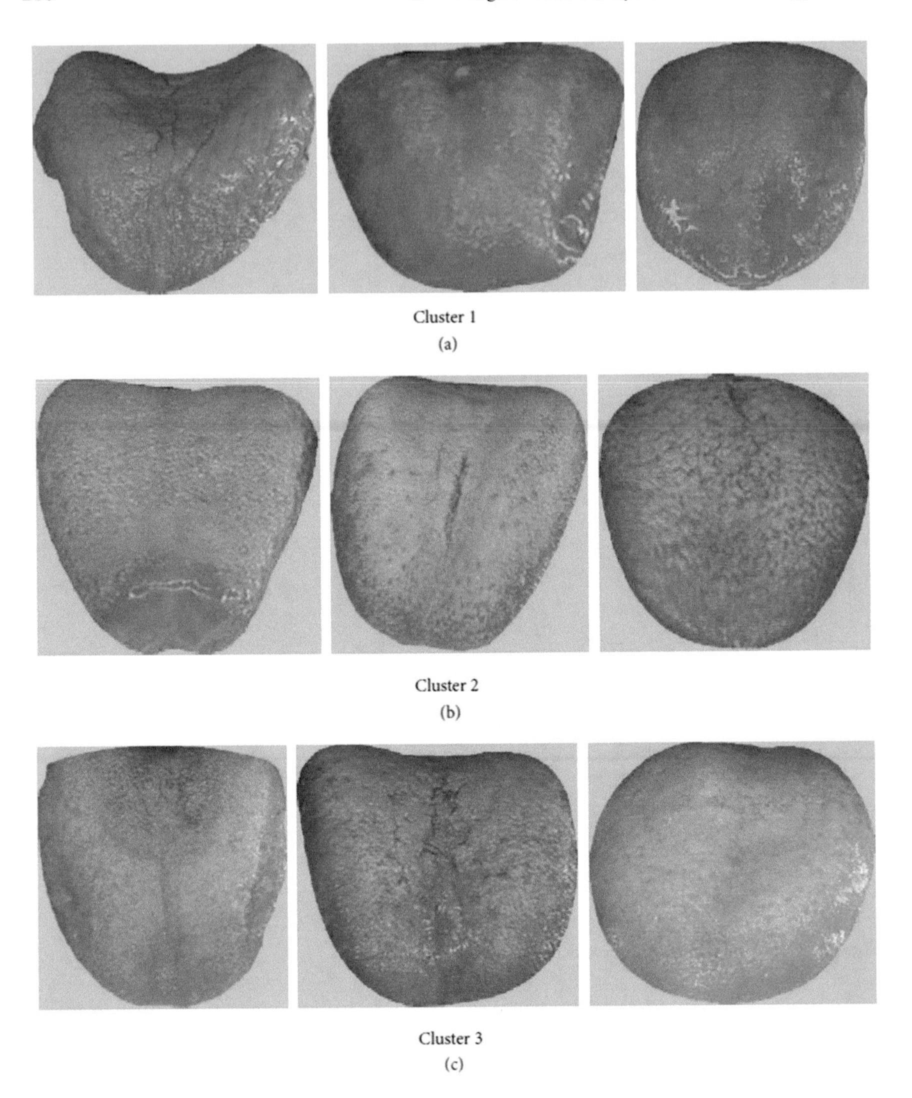

Fig. 11.10 Three typical samples from each cluster

Next, each cluster was examined one by one to determine whether illnesses within it can be classified. This was accomplished by comparing illnesses inside the cluster and removing the illness with the highest classification. The process was repeated until all illnesses had been classified. The same experimental setup described in Sect. 11.4.1 was applied, where half the images were randomly selected for training and test sets. Both *k*-NN and SVM were used as the classifiers along with sequential forward search for feature selection. An illness was considered successfully classified if its average accuracy was greater than or equal to 70%.

Table 11.8 Classification result of the illnesses

Disease ID	Cluster number	k-NN (%)	SVM (%)
1	1	72.53	76.08
2	3	54.87	54.41
3	3	72.97	75.68
4	3	54.87	54.41
5	2	81.45	81.45
6	3	78.61	74.05
7	2	83.33	93.06
8	2	72.02	83.33
9	2	77.78	83.33
10	2	78.71	87.10
11	3	72.82	73.56
12	2	81.45	81.45
13	1	72.53	76.08

The average accuracies stated in the following paragraph represents only SVM. For a complete list of the results please refer to Table 11.8.

Diseases 1 and 13 in Cluster 1 are separable with an average accuracy of 76.08%. In Cluster 2, Disease 7 can be first removed as its classification rate of 93.06% is the highest amongst the six illnesses. Diseases 10, 8, and 9 are subsequently taken out in that order which leaves illnesses 5 and 12 (classification rate of 81.45%). Looking at Cluster 3, Disease 6 with a classification rate of 74.05% is initially removed from the pack. This is followed by Diseases 3 and 11 leaving 2 and 4 which produced the lowest classification result of 54.41%. Table 11.8 summarizes this result. Diseases 1, 3, 5, 6, 7, 8, 9, 10, 11, 12, and 13 achieved an average accuracy greater than 70% and therefore are deemed successfully classified. Typical samples of the successfully classified illnesses are shown in Figs. 11.11, 11.12, 11.13, 11.14, 11.15, 11.16, 11.17, 11.18, 11.19, 11.20, and 11.21.

As part of the future work, we plan on returning to Guangdong Provincial Hospital of Traditional Chinese Medicine and collecting more diseased tongue

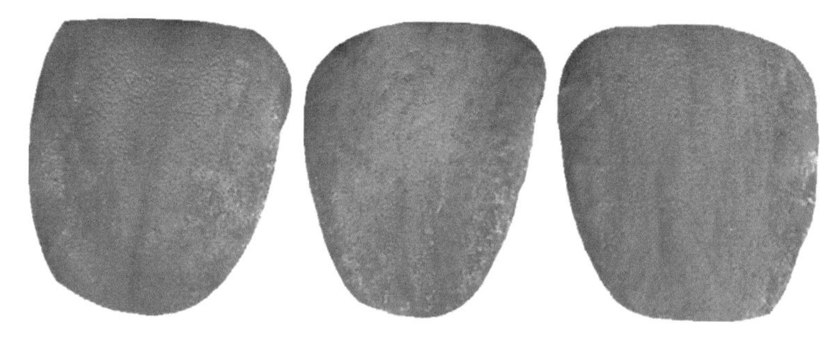

Fig. 11.11 Three typical samples from Disease 1

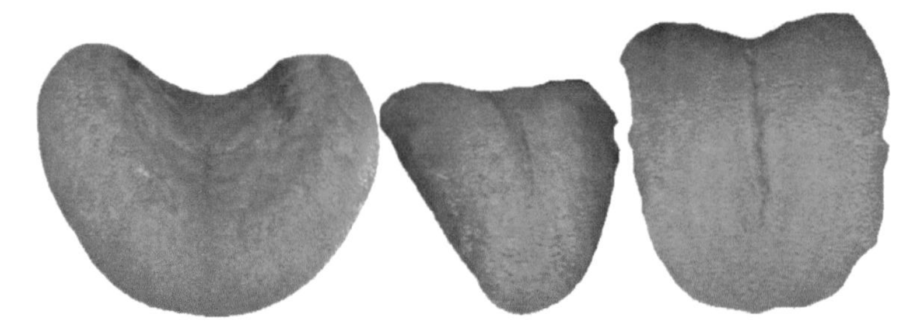

Fig. 11.12 Three typical samples from Disease 3

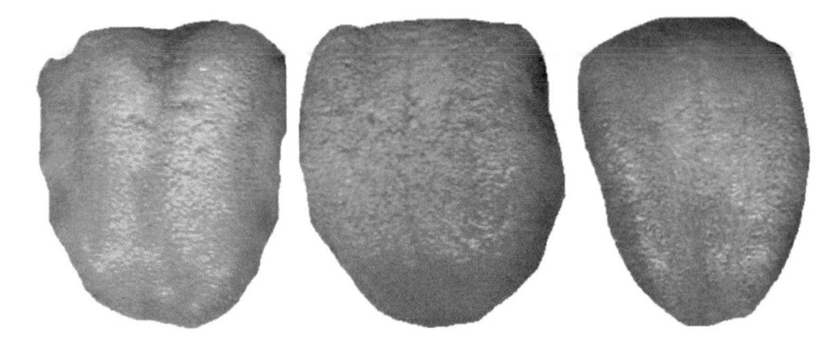

Fig. 11.13 Three typical samples from Disease 5

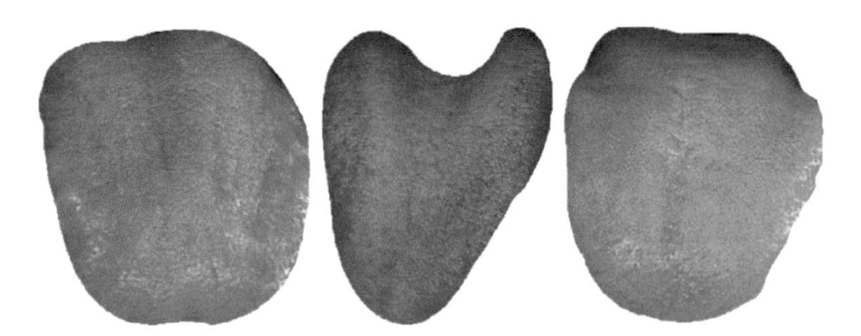

Fig. 11.14 Three typical samples from Disease 6

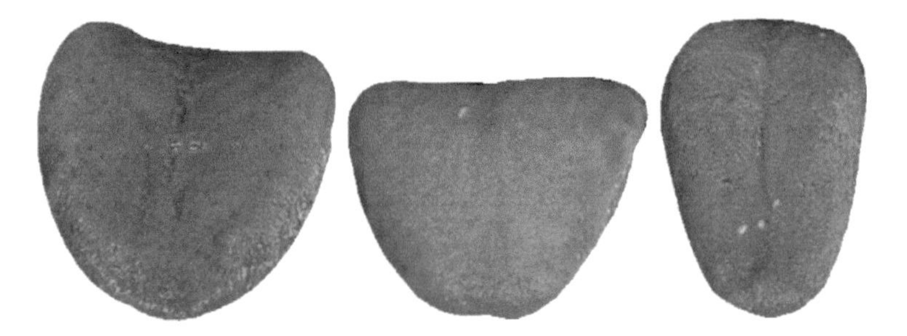

Fig. 11.15 Three typical samples from Disease 7

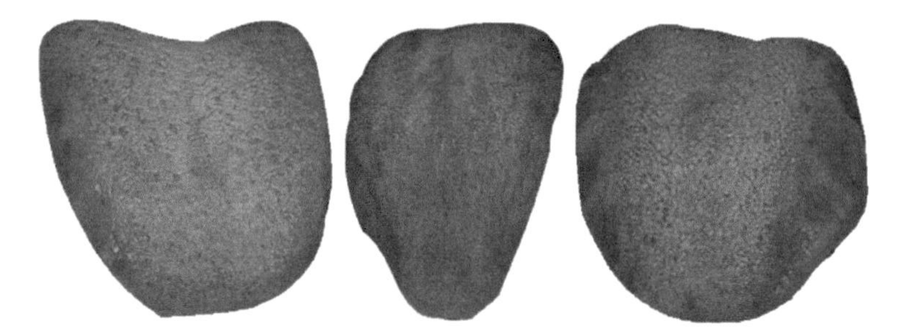

Fig. 11.16 Three typical samples from Disease 8

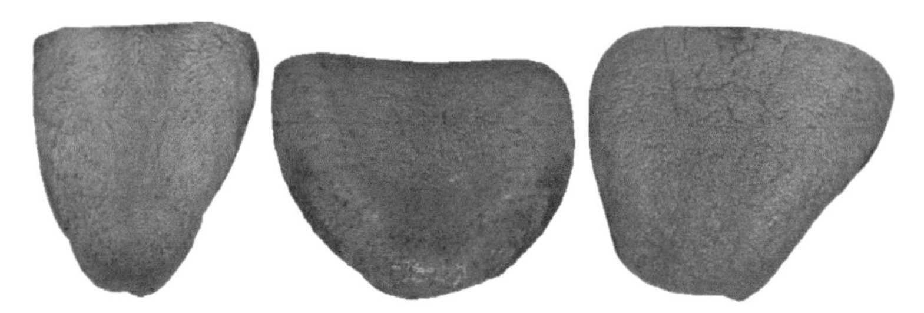

Fig. 11.17 Three typical samples from Disease 9

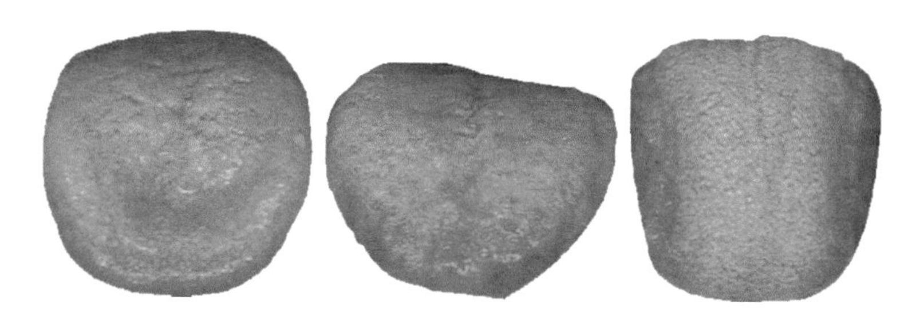

Fig. 11.18 Three typical samples from Disease 10

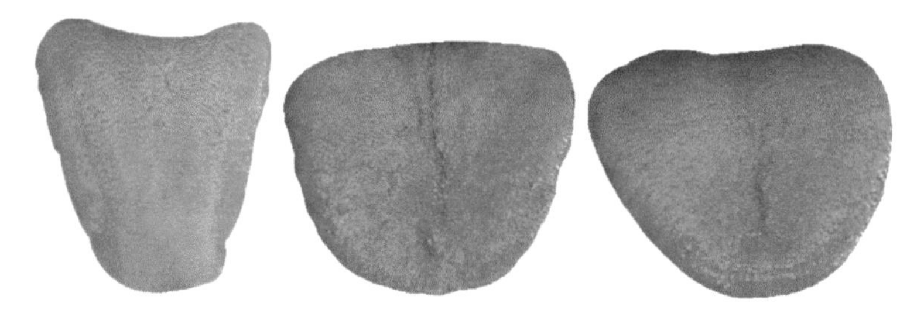

Fig. 11.19 Three typical samples from Disease 11

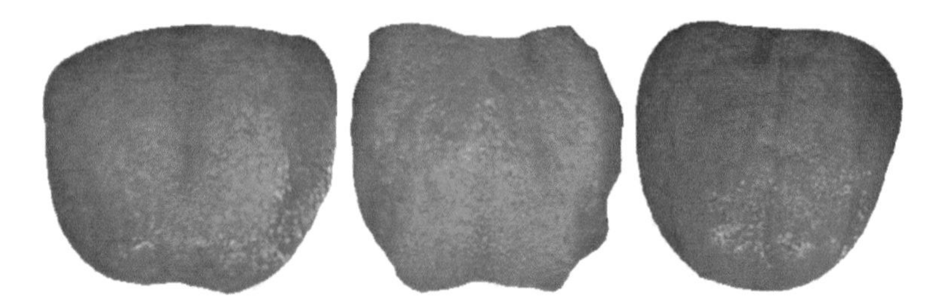

Fig. 11.20 Three typical samples from Disease 12

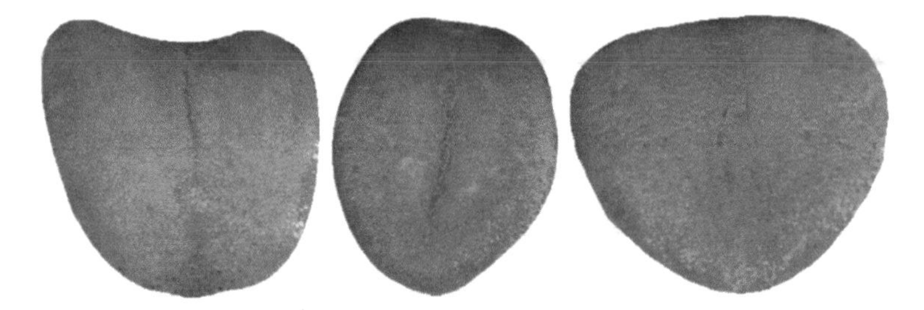

Fig. 11.21 Three typical samples from Disease 13

images. Color features (discussed in Sect. 11.3.2) will be extracted from these new images before combining them with the previous batch. The experimental results in the form of Healthy versus Disease classification and typical disease analysis will be recalculated in order to further validate its statistical accuracy.

11.5 Summary

In this chapter, we propose a tongue color analysis method for tongue image classification. Given a tongue image, the method is capable of distinguishing Healthy versus Disease with an average accuracy of 91.99%. If the image is from Disease, it is further assigned to one of three clusters. From these clusters 11 illnesses can be successfully classified giving a classification rate of at least 70%. The proposed method uses a special capture device with image correction and extracts a tongue color feature vector from each image. This vector consists of 12 color ratios calculated with the tongue color gamut to better characterize each foreground tongue pixel. Testing was carried out on a large dataset collected from Guangdong, China, consisting of 143 Healthy and 902 Disease images (13 specific illnesses with at least 10 samples and a miscellaneous folder). The experimental results showed that there is a relationship between tongue color and the state of the human body, which can be used in medical applications to detect various illnesses. This can potentially lead to a new painless and efficient way to examine patients.

References

Chiu, C. (1996). The development of a computerized tongue diagnosis system. *Biomedical Engineering Applications Basis Communications, 8,* 342–350.
Chiu, C. (2000). A novel approach based on computerized image analysis for traditional Chinese medical diagnosis of the tongue. *Computer Methods and Programs in Biomedicine, 61*(2), 77–89.
Duda, R. O., Hart, P. E., & Stork, D. G. (2012). *Pattern classification,* New York: Wiley.
Kirschbaum, B. (2000). *Atlas of Chinese tongue diagnosis* (Vol. 1), Eastland Press.
Li, B., Huang, Q., Lu, Y., Chen, S., Liang, R., & Wang, Z. (2008). A method of classifying tongue colors for traditional chinese medicine diagnosis based on the CIELAB color space. In *Medical Biometrics* (pp. 153–159), New York: Springer.
Li, C. H., & Yuen, P. C. (2002). Tongue image matching using color content. *Pattern Recognition, 35*(2), 407–419.
Li, N. M., et al. (1994). The contemporary investigations of computerized tongue diagnosis. *The Handbook of Chinese Tongue Diagnosis,* 1315–1317.
Maciocia, G. (1987). *Tongue diagnosis in Chinese medicine,* Eastland press.
Ohta, N., & Robertson, A. (2006). *Colorimetry: fundamentals and applications,* New York: Wiley.
Pang, B., Zhang, D., & Wang, K. (2005a). Tongue image analysis for appendicitis diagnosis. *Information Sciences, 175*(3), 160–176.
Pang, B., Zhang, D., & Wang, K. (2005b). The bi-elliptical deformable contour and its application to automated tongue segmentation in Chinese medicine. *IEEE Transactions on Medical Imaging, 24*(8), 946–956.
Su, W., Xu, Z., Wang, Z., & Xu, J. (2011). Objectified study on tongue images of patients with lung cancer of different syndromes. *Chinese Journal of Integrative Medicine, 17,* 272–276.
Wang, X., & Zhang, D. (2010). An optimized tongue image color correction scheme. *IEEE Transactions on Information Technology in Biomedicine, 14*(6), 1355–1364.
Wang, X., & Zhang, D. (2011). Statistical tongue color distribution and its application. *Health, 2856,* 2566.
Wang, K., Zhang, D., Li, N., & Pang, B. (2001). Tongue diagnosis based on biometric pattern recognition technology. *Pattern Recognition, 10,* 1581918921–1581918949.
Zhang, D. D. (2013). *Automated biometrics: Technologies and systems* (Vol. 7), Berlin: Springer Science & Business Media.
Zhang, D., & Pang, B. (2005). Computerized diagnosis from tongue appearance using quantitative feature classification. *The American Journal of Chinese Medicine, 33*(06), 859–866.
Zhang, H., Wang, K., Jin, X., & Zhang, D. (2005). SVR based color calibration for tongue image (pp. 5065–5070), IEEE.
Zhang, Y., Liang, R., Wang, K., Fan, Y., & Li, N. (2005b). Analysis of the color characteristics of tongue digital images from 884 physical examination cases. *Journal of Beijing University of Traditional Chinese Medicine, 28*(001), 73–75.

Chapter 12
Statistical Analysis of Tongue Color and Its Applications in Diagnosis

Abstract In this chapter, an in-depth analysis of the statistical distribution characteristics of human tongue color with the aim of proposing a mathematically described tongue color space for diagnostic feature extraction is presented. Three characteristics of tongue color space, i.e., the tongue color gamut that defines the range of colors, color centers of 12 tongue color categories, and color distribution of typical image features in the tongue color gamut were investigated in this chapter. Based on a large database, which contains over 9000 tongue images collected by a specially designed noncontact colorimetric imaging system using a digital camera, the tongue color gamut was established in the CIE chromaticity diagram by an innovatively proposed color gamut boundary descriptor using a one-class SVM algorithm. Then, the centers of 12 tongue color categories were defined. Furthermore, color distributions of several typical tongue features, such as red point and petechial point, were obtained to build a relationship between the tongue color space and color distributions of various tongue features. With the obtained tongue color space, a new color feature extraction method was proposed for diagnostic classification purposes, with experimental results validating its effectiveness.

12.1 Introduction

Tongue image analysis, especially its chromatic features provide plenty of valuable diagnostic information reveals disorders or even pathological changes of internal organs in computerized tongue diagnosis systems (Pang, Zhang, Li, & Wang, 2004; Zhang, Pang, Li, Wang, & Zhang, 2005; Chiu, 2000; Maciocia, 1987; Wang, Yang, Zhou, & Wang, 2007). During the past several years, certain achievements have been made in tongue color analysis and diagnostic classification technologies. Nevertheless, many ambiguous and subjective factors exist. For example, due to a lack of knowledge about tongue color distribution in color spaces (CIE*XYZ*, CIE*LAB*, etc.), the range of tongue color and centers for typical color categories have not been objectively defined. Most research on identifying tongue color categories (Huang & Li, 2008; Kakumanu, Makrogiannis, & Bourbakis, 2007) had to

D. Zhang et al., *Tongue Image Analysis*, DOI 10.1007/978-981-10-2167-1_12

be conducted based on samples that were subjectively labeled by TCM (Traditional Chinese Medicine) practitioners. Their obtained results may be unstable and imprecise, or even suffer from limited applicability. In view of this situation, to analyze the statistical distribution characteristics of tongue colors, i.e., a tongue color space, which includes the tongue color gamut (range of tongue colors), centers of typical tongue color categories, and color distribution of typical image features, is of great importance for accurate tongue feature extraction and diagnosis. Furthermore, this fundamental tongue color space may also promote the development of specialized tongue image acquisition devices and image processing algorithms.

Although some research has been done in skin color characterization (Hsu, Abdel–Mottaleb, & Jain, 2002; Jones & Rehg, 2002; Igarashi, Nishino, & Nayar, 2007; Joiner, 2004) and tooth color analysis (Ahn & Lee, 2008; O'Brien, Hemmendinger, Boenke, Linger, & Groh, 1997; Yuan, Brewer, Monaco, & Davis, 2007; Li et al., 2008), there has been no comprehensive study on tongue color distribution analysis. This might be due to two possible reasons: (i) first, there are not enough high quality tongue images. For example, in the pioneering study on tongue color space by Li et al. (Cai, 2002), fewer than 200 images were used, which means that his results were not statistically convincing. Tongue images were usually collected by various digital cameras without strict control of the illuminance and environmental conditions, and a color correction procedure was not involved in the post-processing stage (Chiu, 2000; Pang, Zhang, & Wang, 2005). Hence, most of these images were of poor quality and not applicable. (ii) Second, there is not a "complete" tongue image database that covers people of various health statuses. Most researchers usually focused their research on image samples collected from specific health-status groups, such as appendicitis (Zhang, Liang, Wang, Fan, & Li, 2005), physical examination cases (Xu, Zhang, Li, Tu, & Fei, 2010) and sub-healthy samples (Zhang, Wang, & Lu, 2010). Their databases are consequently nonrepresentative and biased. There is no comprehensive tongue image database, which can cover all health statuses, especially typical disease samples.

Based on a large and high quality tongue image database, this chapter conducts an in-depth analysis of the statistical distribution characteristics of tongue color in order to build a mathematically described tongue color space for feature extraction and diagnostics. As a basis of this study, the image database, which contains over 9000 tongue images and covers various health-status subjects, including healthy, sub-healthy, and over 200 types of diseases, has been collected during the past three years by a specially designed noncontact colorimetric imaging system using a digital camera (Wang & Zhang, 2013; Sch O Lkopf, Platt, Shawe-Taylor, Smola, & Williamson, 2001). Representative colors were then extracted from each image, and combined to form a tongue color distribution in the CIE *x-y* chromaticity diagram. The distribution was then modeled by an innovatively proposed color gamut boundary descriptor using a one-class SVM algorithm (Manevitz & Yousef, 2002; Li, 2011). This generated tongue color gamut can be used to classify tongue-related colors with tongue-unrelated colors. In addition, color center values for 12 tongue color categories were defined based on the obtained tongue color gamut. These color centers were later applied for diagnostic color feature extraction. Moreover, in order to investigate the relationship between tongue features and their corresponding distributions in the tongue color space, several typical tongue features, including red point and petechial point, were detected and subsequently projected to find their corresponding distribution. Finally, based on the investigation of the tongue color space, feature extraction methods were proposed for diagnostic classification purposes, such as classification of healthy and nonhealthy people. Evaluation experiments were conducted to validate the effectiveness of the proposed methods.

The remainder of this chapter is organized as follows. Section 12.2 summarizes tongue image acquisition, color correction, and the composition of the tongue image database. In Sect. 12.3, in order to establish the tongue color space, distribution characteristics of tongue colors are thoroughly described, including the tongue color gamut and its boundary model, typical color centers, and distribution of typical image features. Based on the established tongue color space, Sect. 12.4 presents feature extraction methods and corresponding testing results. Finally, this study is concluded in Sect. 12.5.

12.2 Tongue Image Acquisition and Database

This section describes the tongue image database employed in this study. Section 12.2.1 briefly introduces how the imaging device was designed to ensure the acquisition of high quality and fidelity images. Then, in order to calibrate variations caused by the imaging system components, and to render color images into a device independent sRGB color space, the color correction process is presented in Sect. 12.2.2. Finally, Sect. 12.2.3 provides detailed composition of the tongue image database.

12.2.1 Tongue Image Acquisition Device

There are two essential factors when designing an image acquisition device: (i) illumination, including the illuminant and the environment, and (ii) the imaging camera, including the imaging lens and the CCD (Charge Coupled Device).

According to tongue diagnostic practices, the best illumination for tongue inspection is daylight sunshine in open air (Wang, Yang, Zhou, & Wang, 2007; Wyszecki & Stiles, 1982). Therefore, the commonly used standard illuminant D50 (Green & MacDonald, 2011), which is recommended by CIE (Commission International de l'Eclairage) as a substitute for daylight illumination, was utilized in this device. Also, the illuminant should be small in size and low in power (for safety concerns). After these comprehensive considerations, two OSRAM fluorescent lamps (L8 W-954) were chosen by elaborately comparing a number of products produced by lighting companies (OSRAM, Philips, and GE lighting). These two

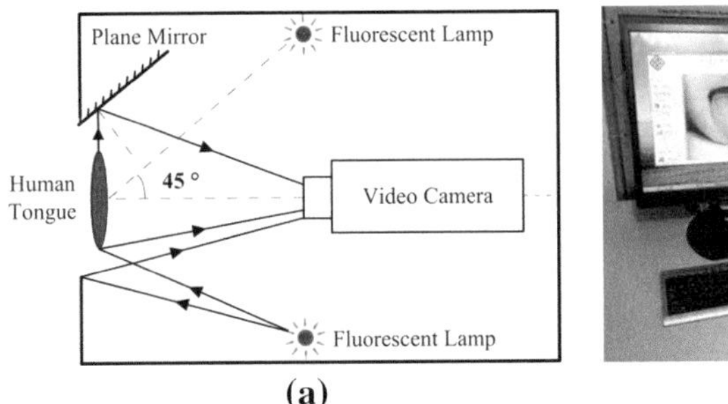

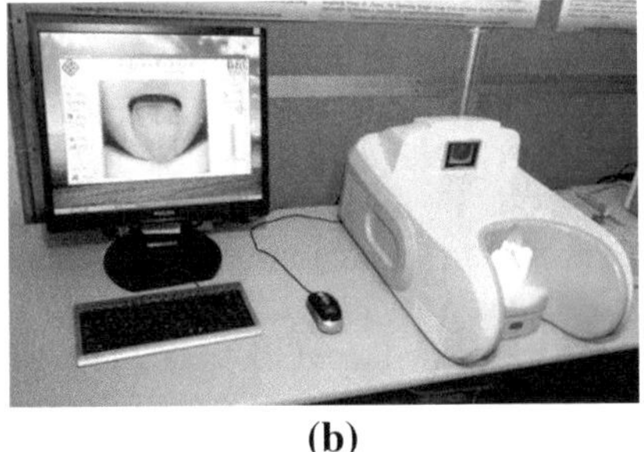

Fig. 12.1 Tongue image acquisition device. **a** Top view of the imaging path and viewing geometry of the tongue imaging device. **b** Appearance of the device and the system interface. © 2016 IEEE. Reprinted, with permission, from Wang, Zhang, Yang, Wang, and Zhang (2013)

lamps provide superb daylight quality and precise color rendering performance (color render index is 90) for tongue image acquisition.

Figure 12.1a shows the schematic diagram for the top view of this device. Both the illuminant and imaging camera are placed inside a semi-closed black box (Fig. 12.1b presents its appearance). The imaging camera is placed in the center of the device, and two fluorescent lamps are placed on either side of the camera. The angle between the incident light and the emergent light is 45°, which is recommended by CIE (Green & MacDonald, 2011).

The imaging camera in the device is a SONY 3-CCD video camera (Sony DXC-390P). Compared to a single CCD camera, a 3-CCD camera can provide superior image quality because it uses three separate CCDs for color measurement. This is a high end industrial camera that can acquire 25 images per second. The image size is 768 × 576 pixels. Since the imaging window size is 10 cm × 8 cm, the resolution of the captured image is larger than 180 dpi, which meets the requirement for tongue texture analysis [The minimum resolution for tongue imaging is 72 dpi (Sch O Lkopf, Platt, Shawe–Taylor, Smola, & Williamson, 2001)].

12.2.2 Color Correction of Tongue Images

Color images produced by digital cameras suffer from device dependent color space rendering, i.e., generated color information is dependent on the imaging characteristics of specific cameras. Furthermore, there are usually noises over the color images due to a slight variation of the illumination. Therefore, in order to render the color image in a high quality manner, color correction is necessary for accurate image acquisition and is often regarded as a prerequisite before further image analysis (Hunt & Pointer, 2011; Wu, Allebach, & Analoui, 2000).

The color correction process usually involves deriving a transformation between the device dependent camera RGB values and device-independent chromatic attributes. Color correction methods are usually divided into two general categories (Luo, Hong, & Rhodes, 2001; Ng, Allebach, Analoui, & Pizlo, 2003; Hardeberg, Brettel, & Schmitt, 1998): (i) physical model-based and (ii) numerical regression-based. For the physical model-based method (Daligault & Glasser, 1991; Quan, Ohta, & Katoh, 2000; Mart I Nez-Verd U, Pujol, Vilaseca, & Capilla, 2003; Vrhel & Trussell, 1999), the spectral sensitivity model of the camera system needs to be precisely measured by a specialized apparatus or mathematically estimated. Without it, the correction performance will dramatically degrade. For the regression-based method (Ng, Allebach, Analoui, & Pizlo, 2003; Cheung, Westland, Connah, & Ripamonti, 2004; Wang & Zhang, 2010), the camera system is treated as a black box, and by the aid of a reference target which contains a certain number of color samples, typical regression algorithms can be utilized to derive a correction transformation between the camera RGB and CIE *XYZ* values. Compared to the model-based method, the regression-based one does not need to precisely estimate the complicated spectral sensitivity model but only requires a group of known target values in RGB and XYZ color spaces. Therefore, it is more common and practical than the previous one.

In this chapter, the numerical regression-based method was adopted and the Munsell Colorchecker 24 was applied as the reference target. Actually, due to the challenging problem of eye-camera metamerism (Wu, Allebach, & Analoui, 2000), the reference target should be the same material as the color samples that need to be predicted (the human tongue body in this study). Though we have tried different methods to achieve such a "tongue calibration target," we have not been able to establish a stable and robust tongue target because the human tongue body is always changing and uncontrollable. We therefore had to apply the commonly used Munsell Colorchecker in this work, and we will continue to improve this part in the future. Furthermore, in a computerized tongue diagnosis system, acquired images should be statistically analyzed by a computer program for feature extraction in order to derive a diagnostic result. Hence, to produce images captured by different devices consistent with each other is equally important as the accurate assessment of the human tongue color. The Munsell color checker-based method ensures that all images captured by different devices are corrected to the same standard (though not the same as the vision of the CIE standard observer). As long as all the tongue images are consistently acquired, the statistical diagnostic results will be reliable and convincible.

Several typical regression algorithms, including polynomial regression, support vector regression, and ridge regression, were compared for their performance accuracy, computational simplicity, and visual acceptability. Finally, the polynomial regression method which has 11 terms was found to be most suitable for the tongue color correction task (Deng & Manjunath, 2001). The experimental result showed that the CIE*LAB* color difference [according to Eq. (12.1)] between estimated values and ground truth values was less than 5 ($\Delta E^*_{ab} < 5$). Here, the color difference of 5 is the acceptable tolerance which was obtained by our conducted psychophysical experiment. In that test, three TCM doctors were individually asked to judge the minimum distinguishable color difference when color samples were shown on tongue images, and the achieved result was around 5. Although this experiment was not rigorously implemented, it could be utilized as a general reference for accuracy assessment. After generation of the transformation matrix, it was applied to the acquired tongue images to transform them into a device independent standard RGB (sRGB) color space. Variations of captured tongue images caused by imaging system components were greatly reduced. More experimental results and explanations can be found in our previous work (Deng & Manjunath, 2001).

$$\Delta E_{ab}^{*} = \sqrt{(L_1^{*} - L_2^{*})^2 + (a_1^{*} - a_2^{*})^2 + (b_1^{*} - b_2^{*})^2} \tag{12.1}$$

12.2.3 Tongue Image Database

In order to analyze the distribution characteristics of tongue colors, a tongue image database satisfying three requirements needs to be built. First, it should include as many images as possible to make the obtained results statistically significant and convincing. Second, acquired images should be of high and consistent quality. Since images captured from the same tongue body by different cameras or under different illumination conditions may vary from each other, our developed high level tongue image acquisition device and its associated color correction process is necessary to meet this demand. Finally, the database should be "complete" enough, i.e., it needs to cover samples captured from subjects of different genders, ages, and especially various health statuses.

Currently, we have a large tongue image database which was collected from 5222 subjects (Over 9000 images) by our dedicated developed device. These subjects were mainly volunteers from healthcare and patient center of Harbin Binghua Hospital and Guangdong Hospital of TCM (Traditional Chinese Medicine). Generally, tongue images were captured in only one session, and each subject was asked to have 12 tongue images taken. However, in order to trace the tongue image changes of the same subject at different disease stages, several subjects (less than 50) were invited to a second or even third session of image collection. All these subjects have been diagnosed (patient subjects) or labeled (healthcare subjects) into different health statuses (healthy, sub-healthily, and various diseases) by western medical professionals in the hospital.

Table 12.1 shows the composition of the tongue image database. In the database over 2780 subjects are patients representing over 200 disease types, 2002 subjects are labeled as subhealthy, and only 440 samples are categorized as healthy. To the best of our knowledge, this is the largest and most comprehensive tongue image database in the research community.

Table 12.1 Composition of the tongue image database

Total	5222 subjects, 1–2 tongue images, and 1 colorchecker image each							
Gender	Male				Female			
	2856				2566			
Health status	Ill			Sub-healthy			Healthy	
	2780 (includes over 200 diseases)			2002			440	
Age group	<10	11–20	21–30	31–40	41–50	51–60	61–70	>70
	6	499	1221	1266	1076	622	269	263

12.3 Tongue Color Distribution Analysis

Based on the tongue image database, this section analyzes the tongue color distribution characteristics. First, Sect. 12.3.1 introduces the generation of the tongue color gamut in the CIE *x-y* chromaticity diagram. The boundary model of this gamut can be utilized for classification of tongue-related colors with tongue-unrelated colors. Moreover, in order to separate common tongue colors from unusual ones, the major tongue color gamut is also presented in this subsection. Second, the definition of 12 tongue color centers is described in Sect. 12.3.2, and thus the tongue colors can be classified into these 12 classes according to their distance to these 12 centers. Third, distributions of typical image features including tongue substance, coating, red point, and petechial point in the tongue color space are introduced in Sect. 12.3.3.

12.3.1 Tongue Color Gamut: Generation and Modeling

Tongue colors are only a subset of the total visible colors. Therefore, to find the range of such a tongue color subset in the gamut of human vision is the first step to understand the properties of tongue colors. This subsection analyzes the tongue color distribution and describes how the tongue color gamut was established in the CIE *x-y* chromaticity diagram. The reason why the CIE *x-y* chromaticity diagram was chosen is due to the fact that this diagram can provide an intuitionistic way to describe all visible colors according to their color stimulus, and thus the relative position of tongue colors and their color composition can be easily observed.

The idea to generate the tongue color gamut is intuitive. As one color value can be represented by a single point on the CIE *x-y* plane, by projecting all pixel colors of the tongue image database onto the CIE *x-y* plane, the tongue color distribution can be achieved. Thereafter, the boundary model of the tongue distribution can be mathematically described by utilizing some fitting or regression algorithms, thus generating the tongue color gamut.

Although the principle of generating the tongue color gamut is not complicated, three essential issues still need to be thoroughly addressed. (i) First, there are thousands of tongue images in the database and the average pixel number for each image is over 10,000 (original image resolution is 768 × 576), and thus the total number of pixel colors are too large to be projected directly on the CIE *x*-*y* plane by current computational and storage resources. Therefore, representative colors for each tongue image need to be extracted to reduce the number of colors. (ii) Second, based on the obtained tongue color distribution, the boundary needs to be mathematically defined to classify whether one color belongs to tongue-related colors (inside the tongue color gamut) or tongue-unrelated colors (outside of the tongue color gamut). Additionally, the boundary of the major tongue color gamut in order to distinguish common and uncommon tongue colors needs to be well described. (iii) Third, as one objective of this study is to build the tongue color gamut as large and complete as possible, testing experiments are also needed to provide for complete verification. These three issues are addressed as follows.

(1) ***Representative Color Extraction***: All tongue colors could be distributed to a set of scattered points when they are projected on the CIE *x*-*y* plane. Obviously, in order to find the maximum range of tongue colors, the outer points are more important than the inner ones. Therefore, colors located on the boundary of the set of scattered points can be regarded as representative colors. In other words, all colors located inside this region would belong to tongue-related colors and may appear on the tongue body. However, this deduction would be true only when colors of the tongue image are continuous, i.e., colors change gradually across the image region and no abrupt changes are observed. This situation seldom happens in real cases. Tongue images usually contain different types of colors, which are mixed together across the image. Thus, the color of tongue images often abruptly and dramatically changes. Therefore, in order to meet this continuous requirement, we propose a segmented image-based representative color extraction method.

Figure 12.2 shows the flowchart for representative color extraction. For each tongue image, after extraction of the tongue body from its back ground, it was segmented into several uniform color blocks according to its color and texture uniformity so as to meet the continuous requirement. The JSEG segmentation method was utilized here (Morovi V C, 2008). Then, for each block all its colors were projected onto the CIE *x*-*y* plane. The representative colors for each block were obtained by searching the boundary points of the scatted point set using a line scanning method. Finally, all colors for each block were combined together as representative colors of the tongue image.

Parameters of the JSEG segmentation method are important for the generation of tongue color distribution. There are three parameters, i.e., the color quantization threshold (q), the number of scales (l), and region merge threshold specific values (m), which mainly affect the number of segmented blocks for a single tongue image. When selecting different parameters, two extreme cases may appear. The first is that the tongue image is segmented by each pixel. This is obviously unacceptable because there are too many blocks and the number of representative colors is not reduced. The other case is that the image is segmented to only one block (actually no segmentation), which it does not meet the continuous requirement. Therefore, we tried to find the relationship between the total number of blocks in the whole database

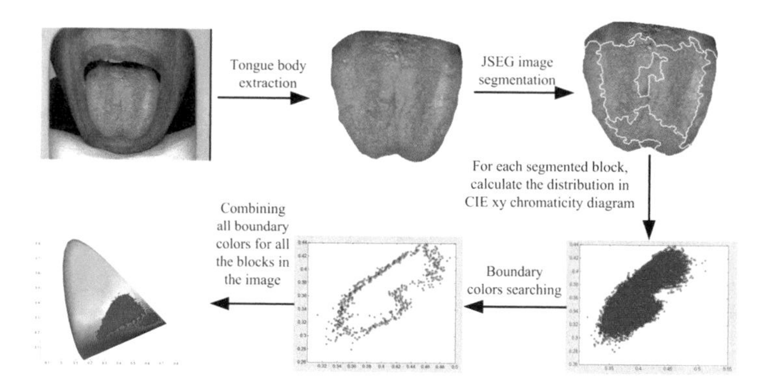

Fig. 12.2 Flowchart for extraction of representative colors. © 2016 IEEE. Reprinted, with permission, from Wang et al. (2013)

with different parameter combinations in order to derive the best block segmentation. This parameter selection experiment was conducted in an alternant way. For instance, when selecting the best color quantization threshold (q), the other two parameters were set to the value first suggested by the author (Morovi V C, 2008). Thus, the relationship between the total block numbers and color quantization threshold was achieved. Figure 12.3 presents the relationship curve. It can be observed that when the quantization threshold increases, the total number gradually decreases, and the inflection point can be chosen as the optimal selection, where $q = 200$. In the same way, the other two parameters were optimally selected as $m = 0.4$ and $l = 3$.

After extracting representative colors of all images by utilizing the above optimized parameters, the tongue color distribution can be achieved by projecting it onto the CIE x-y plane. Figure 12.4a shows it in the CIE chromaticity diagram. The horseshoe-shaped area expresses the gamut of human vision which represents all visible colors. Two observations can be noticed: (i) tongue colors (shown as blue points) only occupy a small region (mainly red and yellow) of the whole area. (ii) Most tongue colors distribute continuously and densely in the center, with outliers sparsely located around it. Figure 12.4b shows the tongue color distribution on the CIE x-y plane. It clearly provides a range of the coordinates for tongue colors, i.e., coordinate x is from 0.25 to 0.55, and y is from 0.15 to 0.55. However, this obtained figure only presents a rough range of tongue colors, and it does not provide the precise boundary to describe the tongue color gamut. Moreover, this figure fails to explicitly illustrate the internal distribution density of tongue colors, which is meaningful for color analysis for diagnostic purposes, i.e., colors sparsely distributed indicate it is unusual to observe them on the tongue body and conveys significant medical clues for diagnosis. Therefore, to find the boundary of the major tongue gamut for identifying normal and abnormal tongue colors is also important.

(2) ***Boundary Modeling by One-Class SVM***: Based on obtained tongue color distribution, this subsection introduces a boundary descriptor for two kinds of tongue color gamuts: the full tongue color gamut to define the range of tongue colors, and the major tongue gamut which defines where most tongue colors are distributed.

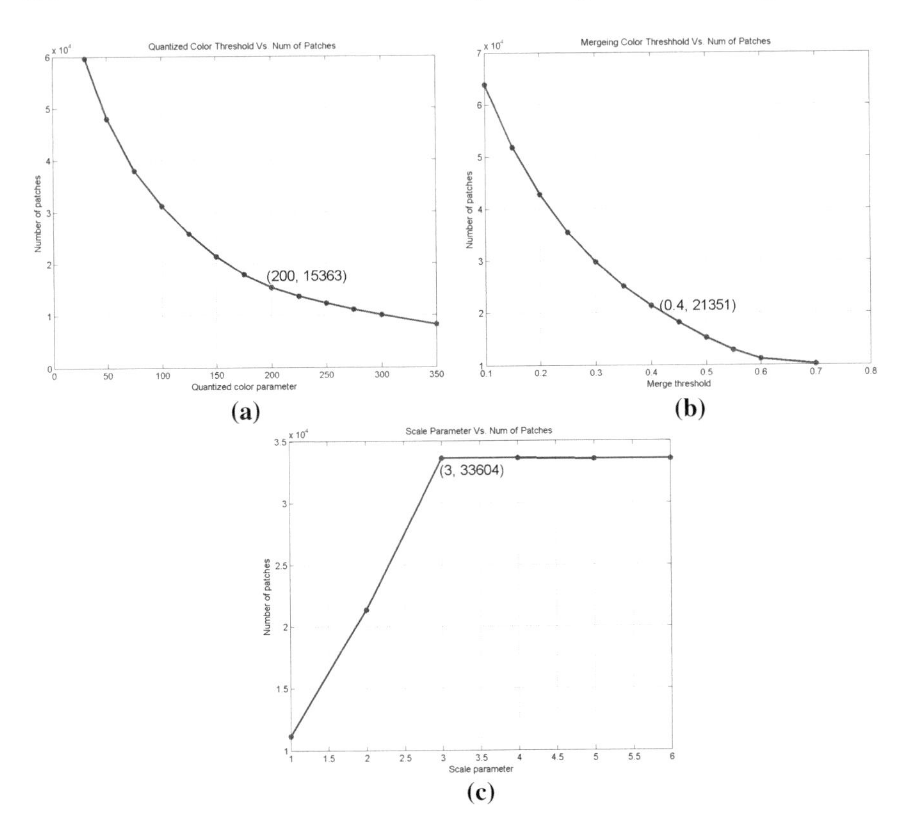

Fig. 12.3 Parameters selection for the JSEG segmentation. **a** Color quantization threshold versus number of blocks. **b** Region merge threshold versus number of blocks. **c** Number of scales versus number of blocks

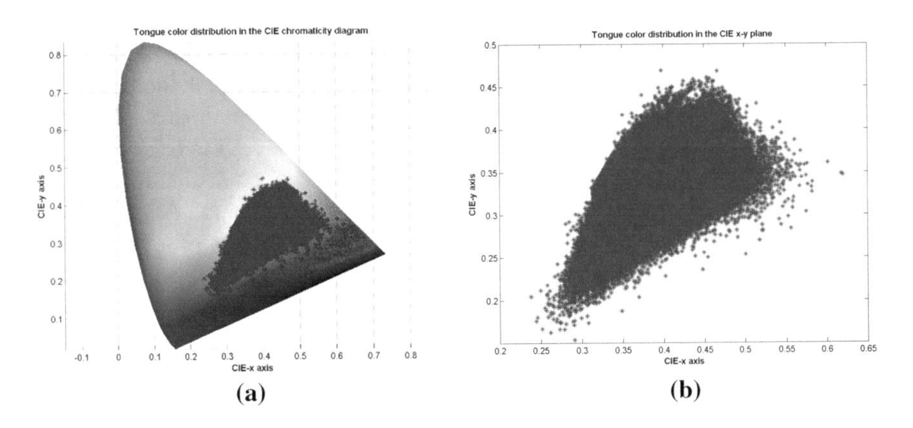

Fig. 12.4 Tongue color distribution in the **a** CIE chromaticity diagram and **b** CIE *x-y* plane. The region covered by tongue colors (blue point) is only a small subset of the gamut of human vision. © 2016 IEEE. Reprinted, with permission, from Wang et al. (2013)

(a) *Down Sampling of the Training Dataset:* After generation of the tongue color distribution, there were still over 1,500,000 representative colors that could be used as training data for model training the tongue color gamut. There are too many samples to be processed by any classification algorithm, and hence they need to be reduced by down-sampling algorithms.

Two kinds of tongue color gamuts, i.e., full gamut and major gamut, are proposed in this study. Therefore, the down-sampling strategy for different gamut training also varies. (i) With regard to the full gamut, it should cover as large and complete an area as possible and thus sparsely distributed color samples should be kept while densely distributed ones should be reduced to retain the shape of the boundary (boundary preserved down-sampling method). (ii) Nevertheless, in terms of the major gamut, since the objective of this gamut is to describe the region where the most tongue colors are distributed, the surrounding sparsely distributed color samples need to be removed while central densely ones need to be retained. In other words, the inherent distribution density is maintained in order to derive the boundary model of the major tongue gamut (the center-preserved down-sampling method). Detailed introduction of these two down-sampling algorithms are provided as follows.

The boundary preserved down-sampling method based on the 2D histogram of the tongue color distribution was proposed to form the full tongue color gamut. Let $C = \{C_i \mid i = 1, 2, \ldots, N^2\}$ represents the histogram, and the bin number for each dimension is set to N = 100. For each square C_i $(i = 1, 2, \ldots, N^2)$, if the number of samples that lie in this bin is Num_i, the new number of samples after reduction is set as:

$$M_i = \begin{cases} \mathrm{Num}_i & \mathrm{Num}_i \leq 10 \\ \mathrm{round}(\log 10(\mathrm{Num}_i) * 10) & \mathrm{Num}_i > 10. \end{cases} \tag{12.2}$$

Here, when Num_i is larger than 10, M_i samples were randomly selected over the Num_i samples, with the remaining samples disregarded. Obviously, this down-sampling method thinned out the number of samples in the dense square while keeping it in the sparse square. By utilizing such an algorithm, the number of training samples was greatly reduced by 97%, and only 53,600 colors were left, while the boundary of the training dataset was approximately preserved.

The center-preserved down-sampling method used to achieve the major tongue gamut is still based on the 2D histogram of the tongue color distribution, with the basic idea of removing surrounding samples which are sparsely distributed. Suppose it represents a preset threshold, for each square, if the original number of samples that lie in this bin is, the new number of samples after reduction is set as:

$$M_i = \begin{cases} 0 & \mathrm{Num}_i \leq S \\ \mathrm{Num}_i & \mathrm{Num}_i > S. \end{cases} \tag{12.3}$$

By tuning the sparsity threshold S, the major tongue gamut with various rates of coverage can be obtained. For example, we may achieve the 99% tongue gamut, which roughly shows where 99% of tongue colors are distributed and where the remaining 1% colors are located.

(b) *Gamut Boundary Description*: For the boundary description of the tongue color gamut, similar research has been done in gamut mapping for color management and device characterization (Kress & Stevens, 1994). Different boundary description methods have been proposed, such as the convex hull (Balasubramanian & Dalal, 1997; Cholewo & Love, 1999), alpha shapes (Morovic & Luo, 1997) and segment maxima (Morovic & Luo 2000; Chang & Lin, 2011). The basic idea of these algorithms is to efficiently cover all training samples by different kinds of geometric shapes. However, the important pre-requisite of these methods is that the training dataset should include samples under all extreme cases (boundary samples) and should exclude any samples which do not belong to this gamut. This is not the case of our task, in which different noisy colors may be included and not all colors have been involved (cannot ensure 100% involvement). Therefore, we utilized a pattern classifier as the gamut boundary descriptor, and the derived classification function can also be regarded as the mathematical description of the boundary. In this study, the one-class SVM algorithm was employed since only one kind of sample (tongue colors) is involved. This algorithm is an extension of the traditional SVM methodology to handle training using only positive information (Manevitz & Yousef, 2002; Li, 2011). In this algorithm, the origin is the only member in the negative class. The objective function of the one-class SVM is defined as follows:

$$\min_{\mathbf{w},b,\xi,\rho} \frac{1}{2}\mathbf{w}^{\mathrm{T}}\mathbf{w} - \rho + \frac{1}{vl}\sum_{i=1}^{l} \xi i \tag{12.4}$$

subject to $\mathbf{w}^{\mathrm{T}}\mathbf{\Phi}(\boldsymbol{X}_i) \geq \rho - \xi i$, $\xi i \geq 0$, $i = 1, \ldots, l$, where $\mathbf{w}$ is a vector orthogonal to the classification hyper sphere, $\mathbf{K}(\mathbf{x}_i)$ represents the kernel function, and $\mathbf{x}_i$ is i-th training sample. ρ represents the preset margin, i.e., the distance between the origin and the hyper sphere. l expresses the number of training samples. $v \in (0, 1)$ is a parameterized constant that controls the fraction of training data that fall outside of the hyper sphere. ξi are slack variables used to "penalize" the rejected samples. By solving the dual problem:

$$\min_{a} \frac{1}{2}\sum_{ij} a_i a_j K(x_i, x_j) s.t\, 0 \leq a_i \leq \frac{1}{vl}, \sum_{i} a_i = 1,$$

we achieved the following decision function:

$$f(x) = \operatorname{sgn}\left(\sum_{i=1}^{l} a_i K(\mathbf{x}_i, \mathbf{x}) - \rho\right) \tag{12.5}$$

Where $K\mathbf{x}_i$, $\mathbf{x}$ represents the kernel function, a_i are obtained coefficients, and ρ represents the preset margin. In this study, the RBF kernel was chosen to train the SVM model because it has only one parameter for model selection and fewer numerical difficulties. The definition of the RBF function is $K(\mathbf{x}_i, \mathbf{x}) = \exp(-\gamma\|\mathbf{x}_i - \mathbf{x}_j\|^2)$.

The LIBSVM toolbox (Schanda, 2007) was employed to implement the algorithm, and all down sampled 53,600 colors extracted from over 9000 tongue images were utilized as the training dataset. Two parameters, gamma (γ) which tunes the training error and which tunes the generalization capability need to be optimized for best performance. In this study, we utilized a fivefold cross validation (CV) method to obtain the best parameters. The whole data set (536,000 colors) was equally randomly divided into 5 subsets. Each time, 1 out of the 5 subsets was used as a test set and the remaining 4 subsets were combined to form the training set. This cross validation process was repeated 5 times and the parameters which achieved the best performance were: $\gamma = 60$ and $1/vl = 0.004$. Figure 12.5a shows the tongue color gamut in the CIE chromaticity diagram. The yellow line is the boundary function line of the SVM model. Figure 12.5b presents the tongue color gamut on the CIE *x-y* plane.

For the major tongue color gamut, one important issue is to find which major tongue color gamut is most meaningful for diagnostic purposes. Since there was no prior knowledge, it was obtained by comparing a series of gamuts which have various rates of color coverage. According to the introduction of the *center-preserved down-sampling method* in Sect. 11.3.1, by tuning the sparsity threshold S, different groups of training samples were obtained to generate these major tongue color gamuts. In this study, gamuts with five rates of coverage, i.e., 100, 99, 98, 97, and 96%, are shown in Fig. 12.6. From this figure, we may observe that three gamuts, i.e., 98, 97, and 96, are close to each other, while the boundary of the 99% color gamut is far from these three gamuts. This illustrates that colors in the 98% gamut are extremely continuous and densely distributed, while colors are distributed sparsely outside the 98% gamut. Therefore, the 98% gamut is more meaningful than the others and will be further studied and applied in the following sections.

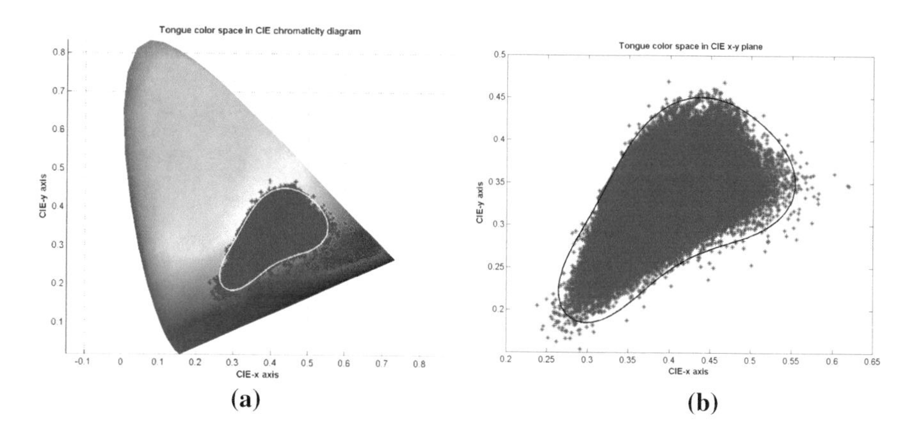

Fig. 12.5 Boundary of the tongue color gamut in **a** CIE chromaticity diagram and on **b** the CIE *x-y* plane. © 2016 IEEE. Reprinted, with permission, from Wang et al. (2013)

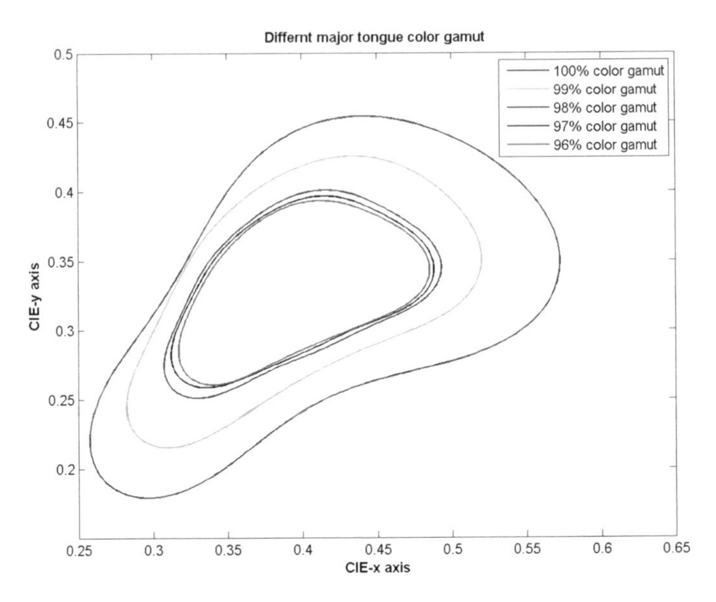

Fig. 12.6 Boundaries of different the major tongue color gamuts in the CIE chromaticity diagram. © 2016 IEEE. Reprinted, with permission, from Wang et al. (2013)

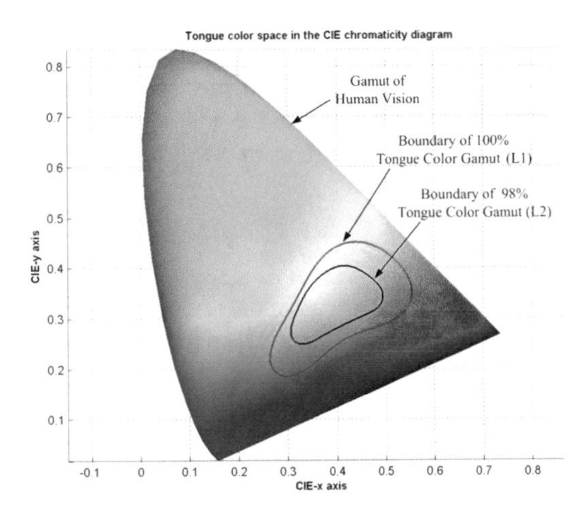

Fig. 12.7 Tongue color gamut in CIE chromaticity diagram. © 2016 IEEE. Reprinted, with permission, from Wang et al. (2013)

In summary, as Fig. 12.7 shows, the tongue color gamut was obtained from the tongue color distribution on the CIE *x-y* plane and enclosed by a boundary line (L1) which was deriven by the one-class SVM method. Line L1 can be defined by:

$$L1(x) = \left\{ x : \sum_{i=1}^{n_1} \omega_i \exp(-\gamma_1^* \|x - x_i\|^2) + b_1 = 0 \right\}, \tag{12.6}$$

where n_1 is the number of support vectors, γ_1 is the parameter of the RBF kernel, b_1 is the offset of the SVM model, and w_i is the coefficient of different support vectors. $\mathbf{x}_i$ represents support vectors, and $\mathbf{x}$ is the color coordinate on the CIE x-y plane. In our proposed tongue color gamut, $b_1 = 65.7178$, $n_1 = 219$, and $\gamma_1 = 60$. Besides the 100% tongue color gamut, the gamut of the 98% tongue colors is enclosed by the boundary line of $L2$ which can be defined as follows:

$$L2(x) = \left\{ x : \sum_{j=1}^{n_2} a_j \exp(-\gamma_2^* \|x - x_j\|^2) + b_2 = 0 \right\} \quad (12.7)$$

where $b_1 = 10.5099$, $b_1 = 44$, and $\gamma_1 = 200$. Based on these two boundary lines, the tongue color gamut can be well defined with each color being classified into different groups, such as tongue-unrelated colors and tongue-unrelated colors, or common tongue colors and rare tongue colors.

(c) *Completeness Verification of the Tongue Color Gamut*: We further tested the completeness of the tongue color gamut by checking whether new tongue colors were distributed inside the boundary. This testing was implemented based on our newly collected 539 images by the designed device which mainly includes images from in patient subjects. Table 12.2 shows the test results. We observed that 99.98% of tested colors were covered by the 100% tongue color gamut, and 98.11% of tongue colors could be found inside of the 98% tongue color gamut. Therefore, the testing results verified the completeness of the tongue color gamut.

12.3.2 Tongue Color Centers

In addition to investigating the tongue color gamut, which defines the range of tongue colors in the CIE chromaticity diagram, further understanding of the tongue color space should be conducted on how tongue colors can be classified into several important and discriminative color categories. This idea is derived from the principle of tongue diagnosis in TCM in which 1–2 main color types are usually extracted from a set of color categories [usually 12 (Wyszecki & Stiles, 1982)], and these extracted color types are then utilized as an important feature for further disease diagnosis. These 12 color categories normally contain: red, light red, deep

Table 12.2 Testing results of two color gamuts using all colors from 539 tongue images

Tongue color gamut	Coverage ratio (%)
100% tongue color gamut	99.98
98% tongue color gamut	98.11

red, blue, light blue, purple, light purple, cyan, yellow, black, gray, and white. The first 8 color categories belong to colors of the tongue substance and the remaining 4 belong to colors of the tongue coating. Based on the principle of TCM, the tongue coating is a layer of fur grime on the surface of the tongue. We call the basement of the tongue body the "tongue substance" and the floating layer the "tongue coating." The tongue has a coating just like the earth has moss. The colors of the tongue substance and coating are important for medical diagnosis. One more issue that needs to be noted is that the name of the tongue color is only used to reflect their relative visual appearance, and they have different color stimuli from pure colors of the same name. For example, the 'red' in tongue color is not the same as the pure red ([255,0,0] in the RGB color model) in our common sense. Figure 12.8 shows tongue images with different color types. (a) mainly includes white (coating) and red (substance), (e) contains gray (coating) and deep red (substance), and (f) is mainly comprised of red (substance).

The identification of different color types of tongue images is normally and subjectively decided by TCM professionals based on their personal medical knowledge or experience. There are no objective and precise definitions for each color category, such as what is the color center value of this 'red' type and how to decide what kind of colors belongs to the'red' type. Standardization research has been done to try to derive the objective color stimulus for the color center of each category by clustering a group of typical color images (Kakumanu, Makrogiannis & Bourbakis, 2007). Their training samples are also labeled by TCM practitioners for each color type. Hence, their obtained results are still subjective and inconvincible. In this subsection, we objectively proposed the definition of the color centers for the 12 color categories, i.e., exact chromatic values of the color centers.

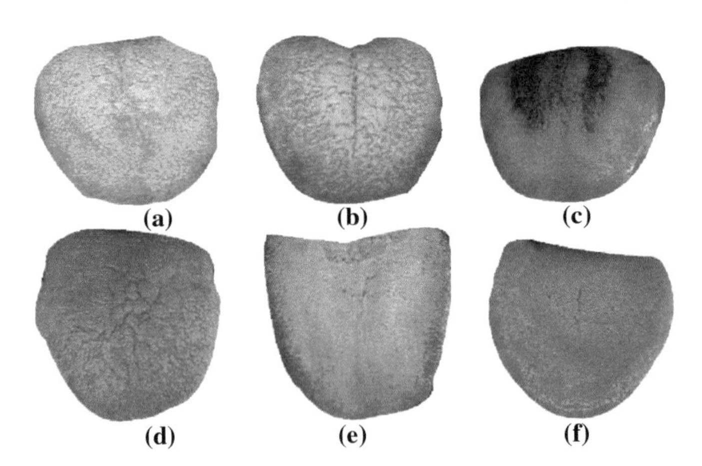

Fig. 12.8 Typical tongue images with various color types. **a** *White* (coating) and *red* (substance), **b** *gray* (coating) and *purple* (substance), **c** *black* (coating) and *deep red* (substance), **d** *yellow* (coating) and *deep red* (substance), **e** *gray* (coating) and *deep red* (substance), **f** *red* (substance). © 2016 IEEE. Reprinted, with permission, from Wang et al. (2013)

The general principle of deriving the color stimulus of each color center is by clustering a set of color samples which are in the same color category. Unlike those training samples which were subjectively labeled by TCM doctors in previous research, a new objective method is proposed to generate the training samples. First, based on the characteristics of the sRGB color space in which all the tongue images are rendered, 12 color centers are predefined to maximize their chromatic and saturation difference. Thereafter, on the basis of these predefined color centers, colors belonging to each color category are utilized as training samples.

These 12 color centers are first predefined to meet the standards in tongue diagnosis of TCM. Based on the identification rule of these 12 color categories, it may be noticed that these colors mainly differ with each other according to their hue and saturation information. For example, red, yellow, and blue are classified by their hue attribute, while red, light red, and deep red are differentiated by their saturation feature. Therefore, these 12 colors should be defined to maximize their chromatic and saturation characteristic. Moreover, based on the knowledge of the sRGB color space (Malacara, 2011) in which all tongue images are rendered, six fundamental colors defined in the sRGB color space, including three primary colors (red, green, and blue) and three secondary colors (yellow, cyan, and purple), have the largest difference in their chromatic feature. Also, colors projected on the line between the white point and the primary colors are the same in hue, but vary in purity (saturation) (Malacara, 2011). Therefore, the definition of the 12 tongue color centers can be obtained by the aid of the sRGB color space.

Figure 12.9 shows the initial position of the predefined 12 color centers in the CIE chromaticity diagram for 10°. The outer horseshoe-shaped line represents the gamut of human vision, and the black triangle enclosed by the R-G-B points stands for the sRGB color space. The white point (P1) of the tongue color gamut is first defined based on the definition of the white point in the sRGB color space. Then it is connected to five points in the sRGB color space (red, yellow, cyan, blue, and purple). Green is not utilized here because such a color is nonexistent in tongue colors. Obviously, these connected five lines intersect with the boundary of the tongue color gamut, where the intersection points can be regarded as centers of typical tongue types. Since most of the tongue colors are distributed in the 98% tongue color gamut, and in order to make the color centers represent more tongue colors, intersection points between connected lines and the 98% tongue color gamut are defined as tongue color centers. This includes Red (P2), Deep Red (P3), Yellow (P4), Cyan (P5), Blue (P6), and Purple (P7). In addition, those less saturated colors are defined between the White point (P1) and their corresponding saturated colors. In this study, mid-points are selected for the light colors (Light Red (P8), Light Purple (P9), and Light Blue (P10)). According to the definition of colors centers, they are defined as far as possible from each other in order to be distinct enough. Also, in this initial definition, Gray (P11) and Black (P12) are monochrome colors, and thus cannot be shown in this figure.

After obtaining these initially selected color centers, their color attributes are further refined according to the tongue color distributions. Tongue colors similar to each defined as color centers, i.e., points distributed near the color centers, are

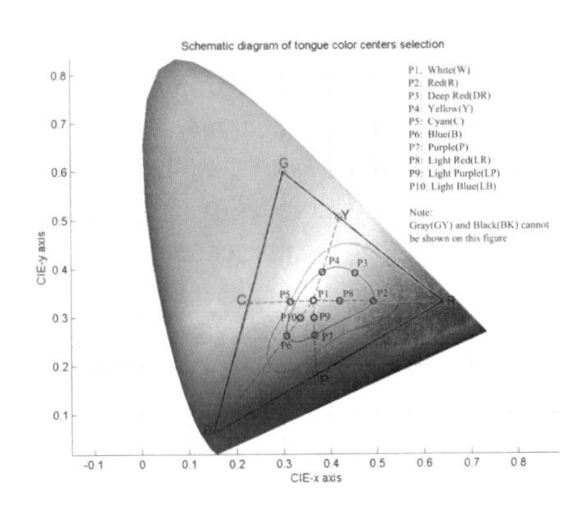

Fig. 12.9 Definition of the tongue color centers in the CIE chromaticity diagram by aid of the sRGB color space. © 2016 IEEE. Reprinted, with permission, from Wang et al. (2013)

clustered to obtain the improved color centers. For example, when refining Purple (P7) and Light Purple (P9), only purplish colors are involved for clustering. In this way, only similar colors are used for clustering thus minimizing the influence of other colors and the final result is more accurate. Finally, the refined 12 color centers and their color squares are shown in Figs. 12.10 and 12.11 Also, RGB and CIE*LAB* values are given in © 2016 IEEE. Reprinted, with permission, from Wang et al. (2013).

Table 12.3.

12.3.3 Distribution of Typical Image Features

The range of tongue colors and the definition of the 12 color centers for the various tongue color categories were presented in the previous section, but the relationship between different parts of the tongue color gamut with various image features was not investigated. The objective of this subsection is to study which image features

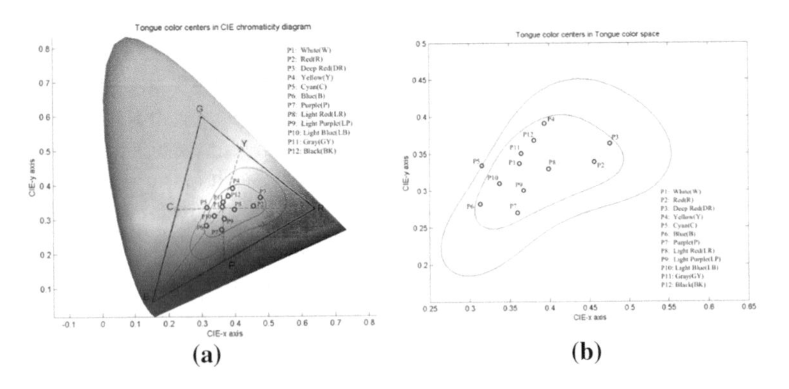

Fig. 12.10 Refined 12 color centers in the CIE chromaticity diagram. **a** Relationship between refined color centers and the sRGB color space. **b** Distribution of the refined 12 color colors in the tongue color space. © 2016 IEEE. Reprinted, with permission, from Wang et al. (2013)

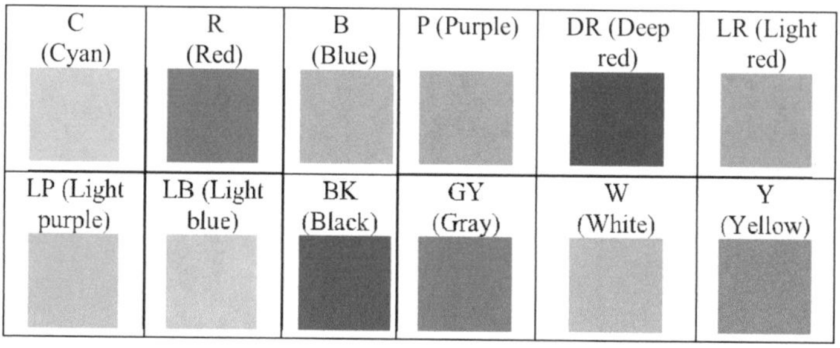

C (Cyan)	R (Red)	B (Blue)	P (Purple)	DR (Deep red)	LR (Light red)
LP (Light purple)	LB (Light blue)	BK (Black)	GY (Gray)	W (White)	Y (Yellow)

Fig. 12.11 Typical 12 color squares with each label on top. © 2016 IEEE. Reprinted, with permission, from Wang et al. (2013)

Table 12.3 RGB and CIE*LAB* values of the 12 colors

Color	[R G B]	[L A B]
C(Cyan)	[188 188 185]	[76.0693 −0.5580 1.3615]
R(Red)	[189 99 91]	[52.2540 34.8412 21.3002]
B(Blue)	[183 165 180]	[69.4695 9.5423 −5.4951]
P(Purple)	[226 142 214]	[69.4695 42.4732 −23.8880]
DR(Deep red)	[136 72 49]	[37.8424 24.5503 25.9396]
LR(light red)	[227 150 147]	[69.4695 28.4947 13.3940]
LP(Light purple)	[225 173 207]	[76.0693 24.3246 −9.7749]
LB(Light blue)	[204 183 186]	[76.0693 7.8917 0.9885]
BK(Black)	[107 86 56]	[37.8424 3.9632 20.5874]
GY(Gray)	[163 146 143]	[61.6542 5.7160 3.7317]
W(White)	[200 167 160]	[70.9763 10.9843 8.2952]
Y(Yellow)	[166 129 93]	[56.3164 9.5539 24.4546]

© 2016 IEEE. Reprinted, with permission, from Wang et al. (2013)

are related to different regions of the tongue color gamut, thereby establishing a correspondence that can be utilized for further feature extraction and diagnostics.

There are normally several types of image features which are important for disease diagnosis, including red point, petechial point, reflection point, shadow point, and abnormal coating. Figure 12.12 shows tongue images having these typical features. The establishment of their corresponding color distributions to these image features is simple and straightforward. First, pixels of these features were manually detected and labeled by TCM professionals. Then, these labeled pixels were projected onto the CIE *x-y* plane, and thus their distribution in the tongue color gamut was found.

Figure 12.13 shows the distribution of all these features. Most colors of the typical tongue coating (labeled as "6") and substance (labeled as "7") are distributed inside of the 98% tongue color gamut, and the tongue coating colors are usually yellowish

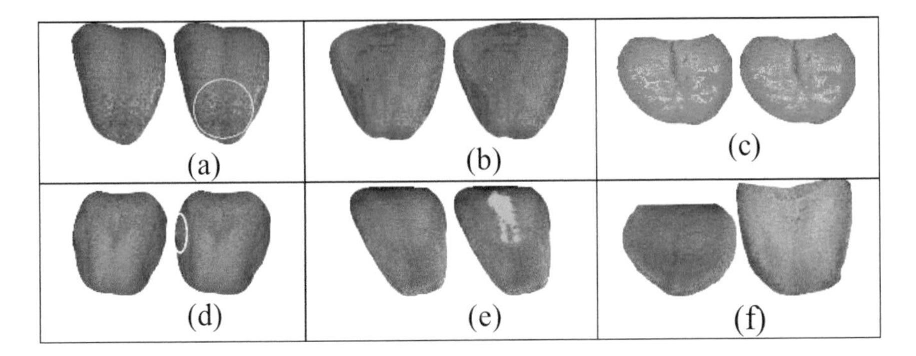

Fig. 12.12 Typical image features. **a** Red point. **b** Petechial point. **c** Reflection point. **d** Shadow point. **e** Abnormal coating and **f** substance and coating. © 2016 IEEE. Reprinted, with permission, from Wang et al. (2013)

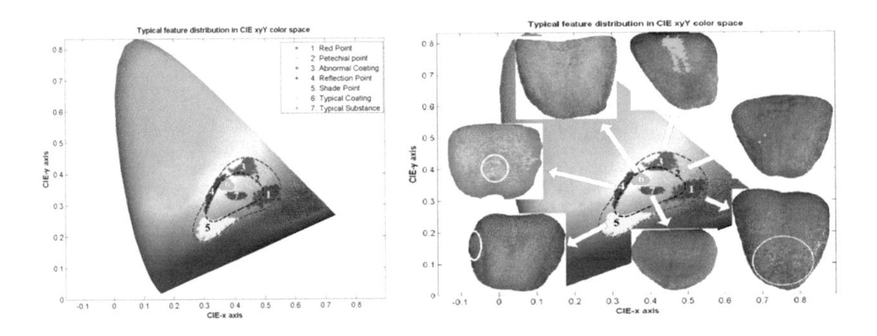

Fig. 12.13 Color distribution of typical image features in the CIE chromaticity diagram. © 2016 IEEE. Reprinted, with permission, from Wang et al. (2013)

while tongue substance colors are normally reddish. However, most noisy or pathological reflective colors are generally distributed in the annular section between the 100% and the 98% tongue color gamuts. For example, colors of red points (labeled as “1”) and petechial points (labeled as “2”) are generally deep red and distributed in the bottom right part. On the other hand, colors which are too yellow are usually abnormal coating colors (labeled as “3”). Colors of noisy features including reflection points and shadow points are also distributed in the 2% regions.

12.4 Color Feature Extraction

Based on the proposed tongue color space, this section describes the tongue color feature extraction method. Every foreground tongue pixel color is first compared to the proposed 12 color centers and assigned to its nearest color. Thus, this forms a 12-dimension ratio vector for each tongue image.

12.4.1 Tongue Color Feature Vector

The general principle of tongue color vector feature extraction is to compare every pixel's color intensity (of the input tongue image) with the 12 colors centers and assign it to the nearest color. Then, the ratio for each color category can be calculated. This feature is a 12-dimension vector and for each dimension the attribute range from 0 to 100%, while the sum of all attributes in this feature vector should equal 100%.

Given a tongue image, image segmentation is first applied to extract all foreground tongue pixels. Then, all foreground tongue pixel colors which are rendered in the sRGB color space are converted to the CIE*XYZ* (Ohta & Robertson, 2006) color space according to the following function:

$$\begin{bmatrix} x \\ Y \\ Z \end{bmatrix} = \Phi_{sRGB \to XYZ} \begin{bmatrix} R \\ G \\ B \end{bmatrix} = \begin{bmatrix} 0.4125 & 0.3576 & 0.1804 \\ 0.2127 & 0.7152 & 0.0722 \\ 0.0193 & 0.1192 & 0.9503 \end{bmatrix} \begin{bmatrix} R \\ G \\ B \end{bmatrix} \quad (12.7)$$

Next, they are transformed to the CIE*LAB* color space by

$$\begin{cases} L^* = 116f(Y/Y_0) - 16 \\ a^* = 500[f(X/X_0) - f(Y/Y_0)] \\ b^* = 200[f(Y/Y_0) - f(Z/Z_0)] \end{cases} \quad (12.8)$$

where $f(x) = \begin{cases} x^{1/3} & (x > 0.008856) \\ 7.787x + 16/116 & (x < 0.008856) \end{cases}$.

In Eq. (12.8), X_0. Y_0, and Z_0 are the CIE*XYZ* tristimulus values of the reference white point. The Lab values are then compared to the 12 color centers (see Table 12.2) by calculating the color difference between them according to Eq. (12.1).

For every input pixel, the nearest color label is assigned to it. After calculating and labeling all input foreground tongue pixels, the total of each color type is summed and divided by the total number of input tongue pixels. Therefore, this ratio of the 12 color categories forms the tongue color vector feature v, where $v = [c_1, c_2, c_3, c_4, c_5, c_6, c_7, c_8, c_9, c_{10}, c_{11}, c_{12}]$ and c_i represents the ratio of the color in Table 12.3.

12.4.2 Typical Samples of Tongue Color Representation

Figures 12.14 and 12.15 show the feature vectors of four typical tongue images. As can be seen in Fig. 12.14, all the pixels are compared to the 12 color centers and labeled by one of them, and then the ratio for each color category is calculated. This image mainly contains yellow and red colors, and the calculated ratios for these two

Color Feature Vector:
[0 15.342 0.015 0.002 2.568 12.077 0.010 0.003 8.125 2.445 1.328 37.920]
C - 0%
R- 15.342%
B - 0.015%
P - 0.002%
DR - 2.568%
LR - 12.07%
LP - 0.010%
LB - 0.003%
BK - 8.125%
GY - 2.445%
W- 1.328%
Y - 37.92%

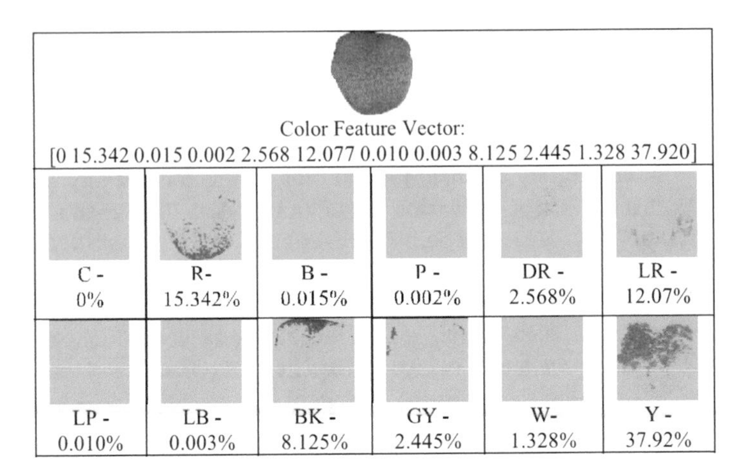

Fig. 12.14 Yellow coating and red substance tongue image sample. The Y, R, and LR colors have large ratios over all the 12 colors. © 2016 IEEE. Reprinted, with permission, from Wang et al. (2013)

Color Feature Vector:
[0 27.728 0.167 0.009 4.351 2.383 0.007 0 20.401 18.180 0.247 0.471]
C - 0%
R - 27.728%
B - 0.167%
P - 0.009%
DR - 4.351%
LR - 2.383%
LP - 0.007%
LB - 0%
BK - 20.401%
GY - 18.180%
W - 0.247%
Y - 0.471%

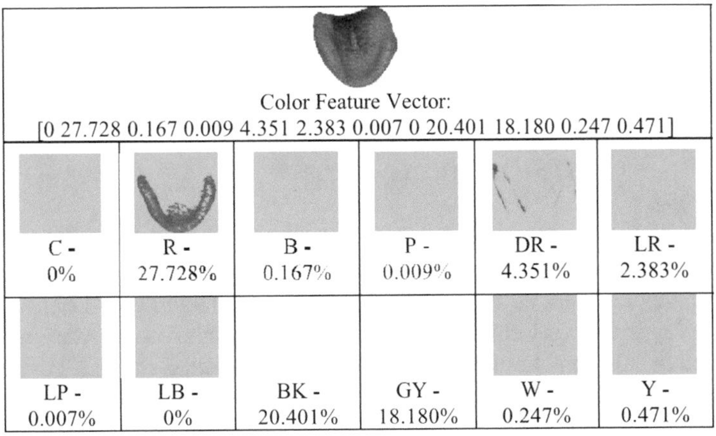

Fig. 12.15 Color feature vector of black (BK) coating and red (R) substance tongue image sample. © 2016 IEEE. Reprinted, with permission, from Wang et al. (2013)

colors are 37.920 and 15.342%, respectively which is in accordance with the observation. Figure 12.15 shows the typical samples of a black coating and a red substance tongue image. The extracted color feature vector can accurately describe the main color component of the tongue image, which can be utilized for further disease diagnosis. We have conducted research on image diagnostic classification using the proposed color feature, and the classification ratio to classify healthy versus nonhealthy is around 80%.

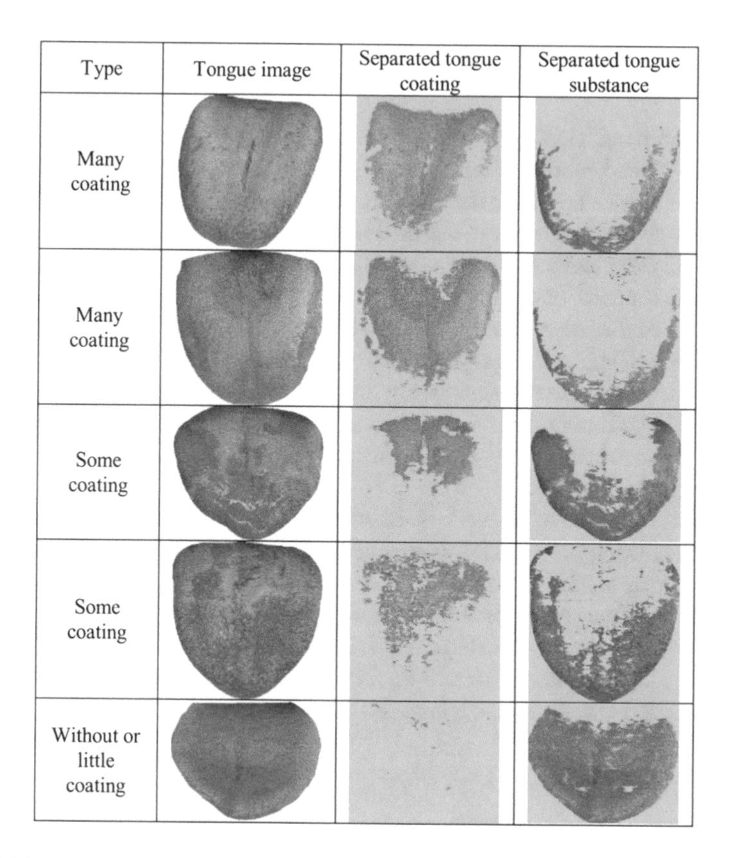

Fig. 12.16 Separation of tongue coating and substance for various types of tongue images including images with many coatings, some coatings, and without or little coating. © 2016 IEEE. Reprinted, with permission, from Wang et al. (2013)

After extracting the color feature vector for each tongue image, the color feature can be used to deal with another classical problem which is the separation of the tongue substance and tongue coating. By separating a tongue image into two parts and identifying the color type of each, the ratio for each color type can be calculated and used as an important clue for disease diagnosis. In this study, each tongue image has been decomposed into 12 colors, with the first 8 colors belonging to the tongue substance and the last 4 colors belonging to the tongue coating. Therefore, we combined all the image pixels of the 8 colors (cyan, red, blue, purple, deep red, light red, light purple, and light blue) as the tongue substance, while image pixels of the 4 remaining colors (black, gray, white, yellow) are the tongue coating. Figure 12.16 shows separated examples for various kinds of tongue images in terms of different amounts of the tongue coating. The performance of the separation by this method has been verified by TCM professionals.

12.5 Summary

This chapter conducted comprehensive and fundamental research on statistical distribution characteristics of tongue colors. A novel color gamut descriptor using a one-class SVM was proposed for mathematically modeling the tongue color gamut. Test results showed that it can cover 99.98% of tongue colors and a large ratio (98.11%) of these colors are densely distributed in a much smaller tongue color gamut (98% gamut). Furthermore, distribution of different typical image features show that most disease-reflection features are located in the 2% region between the 100 and 98% tongue color gamut. This region may be used as an important classification clue for disease diagnosis. By the aid of the proposed tongue color space, especially the definition of 12 color centers, a new color feature extraction method has been proposed and the evaluation results also verified its rationality and possibility for further analysis.

Although we believe this work is the most comprehensive and detailed study of the tongue color space to date, it can be further extended in the following two directions. First, the tongue image database needs to be enlarged to cover as many kinds of tongue images as possible. Second, applications of this tongue color space, such as the development of a dedicated tongue image acquisition device or tongue image analyzing algorithms, should be further studied to promote the development of computerized tongue image analysis.

References

Ahn, J., & Lee, Y. K. (2008). Color distribution of a shade guide in the value, chroma, and hue scale. *The Journal of prosthetic dentistry, 100*(1), 18–28.

Balasubramanian, R., & Dalal, E. (1997). *Method for quantifying the color gamut of an output device* (pp. 110–116), International Society for Optics and Photonics.

Cai, Y. (2002). *A novel imaging system for tongue inspection* (pp. 159–164), IEEE; 1999.

Chang, C., & Lin, C. J. (2011). LIBSVM: A library for support vector machines. *ACM Transactions on Intelligent Systems and Technology (TIST), 2*(3), 27.

Cheung, V., Westland, S., Connah, D., & Ripamonti, C. (2004). A comparative study of the characterisation of colour cameras by means of neural networks and polynomial transforms. *Coloration Technology, 120*(1), 19–25.

Chiu, C. (2000). A novel approach based on computerized image analysis for traditional Chinese medical diagnosis of the tongue. *Computer Methods and Programs in Biomedicine, 61*(2), 77–89.

Cholewo, T. J., & Love, S. (1999). *Gamut boundary determination using alpha-shapes* (pp. 200–204), Society for Imaging Science and Technology.

Daligault, L., & Glasser, J. (1991). *Colorimetric characterization of CCD sensors by spectrophotometry* (pp. 124–130): International Society for Optics and Photonics.

Deng, Y., & Manjunath, B. S. (2001). Unsupervised segmentation of color-texture regions in images and video. *IEEE Transactions on Pattern Analysis and Machine Intelligence, 23*(8), 800–810.

Green, P., & MacDonald, L. (2011). *Colour engineering: achieving device independent colour* (Vol. 30), New York: Wiley.

Hardeberg, J. Y., Brettel, H., & Schmitt, F. J. (1998). *Spectral characterization of electronic cameras* (pp. 100–109): International Society for Optics and Photonics.
Hsu, R., Abdel-Mottaleb, M., & Jain, A. K. (2002). Face detection in color images. *IEEE Transactions on Pattern Analysis and Machine Intelligence, 24*(5), 696–706.
Huang, B., & Lie, N. (2008). Pixel based tongue color analysis. In *Medical Biometrics* (pp. 282–289), New York: Springer.
Hunt, R. W. G., & Pointer, M. R. (2011). *Measuring colour,* New York: Wiley.
Igarashi, T., Nishino, K, & Nayar SK (2007). The appearance of human skin: A survey. *Foundations and Trends{extregistered} in Computer Graphics and Vision, 3*(1), 1–95.
Joiner, A. (2004). Tooth colour: A review of the literature. *Journal of Dentistry, 32,* 3–12.
Jones, M. J., & Rehg, J. M. (2002). Statistical color models with application to skin detection. *International Journal of Computer Vision, 46*(1), 81–96.
Kakumanu, P., Makrogiannis, S., & Bourbakis, N. (2007). A survey of skin-color modeling and detection methods. *Pattern Recognition, 40*(3), 1106–1122.
Kress, W., & Stevens, M. (1994). *Derivation of 3-dimensional gamut descriptors for graphic arts output devices* (pp. 199), Technical Association of the Graphic Arts.
Li, N. (2011). *Tongue diagnostics,* Academy Press.
Li, B., Huang, Q., Lu, Y., Chen, S., Liang, R., & Wang, Z. (2008). A method of classifying tongue colors for traditional chinese medicine diagnosis based on the CIELAB color space. In *Medical Biometrics* (pp. 153–159), New York: Springer.
Lkopf Sch O, B., Platt, J. C., Shawe-Taylor, J., Smola, A. J., & Williamson, R. C. (2001). Estimating the support of a high-dimensional distribution. *Neural Computation, 13*(7), 1443–1471.
Luo, M. R., Hong, G., & Rhodes, P. A. (2001). A study of digital camera colorimetric characterization based on polynomial modeling. *Color: Research and applications, 26*(1), 76–84.
Maciocia, G. (1987). *Tongue diagnosis in Chinese medicine,* Eastland press.
Malacara, D. (2011). *Color vision and colorimetry: Theory and applications,* SPIE.
Manevitz, L. M., & Yousef, M. (2002). One-class SVMs for document classification. *The Journal of Machine Learning Research, 2,* 139–154.
Mart I Nez-Verd U, F., Pujol, J., Vilaseca, & Capilla, P. (2003). *Characterization of a digital camera as an absolute tristimulus colorimeter* (pp. 197–208): International Society for Optics and Photonics.
Morovi V C, J. A. N. (2008). *Color gamut mapping* (Vol. 10), New York: Wiley.
Morovic, J. A. N., & Luo, M. R. (1997). *Gamut mapping algorithms based on psychophysical experiment* (pp. 44–49), Society for Imaging Science and Technology.
Morovic, J., & Luo, M. R. (2000). Calculating medium and image gamut boundaries for gamut mapping. *Color Research and Application, 25*(6), 394–401.
Ng, D., Allebach, J. P., Analoui, M., & Pizlo, Z. (2003). Non-contact imaging colorimeter for human tooth color assessment using a digital camera. *Journal of Imaging Science and Technology, 47*(6), 531–542.
O'Brien, W. J., Hemmendinger, H., Boenke, K. M., Linger, J. B., & Groh, C. L. (1997). Color distribution of three regions of extracted human teeth. *Dental Materials, 13*(3), 179–185.
Ohta, N., & Robertson, A. (2006). *Colorimetry: Fundamentals and applications,* New York: Wiley.
Pang, B., Zhang, D., Li, N., & Wang, K. (2004). Computerized tongue diagnosis based on Bayesian networks. *IEEE Transactions on Biomedical Engineering, 51*(10), 1803–1810.
Pang, B., Zhang, D., & Wang, K. (2005). Tongue image analysis for appendicitis diagnosis. *Information Sciences, 175*(3), 160–176.
Quan, S., Ohta, N & Katoh, N (2000). *Optimization of camera spectral sensitivities* (pp. 273–278), Society for Imaging Science and Technology.
Schanda, J. A. N. (2007). *Colorimetry: understanding the CIE system,* New York: Wiley.
Vrhel, M. J., & Trussell, H. J. (1999). Color device calibration: A mathematical formulation. *IEEE Transactions on Image Processing, 8*(12), 1796–1806.

Wang, Y., Yang, J., Zhou, Y., & Wang, Y.Z., (2007). Region partition and feature matching based color recognition of tongue image. *Pattern Recognition Letters, 28*(1), 11-19.

Wang, X., & Zhang, D. (2010). An optimized tongue image color correction scheme. *IEEE Transactions on Information Technology in Biomedicine, 14*(6), 1355–1364.

Wang, X., & Zhang, D. (2013). A high quality color imaging system for computerized tongue image analysis. *Expert Systems with Applications, 40*(15), 5854–5866.

Wang, X., Zhang, B., Yang, Z., Wang, H., & Zhang, D. (2013). Statistical analysis of tongue images for feature extraction and diagnostics. *IEEE Transactions on Image Processing A Publication of the IEEE Signal Processing Society, 22*(12), 5336–5347.

Wu, W., Allebach, J. P., & Analoui, M. (2000). Imaging colorimetry using a digital camera. *Journal of Imaging Science and Technology, 44*(4), 267–279.

Wyszecki, G., & Stiles, W. S. (1982). *Color science* (Vol. 8), New York: Wiley.

Xu, J., Zhang, Z., Li, L., Tu, L., & Fei, Z. (2010). Research on the tongue color distribution of sub-healthy samples. *Liaoning Journal of Traditional Chinese Medicine, 12.*

Yuan, J. C., Brewer, J. D., Monaco, E. A., & Davis, E. L. (2007). Defining a natural tooth color space based on a 3-dimensional shade system. *The Journal of prosthetic dentistry, 98*(2), 110–119.

Zhang, Y., & Liang, R., Wang, Z., Fan, Y., & Li, F. (2005). Analysis of the color characteristics of tongue digital images from 884 physical examination cases. *Journal of Beijing University of Traditional Chinese Medicine, 28*(001), 73–75.

Zhang, D., Pang, B., Li, N., Wang, K., & Zhang, H. (2005). Computerized diagnosis from tongue appearance using quantitative feature classification. *The American Journal of Chinese Medicine, 33*(06), 859–866.

Zhang, D., Wang, X., & Lu, G. (2010). An integrated portable standardized human tongue image acquisition system. *Chinese Patent, ZL A, 101972138.*

Chapter 13
Hyperspectral Tongue Image Classification

Abstract The human tongue is an important organ of the body, which carries information of the health status. The images of the human tongue that are currently used in computerized tongue diagnosis of traditional Chinese medicine (TCM) are all RGB color images captured with color CCD cameras. However, this conversional method impedes the accurate analysis of the tongue surface because of the influence of illumination and tongue pose. To address this problem, this chapter presents a novel approach to analyze the tongue surface information based on hyperspectral medical tongue images with support vector machines. The experimental results based on chronic Cholecystitis patients and healthy volunteers illustrate its effectiveness.

13.1 Introduction

There are inevitable limitations of tongue images captured by traditional CCD cameras. The principal difficulties are first that when these images are used it is hard to distinguish between the tongue and neighboring tissues that have a similar color in the RGB color space and second it is also difficult to distinguish between the tongue coating and the tongue body. For these reasons, current methods as described in previous chapters, color analysis and segmentation, e.g., perform well ONLY on tongue images acquired under some special conditions and often fail when the quality of the image is less than ideal (Pang, Zhang & Wang, 2005).

Spectroscopy is a valuable tool for so many applications. In remote sensing application, it has been shown that hyperspectral data are effective for material identification in scenes where other sensing modalities are ineffective (Healey & Slater, 1999). In addition, spectral measurements from human tissue have been used for many years for characterization and monitoring applications in biomedicine. In general, the relatively small number of acquisition channels that characterizes multispectral sensors may be sufficient to discriminate among different substance classes (e.g., face, eyes, hair, and backgrounds). However, considering the vast spectral variability for different tissue types, they are less successful when trying to

D. Zhang et al., *Tongue Image Analysis*, DOI 10.1007/978-981-10-2167-1_13

discriminate between different parts of the same object, for example, distinguishing between the tongue coating and the tongue body.

The discriminative capacities of multispectral sensors can be improved using hyperspectral sensors, which are characterized by a very high spectral resolution that usually results in hundreds of observation channels. Such an approach would exploit the interaction of light with human tissue (Tuchin & Tuchin, 2007; Anderson & Parrish, 1981) because the epidermal and dermal layers act as a scattering medium that contains several pigments such as melanin, hemoglobin, bilirubin, and β-carotene. Small changes in the distribution of these pigments cause significant changes in the skin's spectral reflectance (Edwards & Duntley, 1939; Angelopoulo, Molana & Daniilidis, 2001) as has been measured in recent research into the wavelengths of organ reflectance spectra. Moreover, some progress has been made on biomedical engineering application (Vo-Dinh, 2004).

The main information that must be acquired for a diagnosis concerns the tongue body and the tongue coating, and these must be classified for tongue region analysis. This could be done using supervised classification but then there would be a small ratio between the number of available training samples and the number of features. If common statistically based classifiers are used, it is not possible to obtain reasonable estimates of the class conditional hyper-dimensional probability density functions. The classification accuracy decreases when the number of features given as input to the classifier increase over a given threshold (which depends on the number of training samples and the kind of classifier used) (Hughes, 1968). A more promising approach may be found in recent work using support vector machines (SVM) to classify spectral remote sensing images (Roli & Fumera, 2001; Huang, Davis & Townshend, 2002). There are three reasons for this. First, SVM is a more accurate classifier than other widely used pattern recognition techniques, such as the maximum likelihood method and multilayer perceptron neural network classifiers. Second, SVM can carry out classification using only a few training samples. Third, SVM can efficiently and directly analyze hyperspectral data in hyper-dimensional feature space without the need for any feature-reduction procedure (Gualtieri & Chettri, 2000; Melgani & Bruzzone, 2002). The major drawback of SVMs is that they were originally developed to solve binary classification problems. Fortunately, in our work this is no particular handicap since we are dealing with only two classes: the tongue body and the tongue coating.

In this chapter, we propose a novel automatic tongue surface classification method that makes use of hyperspectral medical image analysis and the SVM classifier. Using hyperspectral sensors instead of the traditional CCD, our tongue image acquisition method is in some sense a spectroscopic extension of those proposed in previous chapters. For instance, unlike existing approaches, our method classifies the tongue body and the tongue coating using their hyperspectral properties rather than their color values in the RGB color space.

The rest of this chapter is organized in four sections. Section 13.2 introduces the hyperspectral tongue image capture device. Section 13.3 recalls the mathematical formulation of SVM and describes its application in hyperspectral tongue image classification. Section 13.4 describes two experiments evaluating this approach. Section 13.5 offers some concluding remarks.

13.2 Hyperpectral Images for Tongue Diagnosis

Hyperspectral images (HSI) can be obtained by a special capture device (Du, Liu, Li, Yan, & Tang, 2007) which can record the information of the entire spectrum of each subject point by a sequence of digital images which is called an "image cube." These image cubes consist of a series of optical images recorded at various wavelengths of interest. An example of an image cube is illustrated in Fig. 13.1. Each pixel of the image has two properties: the spectrum property and the luminance property. We analyze these "image cubes" in the spectral range of interest in order to analyze the tongue area. All images were captured in 120 spectral bands with center wavelengths separated by 5 mm over a waveband of 400–1000 nm. A full 120 band hyperspectral image is acquired in about 6 s with 652 × 488 spatial resolution.

In Fig. 13.2, four reflectance spectra were acquired from different locations for one subject in order to compare within-class and between-class variability. It can be

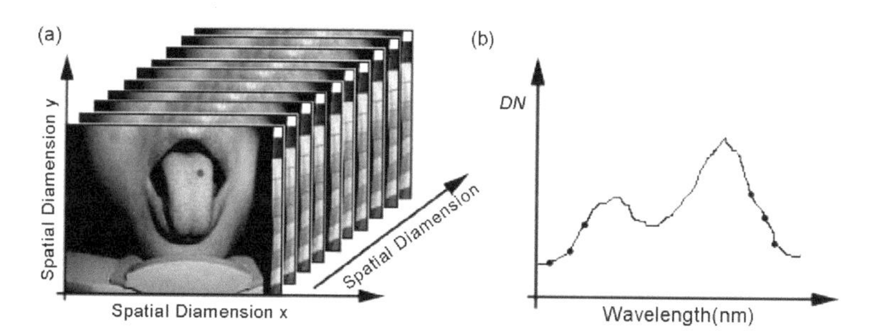

Fig. 13.1 The hyperspectral image cube. (**b**) is the spectrum corresponding to the *red point* in (**a**). Reprinted from Zhi, Zhang, Yan, et al. (2007), with permission from Elsevier

Fig. 13.2 The hyperspectral curves of different subject tongues. Reprinted from Zhi et al. (2007), with permission from Elsevier

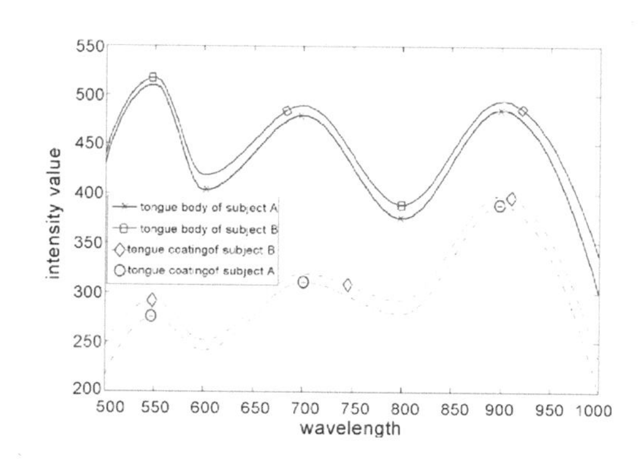

seen in Fig. 13.2 that there are significant differences in both the amplitude and spectral curve shape of the reflectance curves for the different subjects, while the spectral reflectance for one subject remains similar from trial-to-trial.

According to (Pan, Healey, Prasad, & Tromberg, 2003), the raw measurement obtained by the hyperspectral imaging system at spatial coordinate (x, y) and wavelength λ_k is given by

$$I(x, y, \lambda_k) = L(x, y, \lambda_k)S(x, y, \lambda_k)R(x, y, \lambda_k) + O(x, y, \lambda_k), \quad (13.1)$$

where, $L(x, y, \lambda_k)$ is the illumination, $S(x, y, \lambda_k)$ is the system spectral response, $R(x, y, \lambda_k)$ is the reflectance of the viewed subject surface, and $O(x, y, \lambda_k)$ is the offset which includes dark current and stray light. The reflectance $R(x, y, \lambda_k)$ is invariant to the illumination and thus our experiments do not consider illumination variability.

In order to test the feasibility of hyperspectral tongue surface subject classification for tongue diagnosis, we represent each tongue image using spectral reflectance vectors that are extracted from tongue regions. In each tongue region, the spectral reflectance vector $R_t = (R_t(\lambda_1), R_t(\lambda_2), \ldots, R_t(\lambda_l))^T$ is defined for classification, where $t \in (1, 2)$ denotes the tongue coating and the tongue body, respectively, and l is the number of hyperspectral wavebands.

13.3 The Classifier Applied to Hyperspectral Tongue Images

SVM is a popular classifier based on statistical learning theory (Vapnik & Vapnik, 1998). In contrast to traditional learning techniques, SVM does not explicitly depend on the dimensionality of input spaces. This makes it useful for the supervised nonparametric classification of hyperspectral images. There are two types of SVM, linear and nonlinear. The training data of linear SVM may be analyzed as either linearly separable or linearly non-separable. In the following, we describe both of these analyses, beginning with the simpler of the two and follow these with a description of nonlinear SVM. A detailed analysis of the theory of SVM can be found in (Vapnik & Vapnik, 1998; Melgani & Bruzzone, 2004).

13.3.1 Linear SVM: Linearly Separable

Let us assume that the training set $\boldsymbol{X} = (x_1, x_2, \ldots, x_n)$ consists of N vectors from the d-dimension feature space, i.e., $x_i \in R^d (i = 1, 2, \ldots, N)$. A target $y_i = \{1, -1\}$ corresponds to the input vector x_i. If two classes are linearly separable, it is possible to find at least one hyperplane which is defined by a vector $w \in R^d$ (normal to the hyperplane) and a bias $b \in R$ that can separate the two classes without errors. Then we can define a discriminant function associated with the hyperplane:

$$f(x) = w \cdot x + b. \tag{13.2}$$

Then, to find the hyperplane that maximizes the distance between the closest training samples and the separating hyperplane, we estimate w and b, so that $y_i(w \cdot x_i + b) > 0$ $i = (1, 2, \ldots, N)$. The distance can be denoted as $1/\|w\|$. Thus, the geometrical margin between the two classes is given by $2/\|w\|$. By adjusting the hyperplane parameters w and b, we can get

$$\min_{i=1,2,\ldots,N} y_i(w \cdot x_i + b) \geq 1. \tag{13.3}$$

The optimal hyperplane problem can be represented by a Lagrangian formulation, which can be expressed as

$$\begin{cases} \sum_{i=1}^{N} \alpha_i - \frac{1}{2}\sum_{i=1}^{N}\sum_{j=1}^{N} \alpha_i\alpha_j y_i y_j (x_i \cdot x_j) \\ \sum_{i=1}^{N} \alpha_i y_i = 0 \quad (\alpha_i \geq 0,\ i = 1, 2, \ldots, N) \end{cases}, \tag{13.4}$$

where a_i $(i = 1, 2, \ldots, N)$ are Lagrange multipliers, which effectively weight each training sample according to its importance in determining the discriminant function. Accordingly, the discriminant function associated with the optimal hyperplane becomes an equation depending both on the Lagrange multipliers and on the training samples. This function can be expressed as

$$f(x) = \sum_{i \in S} \alpha_i y_i (x_i \cdot x) + b, \tag{13.5}$$

where S is the subset of training samples corresponding to the nonzero Lagrange multipliers a_i. The training samples with nonzero weights are called support vectors.

13.3.2 *Linear SVM: Linearly Non-separable*

Linearly non-separable SVM is used to handle non-separable data and generalized the concept of an optimal separating hyperplane to minimize a cost function. This cost function $\Psi(\cdot)$ is formularized as the following equation:

$$\psi(\omega, \xi) = \frac{1}{2}\|\omega\|^2 + C\sum_{i=1}^{N} \xi_i, \tag{13.6}$$

where the constant C represents a regularization parameter that adjusts the penalty assigned to errors. In other words, the larger the C value, the higher the penalty

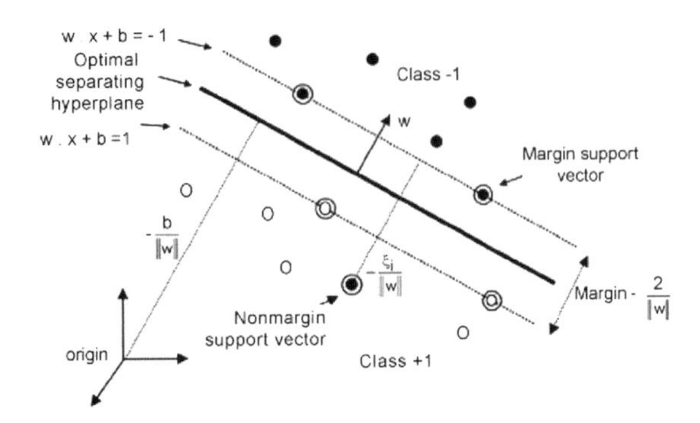

Fig. 13.3 Optimal separating hyperplane in SVM for a linearly non-separable case. *White* and *black circles* correspond with the classes "+1" and "−1," respectively. The support vectors are indicated by *concentric circles* (Melgani & Bruzzone, 2004). Reprinted from Zhi et al. (2007), with permission from Elsevier

associated with misclassified samples. The notation ξi represents the slack variable caused by the non-reparability of the data. In this case, support vectors are either margin support vectors on the hyperplane margin or support vectors that fall on the false side of the margin, as shown in Fig. 13.3.

13.3.3 Non-linear SVM

The non-linear SVM is one of the so-called Kernel methods, which maps the data through a proper non-linear transformation $\phi(\cdot)$ into a higher dimensional feature space $\phi(x) \in R^{d'}$ ($d' > d$), where d and d' are the dimensionalities of the feature vectors. As in linear SVM, to separate sample data in the higher dimension space, we estimate the normal vector $w \in R^{d'}$ and a bias $b \in R$ to find an optimal hyperplane. To avoid the inter-product, which is complex and time consuming, we use the following equation:

$$K(x_i, x) = \phi(x_i) \cdot \phi(x), \tag{13.7}$$

where $K(\cdot)$ is called the kernel function. Thus, the discriminant function $f(x)$ can be formularized as Eq. (13.8), i.e.,

$$f(x) = \sum_{i \in S} \alpha_i y_i K(x_i, x) + b. \tag{13.8}$$

A commonly used kernel function is the Gaussian kernel function, which is defined as

$$K(x_i, x) = \exp\left(-\frac{\|x_i - x\|^2}{2\sigma^2}\right), \tag{13.9}$$

where σ expresses the standard deviation of the Gaussian distribution.

13.4 Experimental Results and Performance Analysis

In this section we describe two experiments, comparing the efficiency and effectiveness of SVM methods with other conventional classifiers and present the ability of SVM for classifying the tongue body and tongue coating based on hyperspectral and RGB images. The hyperspectral medical tongue image dataset used in our experiments consists of a total of 375 images of tongues of 300 patients and 75 healthy volunteers. The images were captured using our hyperspectral image sensor. To measure the area of the tongue, we obtained a series of 400-1000 nm hyperspectral tongue images. Some samples of the image cubes of various tongues are shown in Fig. 13.4. These hyperspectral samples were extracted between 403.7 and 865.2 nm wavelengths.

13.4.1 Comparing Linear and Non-linear SVM, RBFNN, and K-NN Classifiers

The first of our two experiments compared the effectiveness of four classifiers in directly classifying hyperspectral tongue images in the original hyper-dimensional feature space: Linear and non-linear SVM, and two widely used nonparametric classifiers, radial basis functions neural network (RBFNN) and the conventional K-nearest neighbors (K-NN) classifier in terms of classification accuracy and speed.

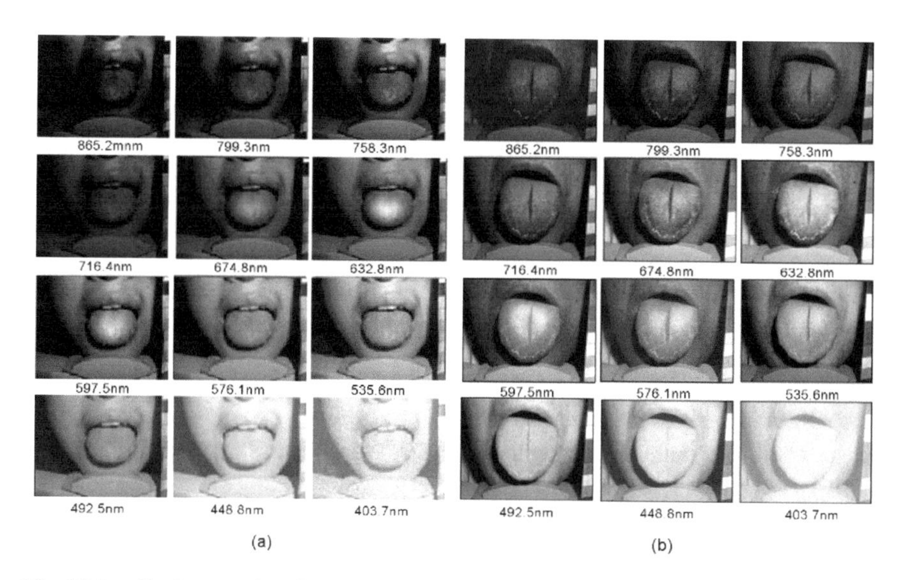

Fig. 13.4 **a** Twelve samples of a hyperspectral tongue image of a healthy man. **b** Twelve sample of a hyperspectral tongue image of a chronic Cholecystitis patient. Reprinted from Zhi et al. (2007), with permission from Elsevier

Table 13.1 Results of a comparison of the classifiers

Methods	Classification accuracy (%)		Computing cost (s)
	w_1	w_2	
Linear SVM	88.74	90.02	1394
Nonlinear SVM	91.27	93.11	596
RBFNN Classifier	87.92	86.74	844
K-NN Classifier	87.66	85.93	691

Reprinted from Zhi et al. (2007), with permission from Elsevier

We selected the RBFNN classifier because, like the SVM method, it is kernel-based, which applies a different strategy based on a "statistical" (rather than a "geometrical") criterion for defining the discriminant hyperplane in the transformed kernel space (Melgani & Bruzzone, 2004).We selected the K-NN classifier which is a very popular classification method in the field of pattern recognition. The experimental platform was a Pentium IV 2.4 MHz with 2 GM of memory.

We used linear SVM without kernel transformation and nonlinear SVM with a Gaussian kernel. For both of these types of SVM, the regularization parameter C must be estimated, since data are not ideally separable. According to Eq. (13.9), the parameter in non-linear SVM σ should be set. In our experiments, we set σ as 0.3 for the optimal classification results. As can be seen in Table 13.1, SVM more accurately and faster classified the hyperspectral tongue images than either RBFNN or K-NN. It can also be seen that non-linear SVM is the most accurate. K-NN has the worst performance as it requires a much larger sample space for training than the SVM methods or K-NN.

13.4.2 Evaluating the Diagnostic Performance of SVM

The second experiment compared the performance of SVM for hyperspectral tongue images with the approach that is used for RGB tongue images, which is the current norm in tongue image analysis systems. The criterion is the ability to diagnose a classic condition of Chinese tongue diagnosis, Cholecystitis, with reference to a set of images manually classified by experts. Chronic Cholecystitis patients present a thick, greasy, yellow tongue coating (Feng & Tianbin, 2002), whereas the tongue of a healthy individual will have little tongue coating or just a thin, white tongue coating. The hyperspectral curves of the tongue body and the tongue coating of both the healthy and unhealthy subjects are shown in Fig. 13.5. It can be seen that the hyperspectral characteristics of the tongue coating and the tongue body are very different between waveband 50 and waveband 100. That is, in the assigned waveband range that we are interested in there is a difference in their hyperspectral curves. Furthermore, the mean values of the spectral curves of the tongue body of both the healthy and unhealthy subjects are about 450. The differences in the average values for the tongue coatings of the healthy and unhealthy

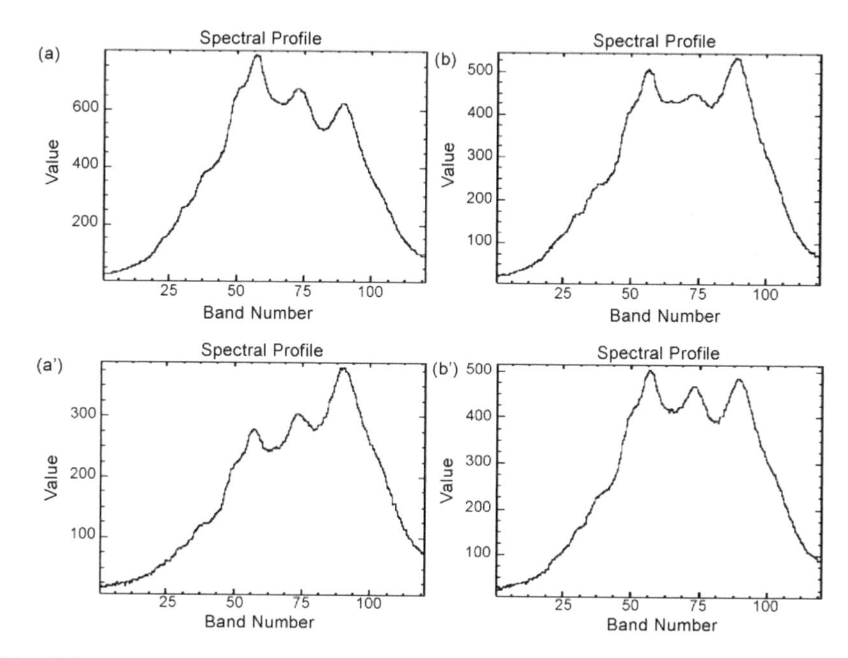

Fig. 13.5 Hyperspectral profiles of the tongue coating and the tongue body. **a** and **b** are the spectral curves of the tongue coating and the tongue body of chronic Cholecystitis patient, respectively. **a**' and **b**' are the spectral curves of the tongue coating and the tongue body of a healthy man. Reprinted from Zhi et al. (2007), with permission from Elsevier

subjects, however, are obvious. It can be seen that the average value of the tongue coating of the chronic Cholecystitis patient is 625, while that of the healthy subject is 295. On the other hand, the standard deviations of the sample values of the tongue coating hyperspectral curves of the chronic Cholecystitis patient and healthy subject are 83.9 and 64.2, respectively, while that of the tongue body of the chronic Cholecystitis patient and healthy subject are 48.7 and 50.6, respectively. It is obviously that the hyperspectral image of the tongue coating has a much larger standard deviation than that of the tongue body. All these facts demonstrate that objects in the same class have similar hyperspectral characteristics.

Table 13.2 reports performance of SVM in HSI and traditional RGB images. We defined the average error rate (AER) to evaluate the classification results. This function can be formularized as follows:

$$\mathrm{AER} = \frac{\mathrm{sum}(\text{classification results} - \text{reference})}{n} \times 100\% \tag{13.10}$$

In this study, the term "reference" in the formula refers to the results obtained by the manual classification of experts. It can be seen that using SVM in HSI can obtain close classification results to the manual ones with an AER of only 0.78% for patients and 0.55% for the healthy subject. However, using SVM in traditional

Table 13.2 The performance of SVM for one of the tongue diagnostic criteria

	The ratio of the areas between the tongue coating and the tongue body		
	SVM in HSI (%)	SVM in RGB (%)	Manual discriminating by experts (%)
Cholecystitis patient A	52.1	39.4	50.9
Cholecystitis patient B	41.7	36.4	40.8
Cholecystitis patient C	38.7	44.1	39.2
Cholecystitis patient D	49.2	52.3	48.7
Healthy subject A	8.1	5.7	7.3
Healthy subject B	3.2	4.5	3.9
Healthy subject C	4.6	3.9	4.2
Healthy subject D	2.9	2.5	2.6

Reprinted from Zhi et al. (2007), with permission from Elsevier

RGB tongue images, the AER is 5.85% for patients and 0.65% for healthy subjects. It is obvious that the SVM in hyperspectral tongue images can obtain a better classification performance for the patients, which is more approximate to the manual discriminating results of tongue surface subjects by experts. These two approaches can obtain similar results for healthy subjects. That is because there is so little tongue coating on the tongue surface of a healthy subject.

13.5 Summary

This chapter presents the utility of hyperspectral medical imaging for tongue diagnosis of Traditional Chinese Medicine. SVM based on the hyperspectral comparison of combinations of tissue types was applied to the images for diagnosis. The experiments consider a database of hyperspectral tongue images from 375 subjects. In order to assess experiments, one was used to compare the performance of some classifiers on analyzing hyperspectral tongue images, and the other was used to evaluate the performance of the hyperspectral approach compared with the traditional RGB approach. The experimental results showed that this method can overcome some limitations of the traditional method for tongue image analysis and provide a better classification performance than that of the traditional method.

References

Anderson, R. R., & Parrish, J. A. (1981). The optics of human skin. *Journal of Investigative Dermatology, 77*(1), 13–19.
Angelopoulo, E., Molana, R., & Daniilidis, K. (2001). Multispectral skin color modeling (pp. 635). IEEE.
Du, H., Liu, Z., Li, Q., Yan, J., & Tang, Q. (2007). A novel hyperspectral medical sensor for tongue diagnosis. *Sensor Review, 27*(1), 57–60.
Edwards, E. A., & Duntley, S. Q. (1939). The pigments and color of living human skin. *American Journal of Anatomy, 65*(1), 1–33.
Feng, I., & Tianbin, S. (2002). *Practicality handbook of tongue diagnosis of TC*. Beijing: Ke Xue Chu Ban She.
Gualtieri, J. A., & Chettri, S. (2000). Support vector machines for classification of hyperspectral data (pp. 813–815). IEEE.
Healey, G., & Slater, D. (1999). Models and methods for automated material identification in hyperspectral imagery acquired under unknown illumination and atmospheric conditions. *Geoscience and Remote Sensing, IEEE Transactions on, 37*(6), 2706–2717.
Huang, C., Davis, L. S., & Townshend, J. (2002). An assessment of support vector machines for land cover classification. *International Journal of Remote Sensing, 23*(4), 725–749.
Hughes, G. P. (1968). On the mean accuracy of statistical pattern recognizers. *Information Theory, IEEE Transactions on, 14*(1), 55–63.
Melgani, F., & Bruzzone, L. (2002). Support vector machines for classification of hyperspectral remote-sensing images (pp. 506–508). IEEE.
Melgani, F., & Bruzzone, L. (2004). Classification of hyperspectral remote sensing images with support vector machines. *Geoscience and Remote Sensing, IEEE Transactions on, 42*(8), 1778–1790.
Pan, Z., Healey, G., Prasad, M., & Tromberg, B. (2003). Face recognition in hyperspectral images. *Pattern Analysis and Machine Intelligence, IEEE Transactions on, 25*(12), 1552–1560.
Pang, B., Zhang, D., & Wang, K. (2005). The bi-elliptical deformable contour and its application to automated tongue segmentation in Chinese medicine. *IEEE Transactions on Medical Imaging, 24*(8), 946–956.
Roli, F., & Fumera, G. (2001). Support vector machines for remote sensing image classification (pp. 160–166). International Society for Optics and Photonics.
Tuchin, V. U. I. V., & Tuchin, V. (2007). *Tissue optics: light scattering methods and instruments for medical diagnosis* (Vol. 13). Bellingham: SPIE press.
Vapnik, V. N., & Vapnik, V. (1998). *Statistical learning theory* (Vol. 1). New York:Wiley.
Vo-Dinh, T. (2004). A hyperspectral imaging system for in vivo optical diagnostics. *IEEE Engineering in Medicine and Biology Magazine, 23*(5), 40–49.
Zhi, L., Zhang, D., Yan, J. Q., et al. (2007). Classification of hyperspectral medical tongue images for tongue diagnosis. *Computerized Medical Imaging & Graphics the Official Journal of the Computerized Medical Imaging Society, 31*(8), 672–678.

Part IV
Tongue Image Analysis and Diagnosis

Chapter 14
Computerized Tongue Diagnosis Based on Bayesian Networks

Abstract Tongue diagnosis is an important diagnostic method in traditional Chinese medicine (TCM). However, due to its qualitative, subjective, and experience-based nature, traditional tongue diagnosis has a very limited application in clinical medicine. Moreover, traditional tongue diagnosis is always concerned with the identification of syndromes rather than with the connection between abnormal tongue appearances and diseases. This is not well understood in Western medicine, and thus greatly obstructs its wider use. In this chapter, we present a novel computerized tongue inspection method aimed at addressing these problems. First, two kinds of quantitative features, chromatic and textural, are extracted from tongue images by using popular digital image processing techniques. Then, Bayesian networks are employed to model the relationship between these quantitative features and diseases. The effectiveness of the method is tested on a group of 455 patients affected by 13 common diseases as well as other 70 healthy volunteers, and the diagnostic results predicted by the previously trained Bayesian network classifiers are reported.

14.1 Introduction

As tongue diagnosis has played a prominent role in the diagnosis and subsequent treatment of disease, it has attracted an increasing amount of attention, both in clinical medicine and in biomedicine. However, traditional tongue diagnosis has its inevitable limitations. First, the clinical competence of tongue diagnosis is determined by the experience and knowledge of the physicians. Second, environmental factors, such as differences in light sources and their brightness, have a great influence on the physicians in obtaining good diagnostic results from the tongue. Finally, traditional tongue diagnosis is intimately related to the identification of syndromes, and it is not very well understood by Western medicine and modern biomedicine. Therefore, it is necessary to build an objective and quantitative diagnostic standard for tongue diagnosis.

D. Zhang et al., *Tongue Image Analysis*, DOI 10.1007/978-981-10-2167-1_14

To address these problems, researchers have been striving to develop methods and systems for computerized tongue diagnosis (Chiu, Lin, & Lin, 1995; Chiu, 1996; Yuen, Kuang, Wu, & Wu, 1999; Watsuji, Arita, Shinohara, & Kitade, 1999; Chiu, 2000; Jiehua, 2001; Li & Yuen, 2002; Nai-Min, 1994; Weng, 1997). Although researchers have made considerable progress in the standardization and quantification of tongue diagnosis, there are still significant problems with the existing approaches. First, some methods are only concerned with the identification of syndromes that are based on sophisticated terms from TCM. Consequently, they are not widely accepted, especially in Western medicine. Second, the underlying validity of these methods and systems is usually based on a comparison between the diagnostic results that are obtained from the methods or systems and the judgments made by skillful practitioners of tongue diagnosis. That is, by using such an approach they cannot hope to avoid subjectivity. Third, only very few samples are used in experiments (usually not more than 120), and this is far from meeting the requirements for obtaining a reasonable result in statistical pattern recognition. Last, many of the developed systems are only dedicated to the recognition of pathological features (such as the colors of the body of the tongue and the furring of the tongue) in tongue diagnosis, and mapping from the images of the tongue to diseases is not considered. This undoubtedly limits the applications of such systems in clinical medicine.

In this chapter, we propose a computerized tongue inspection method based on quantitative features and Bayesian networks. Different from existing approaches, our method is dedicated to the classification of 14 diagnostic categories (13 common diseases and healthy persons) instead of the identification of syndromes. Also, rather than trying to find numeric representations of those qualitative features that originate from traditional tongue diagnosis, we extract two ordinary kinds of quantitative features from tongue images, chromatic and textural features, by using popular image processing techniques. One direct benefit is that the subjectivity of evaluation is eliminated.

14.2 Tongue Diagnosis Using Bayesian Networks

Uncertainty is an inherent issue in nearly all medical problems. The prevailing methods for managing various forms of uncertainty are formalized within a probabilistic framework. The corresponding Bayesian statistics provides a compelling theoretical foundation that coherent subjective beliefs of human experts should be expressible in a probabilistic framework. Bayesian network models provide a practical tool to create and maintain such probabilistic knowledge bases.

A Bayesian network [or Bayesian belief network (BBN)] (Pearl, 1986; Friedman, Geiger & Goldszmidt, 1997) for a problem domain, which is just a set of variables $\{x_1, \ldots, x_n\}$, is a causal probabilistic network that compactly represents a joint probability distribution (JPD) over these variables. The representation consists of a set of local conditional probability distributions, combined with a set of assertions of conditional independence (CI) that allow us to construct the global joint distribution from the local distributions. The decomposition is based on the chain rule of probability, which dictates that

$$p(x_1, \ldots, x_n) = \prod_{i=1}^{n} p(x_i | x_1, \ldots, x_{i-1}) \tag{14.1}$$

For each variable x_i, let $\prod_i \subseteq \{x_1, \ldots, x_{i-1}\}$ (a parent set) be a set of variables that renders x_i and $\{x_1, \ldots, x_{i-1}\}$ conditionally independent. That is,

$$p(x_i | x_1, \ldots, x_{i-1}) = p\left(x_i \prod_i\right). \tag{14.2}$$

Given these sets, a Bayesian network can be described as a directed acyclic graph (DAG) such that each variable $x_1, \ldots, x_n$ corresponds to a node in that graph and the parents of the node corresponding to x_i are the nodes corresponding to the variables in $\prod_i$. Associated with each node x_i are the conditional probability distributions $p(x_i \mid \prod_i)$ -one distribution for each instance of $\prod_i$. Combining (1) and (2), it can be seen that any Bayesian network for $(x_1, \ldots, x_n)$ uniquely determines a joint probability distribution for these variables. That is,

$$p(x_1, \ldots, x_n) = \prod_{i=1}^{n} p\left(x_i \middle| \prod_i\right) \tag{14.3}$$

Bayesian networks have several advantages for data analysis (Heckerman, 1997). First, since the model encodes dependencies among all variables, it readily handles situations where some data entries are missing. Second, a Bayesian network can be used to learn causal relationships, and hence can be used to gain an understanding about a problem domain and to predict the consequences of intervention. Third, because the model has both causal and probabilistic semantics, it is an ideal representation for combining prior knowledge (which often comes in causal form) and data. Fourth, Bayesian statistical methods in conjunction with Bayesian networks offer an efficient and principled approach for avoiding the overfitting of data. Finally, it is found (Henrion, Pradhan, Del Favero, Provan, & O'Rorke, 1996) that diagnostic performance with Bayesian networks is often surprisingly insensitive to imprecision in the numerical probabilities. Knowledge that high levels of precision are not necessary should greatly improve acceptance of these techniques. Many researchers have criticized the use of Bayesian networks because of the need to provide many numbers to specify the conditional probability distributions. However, if rough approximations are adequate, then these criticisms may lose their sting. Thanks to these unique characteristics, BBNs have been widely used in many machine learning applications, and also in medical diagnosis (Tsymbal & Puuronen, 2002; Ogunyemi, Clarke, & Webber, 2000).

For computerized tongue diagnosis, two points should be mentioned when using a BBN as a diagnostic model. First, although Bayesian networks provide a natural and efficient way of representing prior knowledge, we do not employ any such information when constructing our diagnostic model. Consequently, both the graphic structure and the conditional probability tables of the BBN must be estimated from patient case data using statistical algorithms. The reason is twofold. First, humans are often inconsistent in their assessment of probabilities, and demonstrate many forms of bias in their judgments (Tversky & Kahneman, 1974). Similarly, experts are not able to provide probability distributions for a large number of variables in a consistent fashion, although they are usually good at identifying important dependencies that exist across variables in the domain. Thus, it is argued that for the computerized tongue diagnosis application, which involves a large number of variables, obtaining probability estimates from an existing database is often more reliable than eliciting them from human experts. Second, expert knowledge in traditional tongue diagnosis is always concerned with the identification of syndromes instead of with the relationship between tongue appearances and diseases. Therefore, prior knowledge of the relationship between symptoms (abnormal tongue appearances) and diseases in terms of probability distributions is unavailable.

The second point concerning the use of a BBN as a diagnostic model is that, all of the nodes except for the root node (class node) in our model (a Bayesian network classifier) represent quantitative chromatic and textural features obtained by using image processing techniques, which are not directly related to the qualitative pathological features employed in tradition tongue diagnosis. This is consistent with the original intention of our method: the quantification and objectification of traditional tongue diagnosis.

The outline of a computerized tongue diagnosis system that uses a Bayesian network as the feature-matching model is illustrated in Fig. 14.1 Our method is dedicated to the feature extraction and matching processes.

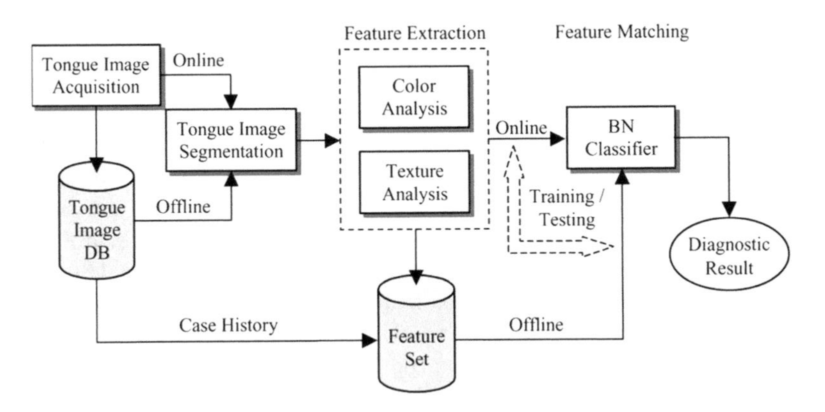

Fig. 14.1 Outline of the computerized tongue diagnosis system. © 2016 IEEE. Reprinted, with permission, from Pang et al. (2004)

14.3 Quantitative Pathological Features Extraction

As mentioned above, the main aim of our method is to diagnose diseases from a set of quantitative features that are extracted using image processing algorithms. However, traditional tongue diagnosis theories on pathological features are all qualitative, and thus subjective, using descriptions such as "reddish purple tongue," and "white, thin, and slippery coating," (Maciocia, 1987). Therefore, how to develop appropriate objective features that are meaningful for diagnosis is an important issue. The most direct way is to find a set of objective measurements, each of which corresponds to a specific qualitative feature in traditional tongue diagnosis, just as many existing methods (Li & Yuen, 2002; Chiu, 2000; Yuen et al., 1999; Takeichi & Sato, 1997) for computerized tongue image analysis usually do. Although direct and simple, these methods suffer from difficulties concerning evaluation standards since they are evaluated by physicians. This leads to a strange situation: methods are purposely devised to replace qualitative features so to avoid subjectivity while they are subjectively evaluated.

Actually, many descriptive features in traditional tongue diagnosis indicate some implicit relations to color and texture related features (for example "reddish purple," "white," "thin," and "slippery"). In order to remain consistent with the original intention of our method, we employ several general chromatic and textural measurements (Pitas, 2000; Reed & Dubuf, 1993) and take no consideration of whether these measurements explicitly correspond to specific qualitative features. Note that some of these features may be neither visible nor understandable by tongue diagnosis practitioners. The correlation and effectiveness of these features in diagnosis are identified in a statistical manner during the training of Bayesian network classifiers.

14.3.1 Quantitative Color Features

A color is always given in relation to a specific color space and the extraction of color features can be performed in different color spaces (Pitas, 2000). A color space is a method by which we can specify, create, and visualize color. A color is usually specified using three coordinates or parameters. These parameters describe the position of the color within the color space being used. Familiar color spaces frequently used in image processing include RGB, HSV, CIE*Yxy*, CIE*LUV*, and CIE*LAB*.

RGB (Red Green Blue) is an additive color system based on trichromatic theory, which is often found in systems that use a CRT to display images. RGB is easy to implement but nonlinear with visual perception. RGB is frequently used in most computer applications since no transform is required to display information on the screen. Consequently, RGB is commonly the basic color space for most applications.

The CIE (the International Commission on Illumination) system is based on the description of color as a luminance component Y, and two additional components X and Z. The magnitudes of the XYZ components are proportional to physical energy, i.e., any color is represented by a positive set of values. The CIEXYZ color space is usually used as a reference color space and is as such an intermediate device-independent color space. Practically, it is often convenient to discuss "pure" color in the absence of brightness. The CIE defines a normalization process to compute two chromaticity coordinates: $x = X/(X + Y + Z)$ $y = X/(X + Y + Z)$. Thus, a color can be specified by its chromaticity and luminance in the form of an xyY(CIEYxy) triple.

The CIEXYZ and RGB systems are far from exhibiting perceptual uniformity. So the CIE standardized two systems based on CIEXYZ, CIELUV and CIELAB, whose main goal is to provide a perceptually equal space. This means that the Euclidian distance between two colors in the CIELUV/CIELAB color space is strongly correlated with human visual perception. CIELUV and CIELAB are device independent but suffer from being quite unintuitive despite the L parameter having a good correlation with perceived lightness.

Different from other color spaces, the HSV color space is an intuitive system in which a specific color is described by its hue, saturation, and brightness values. It is a linear transformation from the RGB space. However, HSV has discontinuities in the value of the hue around red, which make this system noise sensitive. As a result, we use the other four color spaces (RGB, CIEYxy, CIELUV, and CIELAB) for the extraction of quantitative color features.

The color-related measurements used in our method are the mean and standard deviation of the colors of pixels within the whole region of the tongue in the four color spaces. Since both the L channels in CIELUV and CIELAB indicate the sensation of the lightness in the human vision system, we use it only once. Thus, there are a total of 22 different measures as follows. CR_i ($i = 1, 2, \ldots, 11$): Means of each color plane in the four color spaces, and CR_j ($j = 12, 13, \ldots, 22$) standard deviations of each color plane in the four color spaces.

14.3.2 Quantitative Texture Features

Among all statistical methods, the most popular one, which is based on the estimation of the second-order statistics of the spatial arrangement of the gray level values, is the gray-level co-occurrence matrices. A co-occurrence matrix (Haralick, Shanmugam, & Dinstein, 1973) is a square matrix whose elements correspond to the relative frequency of occurrence of pairs of gray level values of pixels separated by a certain distance in a given direction. Formally, the elements of a $G \times G$ gray level co-occurrence matrix $P\mathbf{d}$ for a displacement vector $\mathbf{d} = (\mathrm{d}x, \mathrm{d}y)$ are defined as

$$P_d(g_1, g_2) = \left| \left\{ \begin{array}{l} (a, b) \in N \times N : I(a, b) = g_1, \\ I(a + \mathrm{d}x, b + \mathrm{d}y) = g_2, \\ (a + \mathrm{d}x, b + \mathrm{d}y \ \in \ N \times N) \end{array} \right\} \right|, \quad (14.4)$$

where $I(\cdot, \cdot)$ denotes an image of size $N \times N$ with G gray values, g_1 and g_2 are two gray-level values, and $|\cdot|$ is the cardinality of a set.

In this chapter, two measures of textural features, which are derived from the co-occurrence matrix, are used to extract different textural features from tongue images. These two descriptors are the second-order moment and the contrast measures of the matrix, which are shown as follows:

$$\begin{aligned} W_M &= \sum_{g_1} \sum_{g_2} p^2(g_1, g_2) \\ W_C &= \sum_{g_1} \sum_{g_2} |g_1 - g_2| p(g_1, g_2), \end{aligned} \quad (14.5)$$

where $p(g_1, g_2)$ is a normalized co-occurrence matrix. That is $p(g_1, g_2) = P_d(g_1, g_2)/S$ where S is the total number of pixel pairs (g_1, g_2) across all g_1 and g_2, i.e., $S = \sum_{g_1=0}^{G-1} \sum_{g_1=0}^{G-1} P_d(g_1, g_2)$. W_M measures the smoothness or homogeneity of an image, which will reach its minimum value when all of the $p(g_1, g_2)$ have the same value. W_C is the first-order moment of the differences in the values of the gray level between the entries in a co-occurrence matrix. Both of the textural descriptors are quantitatively calculated. Notice that they have little correlation with the sensation of the human vision system (Reed & Dubuf, 1993). For all the textural measures in the following experiments, we take 64 gray levels (i.e., $G = 64$) and $\mathbf{d} = (6, 6)$.

It is believed (Maciocia, 1987) that different parts of the tongue correspond to different internal organs. The tip of the tongue, for example, reveals heart and lung conditions, and the middle tongue conditions of the spleen and stomach. It does not matter whether this theory is true; the important fact is that there are usually abnormal changes in texture in different parts of the tongue when various diseases are present. Therefore, to represent these possible pathological changes, we calculate the above textural measures for each partition of a tongue. For convenience, we denote each partition of a tongue using a digit: 1–Tip of the tongue; 2–Left edge of the tongue; 3–Center of the tongue; 4–Right edge of the tongue; and 5–Root of the tongue. Thus, we obtain a set of textural measurements for each tongue, which contains a total of 10 textural measures as follows:

$$\left\{ \begin{array}{l} TR_i = W_{M,i} \\ TR_{i+5} = W_{C,i} \end{array} \right. (i = 1, 2, \ldots, 5), \quad (14.6)$$

where $W_{M,j}$ and $W_{C,\ i}$ denote the measurements of W_M and W_C for partition i, respectively.

14.4 Experimental Results

We used the Bayesian Network PowerPredictor, developed by Cheng (Cheng, Bell, & Liu, 1997; Cheng, 2000), to train and test the tongue diagnosis models. The Power Predictor uses a database as input and constructs the Bayesian network classifier, both structure and parameters, as output. The construction process is based on dependence analysis using information theory. The dependency relationships among nodes are measured by using a type of CI test. The learning algorithm uses a three-phase construction mechanism, while at the same time a wrapper algorithm is applied to fight the overfitting problem. Moreover, a natural method for feature subset selection is introduced in the learning process, which can often produce a much smaller Bayesian network classifier without compromising the classification accuracy.

A total of 525 subjects, including 455 patients and 70 healthy volunteers, were involved in the following experiments. There were 13 common internal diseases included (see Table 14.1). The patients were all inpatients mainly from five different departments at the Harbin 211 Hospital, and the healthy volunteers were chosen from students of Harbin Institute of Technology. We took a total of 525 digital tongue images, one for each subject, as the experimental samples. Four typical tongue image samples are shown in Fig. 14.2.

Table 14.1 List of the 13 common diseases and healthy subjects

Disease ID	Disease	Number of subjects
D00	Healthy	70
D01	Intestinal infarction	11
D02	Cholecystitis	21
D03	Appendicitis	43
D04	Pancreatitis	41
D05	Nephritis	17
D06	Diabetes mellitus	49
D07	Hypertension	65
D08	Heart failure	17
D09	Pulmonary heart disease	21
D10	Coronary heart disease	71
D11	Hepatocirrhosis	25
D12	Cerebral infarction	30
D13	Upper respiratory infection	44

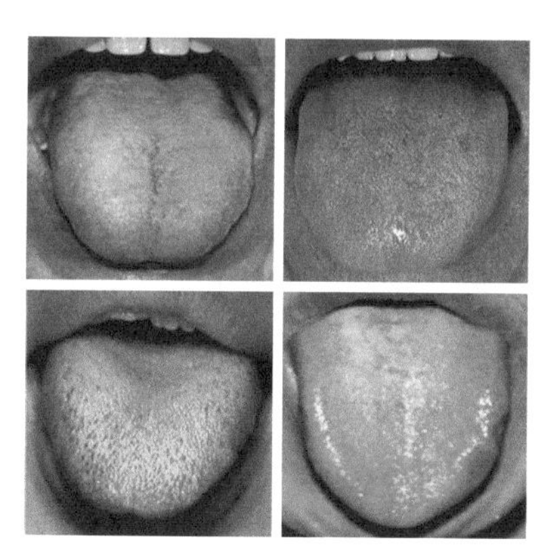

Fig. 14.2 Four tongue image samples of patients suffering intestinal infarction (*upper left*), cholecystitis (*upper right*), appendicitis (*lower left*), and pancreatitis (*lower right*). © 2016 IEEE. Reprinted, with permission, from Pang et al. (2004)

14.4.1 Several Issues

In many projects concerning tongue diagnosis in TCM, the straightforward way to label the samples is to ask TCM doctors to judge them. However, the judgment of tongue diagnosis doctors is always related to syndromes or qualitative features rather than medical diseases. Therefore, these approaches do not solve the problem of the individual empiricism inherent in tongue diagnosis, and the diagnostic results given in this way are too sophisticated to understand. In this research, we used the diagnostic results obtained by using the clinical differential diagnosis methodology as the labels of the tongue images. Since all the subjects in the experiment were inpatients, the diagnoses are highly reliable. During the testing process, the diagnostic results obtained by querying the Bayesian networks were compared with the corresponding labels of the tongue images. This formed an objective evaluation basis for our method.

Another issue concerns the relative small sample size. The weak point of this study and very probably of most attempts to provide medical statistics is the difficulty of gathering both a sufficient number of cases and reliable data for each case. To overcome this problem, we utilized a stratified k-fold cross-validation (CV) technique (Mullin & Sukthankar, 2000) (for all of the experiments, k equals to 10) in all of the following experiments to estimate the accuracy of classifiers. The k-fold CV technique partitions a pool of labeled data, S, into k approximately equally sized subsets. Each subset is used as a test set for a classifier trained on the remaining $k-1$ subsets. The empirical accuracy is given by the average of the accuracies of these k classifiers. When employing a stratified partitioning in which the subsets contain approximately the same proportion of classes as S, we obtain a stratified k-fold CV, which can reduce the estimate's variance.

Next, we used discrete Bayesian networks in the following experiments. The discretization method (Cheng, 2000) of fields (attributes) was "Equal Width," and the number of intervals was set to 5 for all of the fields. Thus, the network parameters–local conditional probability distributions are actually local conditional probabilities. At the same time, in order to demonstrate the superiority of Bayesian network classifiers in tongue diagnosis, we implemented a nearest-neighbor classifier (NNC) for comparison. Similarly, a stratified k-fold CV (k = 10) was used for the evaluation of its accuracy. Thus, each sample in a test subset was assigned to the same label as its nearest labeled sample belonging to the rest of the ($k-1$) subsets. This process was repeated k times on each subset to estimate the overall accuracy.

Finally, in the following experiments, we used a misclassification cost table assuming that all types of misclassification are equally important. This may be not correct in practice, but it does not invalidate the demonstration of the effectiveness of our method in diagnosing diseases.

14.4.2 Bayesian Network Classifier Based on Textural Features

In the first experiment, we trained a Bayesian network classifier based on textural features, called a "texture BNC" (T-BNC). The graphical structure of the learned T-BNC is illustrated in Fig. 14.3. Note that, this BNC structure corresponds to the highest scoring out of tenfold CV iterations. A subset of 5 textural features out of the original feature set (containing a total of 10 textural features) was selected by an underlying feature selection function integrated in the training algorithm. Two of the five surviving features (namely, TR_2 and TR_5) were the measurements of W_M for the left side and root of the tongue. The other three were the measurements of W_C for the tip, left side and root of the tongue, respectively. Obviously, textural measurements related to the tip, sides (although only the measurements for the left side of the tongue were selected, as it was found that both sides have similar values), and root of the tongue are most discriminating for the classification.

The diagnostic results given by the T-BNC are shown in the first column of Table 14.2. The average true positive rate (TPR) was 26.1%, which demonstrates that the textural features utilized in this study are not very discriminating in diagnosing these diseases. Nevertheless, for the identification of appendicitis (D03), pancreatitis (D04), and coronary heart disease (D10), these textural features were more meaningful. Due to the low sensitivity values, we do not list the positive predictive values (PPV) for the T-BNC.

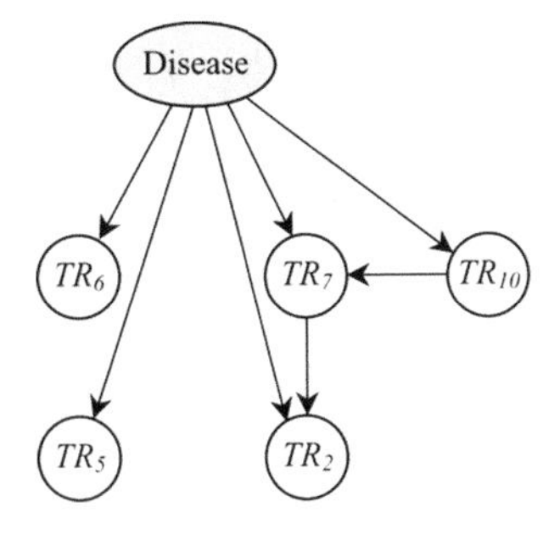

Fig. 14.3 Structure of the T-BNC. © 2016 IEEE. Reprinted, with permission, from Pang et al. (2004)

Table 14.2 Diagnostic results (in percentage) of various Bayesian network classifiers in terms of sensitivity (true positive rate)

Disease ID	Texture BNC	Color BNC	Joint BNC
D00	20.0	50.0	77.1
D01	9.1	45.5	63.6
D02	4.8	42.9	61.9
D03	53.5	86.0	93.0
D04	70.7	90.2	100
D05	5.9	17.6	23.5
D06	4.1	53.1	65.3
D07	3.1	61.5	75.4
D08	5.9	35.3	35.3
D09	4.8	47.6	71.4
D10	64.8	90.1	93.0
D11	12	48.0	64.0
D12	13.3	60.0	80.0
D13	20.5	56.8	70.5
Average	26.1	62.3	75.8

14.4.3 Bayesian Network Classifier Based on Chromatic Features

This section evaluated the suitability of chromatic measures for classification. The graphic structure of the trained model, called a "color BNC" (C-BNC) , is shown in Fig. 14.4. Again, the learned structure also corresponds to the highest scoring in the CV iterations. A subset of 12 chromatic features was selected from the original feature set containing 22 features. Among these surviving measurements, 6 are directly connected to the class node (Disease), which thereafter are called "contribution" nodes. Note that each of the four color spaces used in our experiment includes at least one "contribution" node, and the mean and standard deviation measurements have similar significance for the classification.

The diagnostic results of the color BNC are listed in the second column of Table 14.2 in terms of sensitivity and the first column of Table 14.3 in terms of

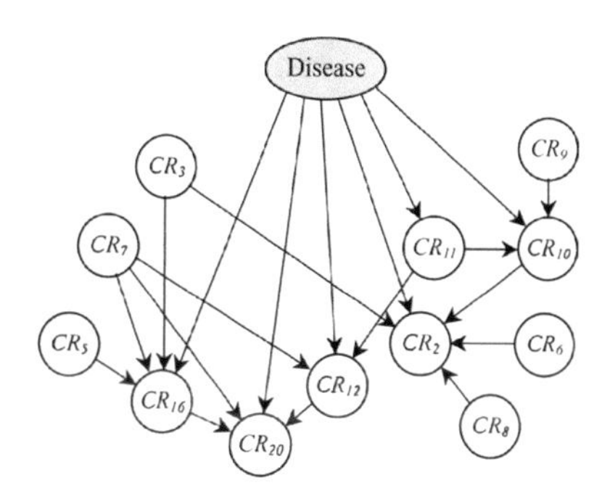

Fig. 14.4 Structure of the C-BNC. © 2016 IEEE. Reprinted, with permission, from Pang et al. (2004)

Table 14.3 Positive predictive values (PPV) of the C-BNC and the J-BNC (in percentage)

Disease ID	Color BNC	Joint BNC
D00	79.5	85.7
D01	100	87.5
D02	100	92.9
D03	60.7	72.7
D04	68.5	75.9
D05	100	80
D06	81.3	84.2
D07	66.7	80.3
D08	100	100
D09	83.3	88.2
D10	37.9	54.5
D11	100	88.9
D12	66.7	75.0
D13	80.6	93.9

PPVs. Obviously, the diagnostic classification capability of the color BNC is significantly better than that of texture BNC: the average TPR of the C-BNC is 62.3%. It should be noticed that the C-BNC gives a very accurate and relatively reliable diagnosis of pancreatitis (D04) with 90.2% TPRs and 68.5% PPVs. The reason for this is that it was found that patients with pancreatitis usually have a distinctively bluish tongue (see Fig. 14.2).

14.4.4 Bayesian Network Classifier Based on Combined Features

Finally, we used both chromatic and textural features to construct a joint BNC (J-BNC) for the classification of these diseases. The graphical structure of the trained J-BNC is illustrated in Fig. 14.5 This structure also corresponds to the

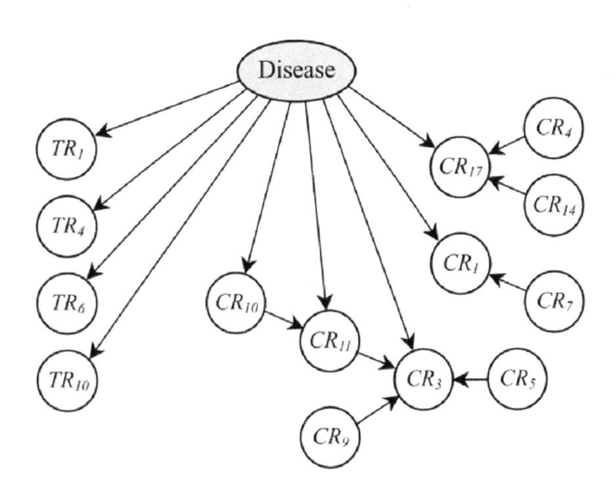

Fig. 14.5 Structure of the J-BNC. © 2016 IEEE. Reprinted, with permission, from Pang et al. (2004)

Table 14.4 Confusion matrix of the J-BNC

		Predicted													
		D00	D01	D02	D03	D04	D05	D06	D07	D08	D09	D10	D11	D12	D13
Actual	D00	**54**			2	3			2			9			
	D01	1	**7**			1		2							
	D02	1		**13**		3						4			
	D03	1			**40**							1			1
	D04					**41**									
	D05	3			1		**4**		1			7		1	
	D06	1			3	1		**32**	3			5		4	
	D07				3				**49**		1	10	2		
	D08	1		1	2			1	1	**6**		5			
	D09				1				1		**15**	3			1
	D10	1			1			1	2			**66**			
	D11				1	1						5	**16**	2	
	D12					1		1	1		1	2		**24**	
	D13		1		1	3	1	1	1			4		1	**31**

Table 14.5 Comparison of J-BNC and NNC on combined features in terms of sensitivity

Disease ID	Joint BNC	NNC
D00	77.1	28.6
D01	63.6	54.5
D02	61.9	33.3
D03	93.0	44.2
D04	100	56.1
D05	23.5	35.3
D06	65.3	18.4
D07	75.4	18.5
D08	35.3	52.9
D09	71.4	52.4
D10	93.0	46.5
D11	64.0	40.0
D12	80.0	20.0
D13	70.5	43.2
Average	75.8	36.2

highest classification scoring in the CV iterations. Out of the 32 features originally taken into consideration, 14 were finally selected among which 9 (5 chromatic features and 4 textural features) were the "contribution" nodes, which were both discriminative and independent. Note that, the four surviving textural features were the measurements of W_M for the tip (TR_1) and right side (TR_4) of the tongue, and the measurements of W_C for the tip (TR_6) and root (TR_{10}) of the tongue. Similar to the T-BNC, textural measurements related to the tip, sides, and root of the tongue are most relevant to the diagnostic classification for the J-BNC. It is interesting that this apparent relationship between diseases and parts of the tongue that was purely learned from statistics has a high degree of accord with the beliefs of traditional tongue diagnosis.

Tables 14.2 and 14.3 show the diagnostic results given by the J-BNC in terms of TPR and PPV. The estimate prediction accuracy was 75.8%, which outperforms both the T-BNC and the C-BNC. Note that for the diagnosis of D00 (healthy), D04 (pancreatitis), D07 (hypertension), and D12 (cerebral infarction), the TPRs and PPVs of the J-BNC were all higher than 75%. For convenience of illustration, the confusion matrix of the J-BNC is given in Table 14.4.

For comparison, we employed a NNC on the combined feature set and utilized the stratified k-fold (k = 10) CV technology to evaluate the classification accuracy. The diagnostic results are given in Table 14.5 in terms of sensitivity. It can be seen that Bayesian network classifiers are quite superior to the NNC with respect to the classification accuracy of tongue images.

14.5 Summary

In this chapter, we proposed a computerized tongue diagnosis method aimed at eliminating the subjective and qualitative characteristics of traditional tongue diagnosis and establishing the relationship between tongue appearance and diseases. Bayesian network classifiers based on quantitative features, namely chromatic and textural measurements, were employed as the decision models for diagnosis. Experiments were carried out on 455 inpatients affected by 13 common internal diseases and 70 healthy volunteers. The estimate prediction accuracy of the joint BNC was as high as 75.8%. In particular, the diagnosis of four groups: healthy, pancreatitis, hypertension, and cerebral infarction had both TPRs and PPVs higher than 75%. The experimental results demonstrated the effectiveness of the method described in this chapter, thus establishing the potential usefulness of computerized tongue diagnosis in clinical medicine.

References

Cheng, J. (2000). *Power predictor system software*. Online Available: http://www.cs.ualberta.ca/~jcheng/bnpp.htm

Cheng, J., Bell, D. A., & Liu, W. (1997). *Learning belief networks from data: An information theory based approach* (pp. 325–331), ACM.

Chiu, C. (1996). The development of a computerized tongue diagnosis system. *Biomedical Engineering Applications Basis Communications, 8,* 342–350.

Chiu, C. (2000). A novel approach based on computerized image analysis for traditional Chinese medical diagnosis of the tongue. *Computer Methods and Programs in Biomedicine, 61*(2), 77–89.

Chiu, C. C., Lin, H. S., & Lin, S. L. (1995). A structural texture recognition approach for medical diagnosis through tongue. *Biomedical Engineering Applications Basis and Communications, 7*(2), 143–148.

Friedman, N., Geiger, D., & Goldszmidt, M. (1997). Bayesian network classifiers. *Machine Learning, 29*(2–3), 131–163.

Haralick, R. M., Shanmugam, K., & Dinstein, I. H. (1973). Textural features for image classification. *IEEE Transactions on Systems, Man and Cybernetics, 6,* 610–621.

Heckerman, D. (1997). Bayesian networks for data mining. *Data Mining and Knowledge Discovery, 1*(1), 79–119.

Henrion, M., Pradhan, M., Del Favero, B., Provan, G., & O'Rorke, P. (1996). *Why is diagnosis using belief networks insensitive to imprecision in probabilities?* (pp. 307–314), Morgan Kaufmann Publishers Inc.

Jiehua, Z. (2001). Towards the standardization of tongue diagnosis: an image processing approach. *Chinese Journal of Biomedical Engineering, 20*(2), 132–137.

Li, C. H., & Yuen, P. C. (2002). Tongue image matching using color content. *Pattern Recognition, 35*(2), 407–419.

Maciocia, G. (1987). *Tongue diagnosis in Chinese medicine,* Eastland press.

Mullin, M. D., & Sukthankar, R. (2000). *Complete cross-validation for nearest neighbor classifiers* (pp. 639–646).

Nai-Min, L. I. (1994). *The handbook of Chinese tongue diagnosis*. Xue-Yuan Publishing.

Ogunyemi, O., Clarke, J. R., & Webber, B. (2000). *Using Bayesian networks for diagnostic reasoning in penetrating injury assessment* (pp. 115–120), IEEE.

Pang, B., Zhang, D., Li, N., et al. (2004). Computerized tongue diagnosis based on Bayesian networks. *IEEE Transactions on Bio-Medical Engineering, 51*(10), 1803–1810.

Pearl, J. (1986). Fusion, propagation, and structuring in belief networks. *Artificial Intelligence, 29*(3), 241–288.

Pitas, I. (2000). *Digital image processing algorithms and applications,* New York: Wiley.

Reed, T. R., & Dubuf, J. H. (1993). A review of recent texture segmentation and feature extraction techniques. *CVGIP: Image understanding, 57*(3), 359–372.

Takeichi, M., & Sato, T. (1997). Computerized color analysis of "xue yu" (blood stasis) in the sublingual vein using a new technology. *The American journal of Chinese medicine, 25*(02), 213–219.

Tsymbal, A., & Puuronen, S. (2002). *Ensemble feature selection with the simple Bayesian classification in medical diagnostics* (pp. 225–230), IEEE.

Tversky, A., & Kahneman, D. (1974). Judgment under uncertainty: Heuristics and biases. *Science, 185*(4157), 1124–1131.

Watsuji, T., Arita, S., Shinohara, S., & Kitade, T. (1999). *Medical application of fuzzy theory to the diagnostic system of tongue inspection in traditional Chinese medicine* (pp. 145–148), IEEE.

Weng, L. (1997). *The illustrations of clinical tongue diagnosis and disease treatments,* Xue-Yuan Publishing.

Yuen, P. C., Kuang, Z. Y., Wu, W., & Wu, Y. T. (1999). Tongue texture analysis using opponent color features for tongue diagnosis in traditional Chinese medicine. In *Proceedings of TAMV* (pp. 21–27).

Chapter 15
Tongue Image Analysis for Appendicitis Diagnosis

Abstract Medical diagnosis using the tongue is a unique and important diagnostic method of traditional Chinese medicine (TCM). However, the clinical applications of tongue diagnosis have been limited due to three factors: (1) tongue diagnosis is usually based on the capacity of the eye for detailed discrimination. (2) the correctness of tongue diagnosis depends on the experience of physicians, and (3) traditional tongue diagnosis is always dedicated to the identification of syndromes rather than diseases. To address these problems, in this chapter, we present a tongue-computing model (TCoM) for the diagnosis of appendicitis based on quantitative measurements that include chromatic and textural metrics. These metrics are computed from true color tongue images using appropriate techniques of image processing. When our approach was applied to clinical tongue images, the results of the experiments were encouraging.

15.1 Introduction

Benefiting from the study in the last chapter we focus on the diagnosis of special diseases. Hence we present in this chapter a computerized tongue inspection approach, which is called a tongue-computing model (TCoM), for the diagnosis of a special disease, appendicitis. Compared with existing models and approaches, the TCoM has several outstanding characteristics. First, it is not concerned with the identification of syndromes that are very popular in TCM. Instead, it establishes a mapping from quantitative features to a specific disease (e.g., appendicitis). Consequently, the TCoM is actually mostly independent of TCM, except that it is related to tongue diagnosis. Second, the underlying validity of the TCoM is based on diagnostic results using Western medicine. The measurements of the chromatic and textural properties of a tongue, which are obtained via image processing techniques, are compared with the corresponding diagnostic results from using Western medicine, instead of the judgment of a TCM doctor. This forms the objective basis of the TCoM and such an approach could expedite its use in clinical applications. Last, all of the images of the tongue in our experiments (912 samples)

D. Zhang et al., *Tongue Image Analysis*, DOI 10.1007/978-981-10-2167-1_15

were selected from a tongue image database that contains more than 12,000 samples. And therefore, the diagnostic results that are presented in this chapter are statistically very reliable.

The rest of this chapter is organized in five sections. In Sect. 15.2 we describe the main features used by the model as well as their extraction methods. Then, we briefly introduce a filter for identifying filiform papillae in Sect. 15.3 The experimental results and quantitative evaluations are shown in Sects. 15.4 and 15.5 offers some concluding remarks.

15.2 Chromatic and Textural Features for Tongue Diagnosis

15.2.1 The Image of the Tongue of a Patient with Appendicitis

Appendicitis is an acute abdominal disease. The main abnormal changes that are shown in the images of the tongue of the patients with appendicitis include three aspects: the color of the body of the tongue and its coating, the texture of the tongue and its coating, and, in particular, the pathological changes at the tip of the tongue (see Fig. 15.1). The color of the tongue substance could be light red, red, or dark red, according to how serious the problem has become. Also, abnormal changes in the coating indicate the severity of the appendicitis. Its color could be white or yellow, and the coating may be thin or thick, or it might have a greasy appearance or a combination of these properties. Moreover, the most important sign of appendicitis in an image of the tongue is that there are lots of prickles on the tip of the tongue, whose color is usually distinctly red. A typical image of a tongue from a patient with appendicitis is shown in Fig. 15.2 together with an image of a normal tongue for comparison.

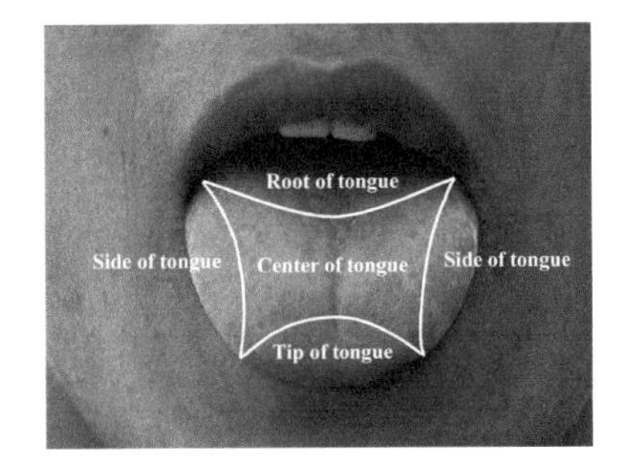

Fig. 15.1 The partition of a tongue. Reprinted from Pang, Zhang, and Wang (2005), with permission from Elsevier

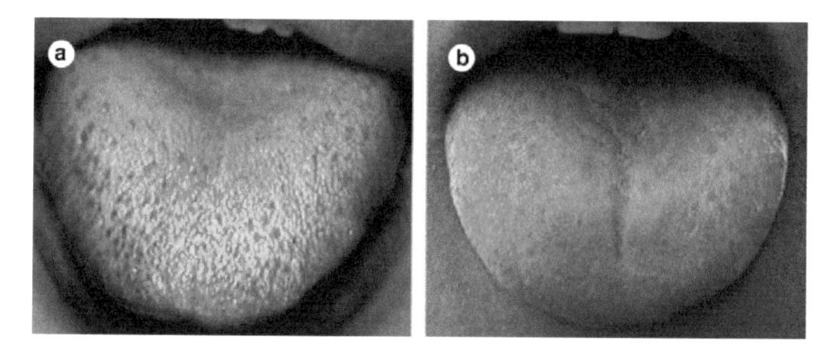

Fig. 15.2 **a** A typical image of the tongue from a patient with appendicitis, and **b** a typical normal tongue image. Reprinted from Pang et al. (2005), with permission from Elsevier

15.2.2 Quantitative Features of the Color of the Tongue

The color always has to be given relative to a specific color space. The extraction of the features of the color can be performed in different color spaces, which usually include RGB, HSV, CIEYxy, CIELUV, and CIELAB. Different from the other color spaces, the HSV color space is an intuitive system in which a specific color is described by its hue, saturation, and brightness values. This color space is often used in software systems to aid in interactive selection and manipulation of color. However, the HSV space has discontinuities in the value of the hue around the red, which make this approach sensitive to noise. Therefore, in our system we use the remaining four color spaces (RGB, CIEYxy, CIELUV, and CIELAB) for the extraction of quantitative features of the color.

The metrics for color that are used in our algorithms are the means and standard deviations of the colors of each pixel within a region of the tongue, using all of the four color spaces. Thus, there are a total of 22 different metrics in four color spaces as follows.

CM_i ($i = 1, 2, \ldots, 10, 11$): Mean of each plane of color in the four color spaces, and CM_i ($i = 12, 13, \ldots, 22$): Standard deviations of each plane of color in the four color spaces.

Since both of the L channels in CIELUV and CIELAB indicate the sensation of the lightness in the human vision system, we only use it once in the calculation of the features of the color.

15.2.3 Quantitative Features of the Texture of the Tongue

Methods for extracting the features of the texture can be roughly categorized as follows: feature-based, model-based, and structural. In feature-based methods, some characteristic or characteristics of the textures are chosen and regions are sought in which these characteristics are relatively constant (or the boundaries between the

Table 15.1 Numbers indicating different partitions of a tongue

1	Tip of the tongue
2	Left edge of the tongue
3	Center of the tongue
4	Right edge of the tongue
5	Root of the tongue

Reprinted from Pang et al. (2005), with permission from Elsevier

regions). In this chapter, two feature-based texture operators, which are derived from the co-occurrence matrix, are implemented to extract different textural features from images of the tongue. These two descriptors are the second moment and the contrast metrics based on a co-occurrence matrix, which are shown as follows:

$$\begin{aligned} W_M &= \sum_{g_1}\sum_{g_2} P^2(g_1, g_2) \\ W_C &= \sum_{g_1}\sum_{g_2} |g_1 - g_2| P(g_1, g_2) \end{aligned} \tag{15.1}$$

where $P\,(g_1,\,g_2)$ is a co-occurrence matrix and g_1 and g_2 are two values of the gray level. W_M measures the smoothness or homogeneity of an image that will reach its minimum value when all of the $P\,(g_1,\,g_2)$ have the same value. W_C is the first moment of the differences in the values of the gray level between the entries in the co-occurrence matrix. Both of the textural descriptors are quantitatively calculated and have little correlation with the sensation of the human vision system.

It has been found in clinical practice (Li, Wang & Li, 1987; Chen & Bei, 1991) that there is some relation between abnormal changes of different parts of the tongue and diseases. That is, different diseases may cause pathological changes to different parts of the tongue. Therefore, we calculate the above two textural metrics for each partition (see Fig. 15.1) of a tongue. For convenience, we denote each partition of a tongue with a number, as shown in Table 15.1 Thus, we obtain a set of textural features for each tongue, which contains 10 textural metrics as follows.

$$\begin{cases} TM_i = W_{M,i} \\ TM_{i+5} = W_{C,i} \end{cases} \quad (i = 1, 2, \ldots, 5) \tag{15.2}$$

where $W_{M,i}$ and $W_{C,i}$ denote the measurements of W_M and W_C for each partition, respectively.

15.3 Identification of Filiform Papillae

15.3.1 Typical Figures and Statistics of Filiform Papillae

A typical pathological change in the tongue of a patient suffering from appendicitis is that there are lots of "prickles" on the tip of the tongue. Actually, these "prickles" are

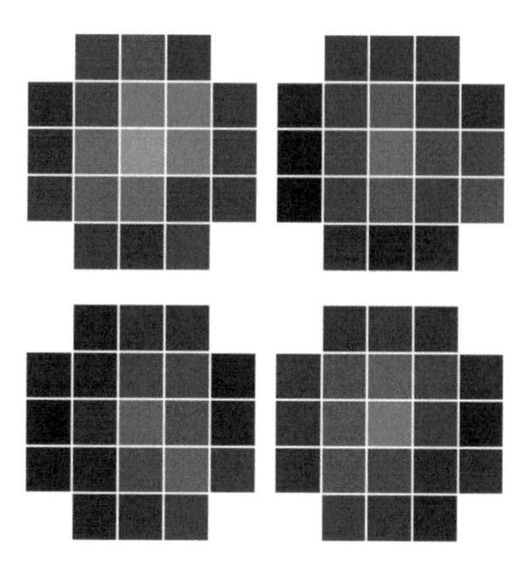

Fig. 15.3 Samples for the intensity distribution of filiform papilla. Reprinted from Pang et al. (2005), with permission from Elsevier

hyperplastic filiform papillae. Under normal conditions, the filiform papillae, which are flat and not easily seen, are distributed evenly over the whole surface of the tongue (see Fig. 15.3b). However, under the conditions of some diseases, such as appendicitis, there are usually abnormal changes in the filiform papillae (Li et al., 1987). For example, when a patient suffers from appendicitis, the filiform papillae on the tip of the tongue always become hyperplastic, as shown in Fig. 15.4a. (Note the white prickles on the tip of the tongue, which are protuberances from the surface of the tongue.)

Thus, to achieve a better diagnosis of appendicitis, the identification of the filiform papillae is very important. Instead of using the general description of filiform papillae (such as "protuberant prickles"), which is based on the human vision system, we must obtain a quantitative measurement of the filiform papillae in a specific plane of color. We have found that filiform papillae are most obvious in the blue plane of a true color image. At the same time, a filiform papilla is usually a very small feature in an image of the tongue that is sampled using our capturing system. So a square template, which we call a filiform papilla template (FPT), of 5×5 pixels is enough to cover a filiform papilla (although the four pixels at the corners of the template are not included). Therefore, we record the distribution of the intensity (in the blue plane) within the template for each filiform papilla, and we obtain a quantitative measurement of the filiform papillae. Figure 15.5 illustrates four examples of our results.

Fig. 15.4 The statistics for the average values of the relative intensity in a FPT. Reprinted from Pang et al. (2005), with permission from Elsevier

	5.8	6	5.8	
5.8	7	8	7	5.8
6	8	10	8	6
5.8	7	8	7	5.8
	5.8	6	5.8	

FPF_8.4-0.6

	-0.5	-0.4	-0.5	
-0.5	0.2	0.8	0.2	-0.5
-0.4	0.8	1.0	0.8	-0.4
-0.5	0.2	0.8	0.2	-0.5
	-0.5	-0.4	-0.5	

FPF_4.1-0.6

	-0.3	-0.2	-0.3	
-0.3	0.0	0.4	0.0	-0.3
-0.2	0.4	1.0	0.4	-0.2
-0.3	0.0	0.4	0.0	-0.3
	-0.3	-0.2	-0.3	

Fig. 15.5 The proposed filiform papilla filters (FPF). Reprinted from Pang et al. (2005), with permission from Elsevier

The statistics for the average values of the relative intensity in a FPT, which is centered at a filiform papilla, are shown as follows:

Note that this template is centrosymmetric, and for convenience we use a variable vector to represent the template as follows:

$$V = \{v_i | i = 1, 2, \ldots, 5\} \tag{15.3}$$

To be more specific, V is evaluated by {10, 8, 7, 6, and 5.8} in this case.

15.3.2 *Filter for Filiform Papillae*

Based on the statistics of the filiform papillae that were established in the previous section, we can design a filter to highlight all of the filiform papillae and repress other pathological signs (such as the white coating, spots, and fungiform papillae). However, developing such a filter is difficult due to the following two factors.

Theoretically, to highlight a filiform papilla we can develop a centrosymmetric filter, T, of size 5 × 5 pixels, with its elements satisfying the following equations:

$$T = \arg\max\left\{\sum_i (t_i \cdot v_i)\right\} \tag{15.4}$$

$$S_T = \sum_i t_i = 0 \tag{15.5}$$

where $T = \{t_i \mid i = 1, 2, \ldots, 5\}$ is the vector of the centrosymmetric filter, expressed in a similar way to the filiform papilla template, and v_i is defined in Eq. (15.3). Unfortunately, this equation is so ill conditioned that no meaningful solution can be obtained.

Moreover, in addition to the ability to highlight all filiform papillae, the filter is also required to repress other pathological details. That is, it should be designed to increase as much as possible the difference between a filiform papilla and any other pathological features. However, in practice, this is very difficult to achieve because there are so many kinds of pathological details. At the same time, there are lots of possible distributions in intensity for each kind of pathological detail. Therefore, no reliable statistics can be obtained.

In this chapter, we make use of both statistical and empirical methods to find a reasonable solution to this problem. After many experiments, we produced two filters, which we call filiform papilla filters (FPF), which are denoted by FPF_8.4–0.6 and FPF_4.1–0.6, as follows:

To highlight the filiform papillae, we convolve the blue plane of an original image using the two FPF filters. Then, each point with a resultant value of the convolution greater than a threshold is marked as a hyperplastic filiform papilla. In practice, the threshold can be zero.

Because of the interference from other pathological details, many spurious filiform papillae are found. This is especially the case for fungiform papillae and spots, which have very different distributions of intensity compared with a filiform papilla but usually produce similar results when filtered by a FPF. This unwanted result originates from the method used to seek solutions to Eqs. (15.4) and (15.5), which are ill conditioned.

To address this problem, we introduce a secondary filtering operation that is based on the results obtained from the FPF. The key point of using the second filtering operation is to take into account the essential characteristic of a hyperplastic filiform papilla: In the distribution of the intensity within a FPT, the pixels take on much larger values at the center than in the nearby surroundings.

15.4 Experimental Results and Analysis

We developed a prototype of our approach, which was applied to 912 (456×2) samples chosen from our database of over 12,000 clinical images of the tongue. These samples were gathered using a specially designed light-tight capturing device that was composed of a 3-CCD (charge coupled device) digital camera and two standard D65 lights. The camera was carefully calibrated (white balancing) using a white color plate and its preferences were afterwards kept unchanged. This ensured a stable imaging condition. The subjects were all in-patients mainly from five departments of internal medicine at the Harbin 211 Hospital.

The experimental samples include 114 images from tongues affected by appendicitis and 798 samples from tongues affected by 13 other familiar diseases, such as pancreatitis, hypertension, and diabetes. These samples were captured from 456 patients (two samples from each person), and they were divided into two sets: the training set and test set. In this section, we present the experimental results for the diagnosis of appendicitis.

The results presented in this section are divided into three parts. The first part evaluates the performance of the color metrics in each color space (RGB, CIEYxy, CIELUV, and CIELAB). The second part evaluates the performance of textural metrics in different partitions of the tongue. Based on the results in the first two parts, we eliminated those metrics that did not perform well. The third part reports the performance of a combined metric that includes the surviving metrics from the first two experiments.

It can be seen that our approach actually includes a procedure for feature selection involving the evaluation of the performance of color and texture related metrics. To provide a quantitative measurement in order to evaluate the capability of the different metrics in differentiating appendicitis from other diseases, we introduced a new measurement, called *grade of differentiation* (GOD), which can be calculated as follows:

$$\mathrm{GOD}_i = \left| \frac{A_{i,\mathrm{mean}} - O_{i,\mathrm{mean}}}{A_{i,\mathrm{mean}}} \right| \tag{15.6}$$

where $A_{i,\mathrm{mean}}$ is the mean of metric i, which is evaluated for the samples with appendicitis, and $O_{i,\mathrm{mean}}$ is the mean of metric i, which is evaluated for all of the other samples.

Finally, for the classification of an image of the tongue (to determine whether it is associated with appendicitis or not) based on the set of metrics, we first used a so-called nearest distance rule for the classification of each metric. Then, we employed the consensus of all of the metrics in the set to obtain each conclusion.

15.4.1 Evaluation Basis for Diagnosis

In many pattern recognition and matching problems, such as identification and verification of identities, it is easy to define the criteria of the evaluation. That is, each testing and training sample is labeled. In many projects that focus on tongue diagnosis in traditional Chinese medicine, the straightforward way to label the samples is to ask doctors of TCM to judge them. Since this is usually the evaluation criterion of the matching, such approaches do not avoid subjectivity. In this research, the evaluation of the diagnosis is based on the diagnostic results from Western medicine. We used the relationship between the measurements of the chromatic and textural properties of a tongue (obtained via image processing techniques) and the diagnostic results of the corresponding patient. This provides an objective evaluation of our approach.

15.4.2 Performance of Metrics for Color

The objective of this section is to discover which metrics do not perform well for diagnosis of appendicitis. Figure 15.6 shows the results for the GODs of different metrics (means) in four color spaces (as defined in Sect. 15.2.2). For the

Table 15.2 Diagnostic results of appendicitis using chromatic metrics (number of correct and false classifications to total number)

	CM1-CM22	CM8-CM14, CM16, CM18
Correct/total	32/57	38/57
False/total	142/399	126/399

Reprinted from Pang et al. (2005), with permission from Elsevier

measurement of the mean, the metric that gave the best performance was CM11 (the **B** chromatic plane in the CIELAB space), whereas the metric that gave the worst performance is CM2 (the **B** plane in the RGB space). Moreover, all of the metrics that are related to lightness or brightness (CM4 and CM7) exhibited poor performance. However, the four chromatic metrics in the two CIE perceptual uniform color spaces (CM8-CM11) performed exceptionally well.

Figure 15 illustrates the results of the GODs of different metrics (standard deviation) in the four color spaces. The best performing metrics were CM12 (deviation of R in the RGB space) and CM18 (deviation of L in the CIELUV/AB space), whereas the worst performing metric was CM15 (deviation of Y in the CIEYxy space). A very interesting contrast can be seen for the four chromatic channels that correspond to CM19-CM22 in Fig. 15 that had a very poor performance, whereas they performed well in Fig. 15.

The diagnostic results of appendicitis based on the 22 chromatic metrics and a subset, which was selected according to the performance presented in this section, of the total chromatic metrics are shown in Table 15.2. It can be seen that, the ratios of the correct classification were 56.14%, when using all chromatic metrics and rose

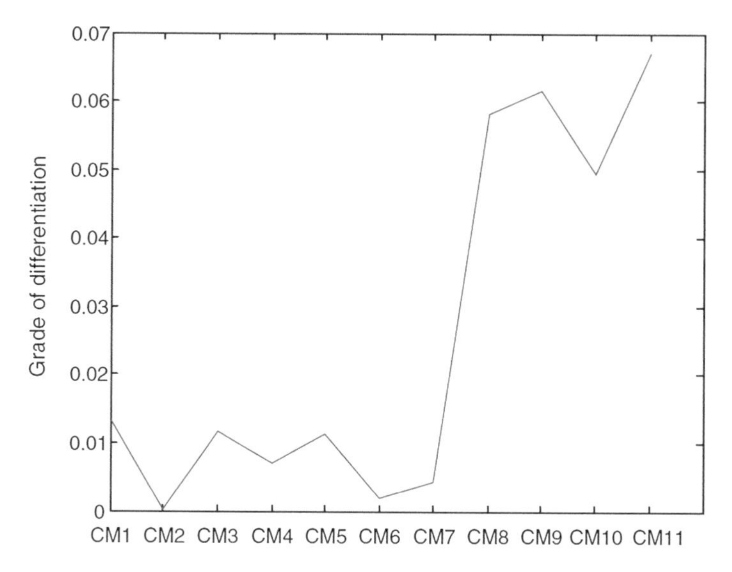

Fig. 15.6 GODs of the means in the four color spaces. Reprinted from Pang et al. (2005), with permission from Elsevier

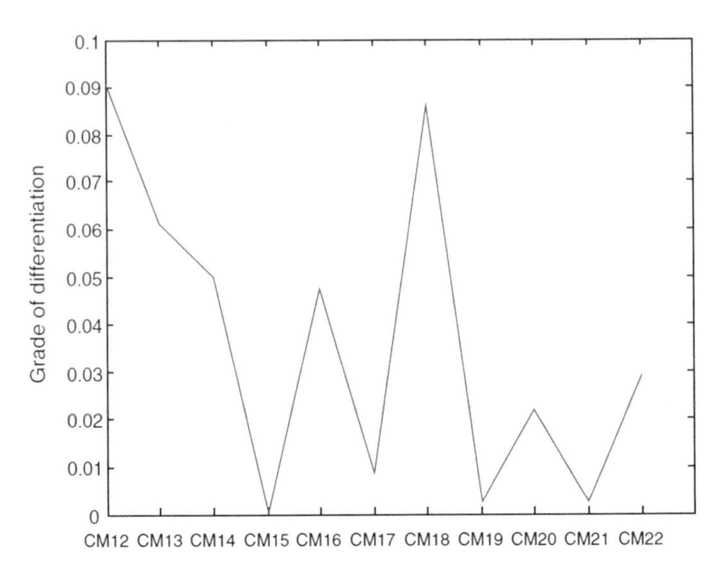

Fig. 15.7 GODs of the standard deviations in the four color spaces. Reprinted from Pang et al. (2005), with permission from Elsevier

to 66.67%, when a subset of these metrics was used. Also, the values of FAR decreased through this feature selection (Figs. 15.6 and 15.7).

15.4.3 Performance of Textural Metrics

This section evaluates the suitability of different textural metrics for diagnosing appendicitis. Two kinds of textural features (W_M and W_C) are implemented for five partitions of the tongue, providing a total of 10 different metrics whose GODs are shown in Fig. 15. It can be seen that all of the metrics of W_M provided a much better performance than those of W_C. TM5 (W_C measurement of the root of the tongue) provided the best performance. Such a difference might be the result of the different degrees to which W_M and W_C correspond to the perception of the human vision system to a specific texture, especially in an image of the tongue.

A problematic result was the relatively low value of GOD for the W_M measurement at the tip of the tongue, as shown in Fig. 15. Actually, because of the existence of hyperplastic filiform papillae, the picture of the tip of a tongue affected by appendicitis is very different from other diseases. However, all of the textural metrics that were introduced in this chapter failed to report such a difference. To solve this problem, in the next section we apply the FPF approach to reliably identify the hyperplastic filiform papillae.

Table 15.3 shows the diagnostic results of appendicitis by all using the textural metrics and a subset of these metrics, respectively. Similar to the case of the

Table 15.3 Diagnostic results of appendicitis using textural metrics (number of correct and false classifications to total number)

	TM1–TM10	TM1–TM5
Correct/total	41/57	47/57
False/total	215/399	176/399

Reprinted from Pang et al. (2005), with permission from Elsevier

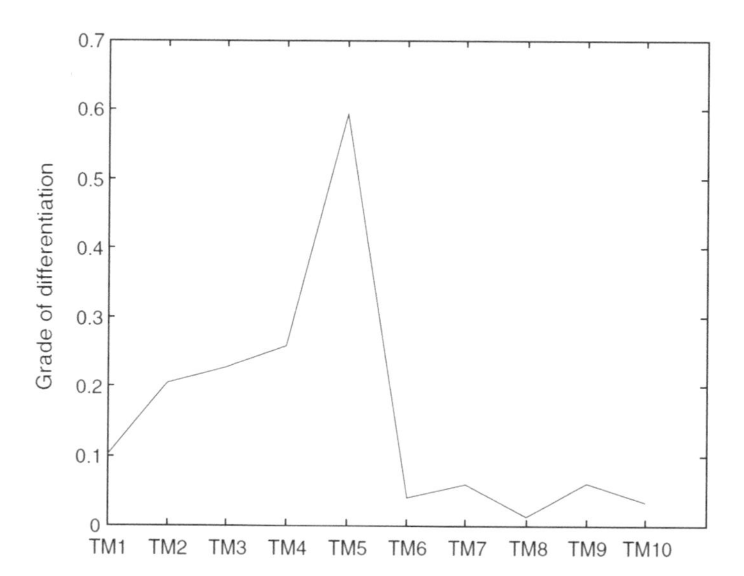

Fig. 15.8 GODs of textural measurements in different partitions of the tongue. Reprinted from Pang et al. (2005), with permission from Elsevier

chromatic metrics, the feature selection also improved the performance. Note that, although the ratios of correct classification increased, compared with those using chromatic metrics, the ratios of false classification also increased (Fig. 15.8).

15.4.4 Performance of the FPF

The results in the previous section showed that the metrics W_M and W_C do not perform well in the identification of hyperplastic filiform papillae. In this section, we used the FPF, which was defined in Sect. 15.3.2, to address this problem.

The first example is shown in Fig. 15, which shows the results of applying the FPFs (including FPF_8.4–0.6 and FPF_4.1–0.6) to two images of a tongue, which has many hyperplastic filiform papillae on the tip of the tongue because it is affected by appendicitis. It can be seen that both of the FPFs successfully located abnormal filiform papillae. However, they also located some spurious filiform papillae. In

Table 15.4 Diagnostic results of appendicitis using the combined metrics (number of correct and false classifications to total number)

	Combined metrics
Correct/total	53/57
False/total	34/399

Reprinted from Pang et al. (2005), with permission from Elsevier

both cases, the FPF_4.1–0.6 filter provided better performance compared with the FPF_8.4–0.6 filter. The FPF_4.1–0.6 can eliminate many of the other pathological details, such as spots, lighter reflecting points (caused by saliva), and partial fungi form papillae. However, the results from this filter are still far from meeting our requirements for an approach for the diagnosis of appendicitis using the tongue.

To address this problem, we made use of the secondary filtering process (which was introduced in Sect. 15.3.2) and the preceding convolving procedure using the FPF. Hereafter, we call this method *dual filtering*. The results of applying dual filtering are illustrated in Fig. 15, where the results of using the FPF are also shown for comparison. As demonstrated in Fig. 15, the dual filtering approach exhibits superior performance in the identification of abnormal filiform papillae compared with using a single FPF.

A reliable identification of filiform papillae will significantly increase the accuracy of the diagnosis of appendicitis. Accordingly, we used a set of metrics that includes the surviving metrics from the first two experiments and a new metric determined from the dual filtering, to further improve the performance of the TCoM for the diagnosis of appendicitis. It can be seen from the diagnostic results, shown in Table 15.4, that the accuracy of the diagnosis of appendicitis was considerably

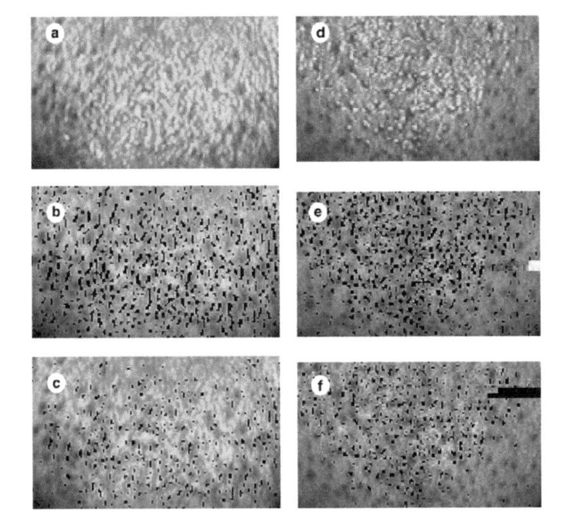

Fig. 15.9 Two examples of the identification of filiform papillae (marked in *black*) by FPF filtering. **a**, **d** The original tongue images; **b**, **e** are the results using FPF_8.4–0.6 filter; **c**, **f** are the results using FPF_4.1–0.6. Reprinted from Pang et al. (2005), with permission from Elsevier

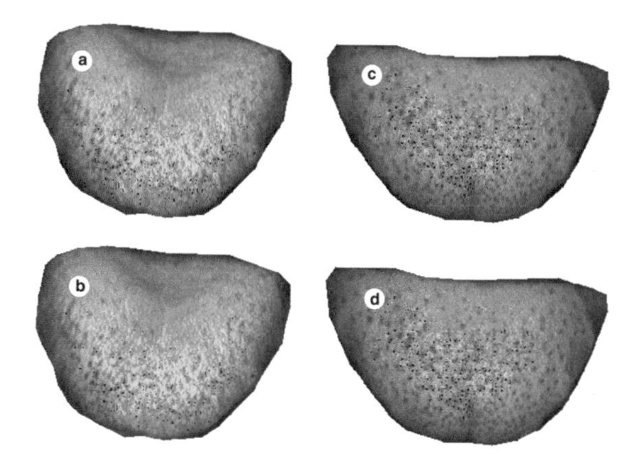

Fig. 15.10 Comparison of FPF filtering and dual filtering on the identification of filiform papillae (filiform papillae are marked in black). (**a**, **c**) The results using FPF filtering; (**b**, **d**) are the results using dual filtering. Reprinted from Pang et al. (2005), with permission from Elsevier

improved: the ratio of the correct classification increased to 92.98% and that of the false classification decreased to 8.52% (Figs. 15.9 and 15.10).

15.5 Summary

In this chapter, we proposed a distinct computerized tongue diagnosis approach, which is called a tongue-computing model (TCoM), for the diagnosis of appendicitis based on a quantitative analysis of the pathological changes on the surface of a tongue. Both chromatic and textural features were used to build the mapping from a tongue image to corresponding diseases in a statistical way. Experiments were implemented on a large tongue image database, and the results were promising.

The main contribution of this research is that, this is the first time, to the best of our knowledge a computerized tongue image analysis approach is proposed for the building of mapping from tongue signs to Western medicine defined diseases. This will undoubtedly boost the modernization process of the traditional tongue diagnosis and, more importantly, shorten the gap between tongue diagnosis and clinical application.

References

Chen, Z.L., & Bei, R.P. (1991). *Tongue Furring and Diseases*. People's Sanitation Publishing House.

Li, N.M., Wang, Y.F., & Li, Z.C. (1987). *Diagnosis through Inspection of the Tongue*. Heilongjiang Science and Technology Press.

Pang, B., Zhang, D., & Wang, K. (2005). Tongue image analysis for appendicitis diagnosis. *Information Sciences, 175*(3), 160–176.

Chapter 16
Diagnosis Using Quantitative Tongue Feature Classification

Abstract This chapter focuses on relationships between diseases and the appearance of the human tongue in terms of quantitative features. The experimental samples are digital tongue images captured from three groups of candidates: one group in normal health, one suffering with appendicitis, and a third suffering with pancreatitis. For the purposes of diagnostic classification, we first extracted chromatic and textural measurements from the original tongue images. A feature selection procedure then identified the measures most relevant to the classifications, based on the three tongue image categories. The study in this chapter validates the use of tongue inspection by means of quantitative feature classification in medical diagnosis.

16.1 Introduction

Recently, there have been a number of responses to the nonobjective problem (Chiu, 1996; Li & Yuen, 2002; Li et al., 1994; Takeichi & Sato, 1997; Watsuji, Arita, Shinohara, & Kitade, 1999; Weng, 1997; Cai, 2002; Jiehua, 2001), but they have at least one of three significant weaknesses. First, some approaches (Takeichi & Sato, 1997; Watsuji et al., 1999) are limited in that they identify only syndromes defined in sophisticated terms from TCM, making them hard to place within the framework of Western medicine. Second, these approaches are usually validated by comparing the system-derived diagnoses and the diagnoses of skilled tongue diagnosis practitioners. Such a validation is itself essentially subjective. Finally, many of the systems (Chiu, 2000; Li & Yuen, 2002; Watsuji et al., 1999; Weng, 1997; Jiehua, 2001) are dedicated to the recognition of pathological features such as colors or furring of the tongue that are not capable of being mapped from the appearance of the tongue to the diagnosis of specific diseases.

In this chapter, we focus on the investigation of the relationship between the appearance of the tongue, in terms of quantitative features and clinical diseases. This kind of mapping from exterior signs (features) to interior causes (diseases) can be dealt with using techniques from biometrics (Zhang, 2013), which have typically

D. Zhang et al., *Tongue Image Analysis*, DOI 10.1007/978-981-10-2167-1_16

been used to identify persons by their biological features. We introduce modern biometric techniques into traditional tongue inspection (TI) to classify three diagnostic categories, normal, appendicitis, and pancreatitis, based on quantitative features of the tongue.

16.2 Tongue Image Samples

The tongue image samples used in this study were attained using an online capturing device designed by our research center, that consists of two D65 lights, a lens, a CCD sensor board, and a video frame grabber that produces high-quality digital images (Patent No: 02132458.1, China). The captured tongue images were checked by expert TCM tongue diagnosticians and were found to satisfy their requirements.

Tongue images were captured from three diagnostic groups: normal, appendicitis, and pancreatitis. The normal group was drawn from healthy student volunteers at the Harbin Institute of Technology. The appendicitis and pancreatitis groups were drawn from inpatient volunteers suffering from those diseases in the general surgical department at the Harbin 211 Hospital. The digital tongue image samples of these last two groups were captured in the acute stage of the disease, at which point the appearance of the tongue is usually more representative.

The appearance of the tongue in each category is in general quite distinct relative to the other two categories (Fig. 16.1). For example, a normal tongue (Fig. 16.1a) has vitality, its color is vibrant and vital, its body is pale red and appears fresh, and its coating is thin and white. The tongue of an appendicitis patient (Fig. 16.1b) differs in that, depending on the seriousness of the disorder, its tongue body is light red, red or dark red, and its coating is white or yellow and is usually thick. Another important tongue sign indicating appendicitis is the appearance of numerous distinct red prickles on the tip of the tongue. The tongue of a person suffering from pancreatitis (Fig. 16.1c) is distinctive in that the body of the tongue is usually bluish or bluish purple.

16.3 Quantitative Chromatic and Textural Measurements

Once qualitative descriptive diagnostic features were identified, it was necessary to develop quantitative measures that would be meaningful to the diagnosis of appendicitis and pancreatitis. Initially, one notes the subjective qualities of the standard descriptions: "pale red," "thick coating," "bluish purple," "thin," "prickles," yet we also note that many of these descriptions also relate to color- and

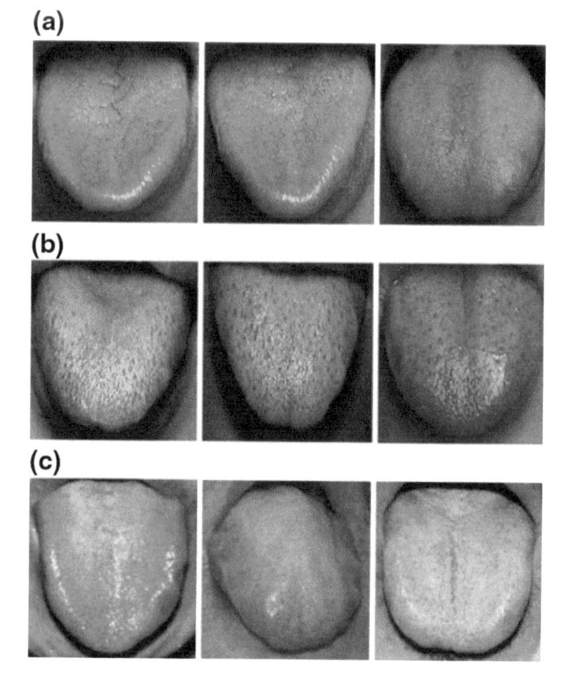

Fig. 16.1 Typical samples of digital tongue images **a** Normal **b** Appendicitis, and **c** Pancreatitis. Zhang, Pang, Li, et al. (2005), Copyright (2005), with permission from OSA

texture-related features. On this basis, we employed several general chromatic and textural measurements (Castleman, 1996; Reed & Dubuf, 1993) without considering whether these measurements would correspond well to specific qualitative features (for more on this, see the Discussion section). A subsequent feature selection procedure allowed the identification of a diagnostically useful subset of quantitative features.

The color- and texture-related measurements used in our method are the means and standard deviations of the values of pixels within the whole region of the tongue in each spectral channel of four color spaces (Castleman, 1996): RGB, CIEYxy, CIELUV, and CIELAB. RGB (Red Green Blue) is an additive color system based on tri-chromatic theory that is commonly the basic color space for most applications. The other three color spaces are all defined by the International Commission on Illumination (CIE). The CIEYxy triple is composed of a luminance component Y, and two additional normalized chromaticity coordinates x and y. The CIELUV and CIELAB are color systems that have a better correlation with human visual perception. The L component indicates the sensation of lightness while the UV and AB pairs are additional chromaticity elements.

Since both of the L channels in CIELUV and CIELAB refer to light perception in the human vision system, we use it only once. Thus, there are 11 chromatic (means) and 11 textural (standard deviations) measurements constituting 22 different features. These quantitative features together form a chromatic–textural feature space for the classification.

16.4 Feature Selection

A feature space of 22 dimensions includes too many parameters for efficient classification, especially for visualization. Fortunately, some of these chromatic–textual features are highly correlated. For example, RGB values can be transformed into CIEXYZ tristimulus values by a conversion matrix, and vice versa. It is possible, then, before the diagnostic classification process, to use feature selection to remove a number of redundant features, producing, we hope, a subspace of extremely lower dimensionality. A subspace of, for example, just three or even two dimensions would allow all of the samples to be correctly classified using a separating vector, i.e., to be linearly separable. A direct benefit of this kind of dimension reduction is a clear visualization.

Basically, we need to identify those features, from a total of 22 chromatic textural features, which are most relevant to the classification. First, we divided the single three-category classification problem into three two-category classification problems normal versus pancreatitis, appendicitis versus pancreatitis, and appendicitis versus normal. We then determined the contribution of each feature to a classification (for example, normal versus appendicitis) by calculating a quantitative measure, the grade of discrimination (GOD). For the purposes of a classification, a feature's GOD is defined as the variance-normalized distance between two class means (centers). Next, for each classification, we selected features in a descending order with respect to their GODs until the two classes under consideration were linearly separable in the resulting subspace formed by the selected features. We repeated this feature selection process for each of the three two-category classifications.

16.5 Results and Analysis

There were a total of 138 experimental sample digital tongue images: 56 normal samples, 53 appendicitis samples, and 29 pancreatitis samples. For each sample, we first computed all of the chromatic–textural features and then used the feature selection process to identify the most relevant features for each of the three classifications. The experimental results indicated that both normal and appendicitis digital tongue images can be linearly separated from pancreatitis digital tongue images (Figs. 16.2 and 16.3) using the two highest scorings, with respect to the GODs, chromatic features means of CIE*y* and CIEV. The results also showed that normal and appendicitis digital tongue images are linearly separated using the three highest scoring chromatic–textural feature standard deviations of CIEA, CIEB, and L (Fig. 16.4). These results have a high degree of accordance with our own common observations: that some diseases produce mainly chromatic and textural changes in the appearance of the tongue.

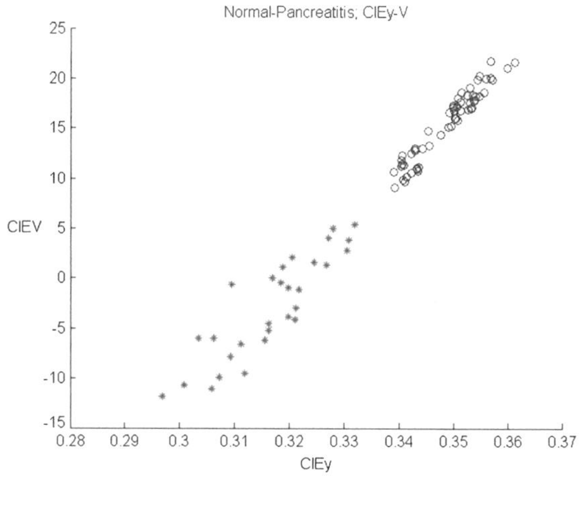

Fig. 16.2 Chromatic analysis I (*open circle* normal and *asterisk* pancreatitis). Shown here are two projections of the chromatic features (mean values) of the normal and pancreatitis samples to the y color plane of the CIEYxy color space and the V color plane of the CIELUV color space. The samples closely clustered according to the two categories. Zhang et al. (2005), Copyright (2005), with permission from OSA

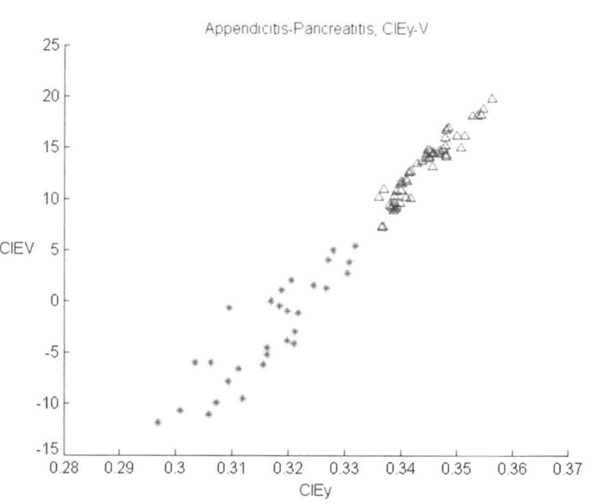

Fig. 16.3 Chromatic analysis II (*open triangle* Appendicitis and *asterisk* Pancreatitis). Shown here are two projections of the chromatic features (mean values) of the appendicitis and pancreatitis samples to the y color plane of the CIEYxy color space and the V color plane of the CIELUV color space. The samples closely clustered according to the two categories. Zhang et al. (2005), Copyright (2005), with permission from OSA

16.6 Summary

This research was originally inspired by the ideas of traditional Chinese medicine, which advocates diagnosing from the appearance of the tongue. Traditional TI techniques qualitatively and entirely subjectively define and describe the relationships between syndromes and abnormal tongue signs. Using quantitative feature classification, our research has shown that there is in fact a quantifiable connection between some disease states and the appearance of the tongue.

Given that traditional TI theories of pathological features are all qualitative and thus subjective (Maciocia, 1987), it would be of value to develop, where possible, quantitative measures that are diagnostically useful. The most direct approach would be to identify a set of objective measurements corresponding to a specific

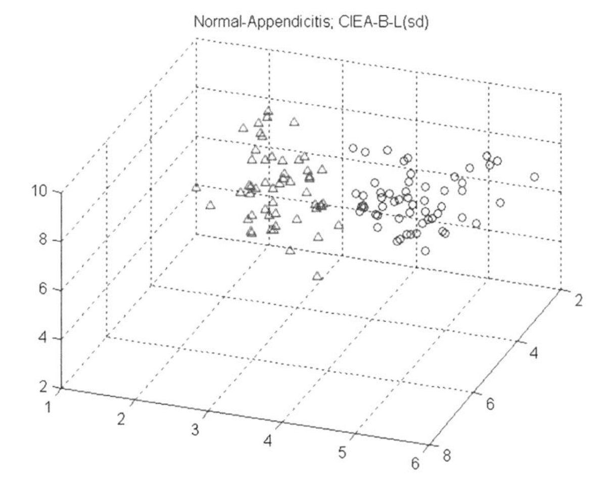

Fig. 16.4 Chromatic–textural analysis (*open circle* Normal and *open triangle* Appendicitis). Shown here are three projections of the chromatic–textural features (standard deviation values) of the normal and appendicitis samples to the A and B color planes of the CIELAB color space and the L plane (indicating the brightness sensation of the human vision system). The samples closely clustered according to the two categories. Zhang et al. (2005), Copyright (2005), with permission from OSA

qualitative feature in traditional tongue diagnosis. This is the usual approach of current computerized tongue image analysis (Chiu, 2000; Chiu, Lin & Lin, 1995; Li & Yuen, 2002; Watsuji et al., 1999; Jiehua, 2001). Although direct and simple, these approaches are difficult to evaluate, in that the underlying validity of these approaches is based on practitioner judgments. This is clearly somewhat circular: approaches are purposely devised to avoid subjectivity by replacing qualitative descriptions with quantitative measures, yet are then subjectively evaluated. In this study, however, we employed several general chromatic and textural measurements, but did not consider whether these measurements match specific qualitative features.

In this chapter, we described a method for using quantitative feature classifications to diagnose two common diseases from the appearance of the human tongue. We also identified in ranked order the measures that contribute to these classifications and the minimal sets that can linearly classify our samples into their diagnostic categories. To the best of our knowledge, this is the first application of biometric techniques for the diagnostic classification of diseases using quantitative features derived from digital tongue images. This study somewhat justifies the validity of our belief that we can diagnose diseases from tongue appearance.

References

Cai, Y. (2002). A novel imaging system for tongue inspection (pp. 159–164). IEEE; 1999.

Castleman, K. R. (1996). Digital image processing. *Curve and Surface Fitting*, 501–507.

Chiu, C. (1996). The development of a computerized tongue diagnosis system. *Biomedical Engineering Applications Basis Communications, 8,* 342–350.

Chiu, C. (2000). A novel approach based on computerized image analysis for traditional Chinese medical diagnosis of the tongue. *Computer Methods and Programs in Biomedicine, 61*(2), 77–89.

Chiu, C. C., Lin, H. S., & Lin, S. L. (1995). A structural texture recognition approach for medical diagnosis through tongue. *Biomed. Eng. Appl. Basis Commun, 7*(2), 143–148.

Jiehua, Z. (2001). Towards the standardization of tongue diagnosis: an image processing approach. *Chinese Journal of Biomedical Engineering, 20*(2), 132–137.

Li, C. H., & Yuen, P. C. (2002). Tongue image matching using color content. *Pattern Recognition, 35*(2), 407–419.

Li, N. M., et al. (1994). The contemporary investigations of computerized tongue diagnosis. *The Handbook of Chinese Tongue Diagnosis*, 1315–1317.

Maciocia, G. (1987). *Tongue diagnosis in Chinese medicine*. Eastland press.

Reed, T. R., & Dubuf, J. H. (1993). A review of recent texture segmentation and feature extraction techniques. *CVGIP: Image understanding, 57*(3), 359–372.

Takeichi, M., & Sato, T. (1997). Computerized color analysis of "xue yu"(blood stasis) in the sublingual vein using a new technology. *The American journal of Chinese medicine, 25*(02), 213–219.

Watsuji, T., Arita, S., Shinohara, S., & Kitade, T. (1999). Medical application of fuzzy theory to the diagnostic system of tongue inspection in traditional Chinese medicine (pp. 145–148). IEEE.

Weng, W. L. (1997). The development of modern tongue diagnosis. *The illustrations of clinical tongue diagnosis and disease treatments, Shed-Yuan Publishing, Peking*, 26–49.

Zhang, D. D. (2013). *Automated biometrics: Technologies and systems* (Vol. 7). Springer.

Zhang, David, Pang, Bo, Li, Naimin, et al. (2005). Computerized diagnosis from tongue appearance using quantitative feature classification. *American Journal of Chinese Medicine, 33* (6), 859–866.

Chapter 17
Detecting Diabetes Mellitus and Nonproliferative Diabetic Retinopathy Using CTD

Abstract Diabetes mellitus (DM) and its complications leading to diabetic retinopathy (DR) will soon become one of the twenty-first century's major health problems. This represents a huge financial burden to healthcare officials and governments. To combat this approaching epidemic, this chapter presents a noninvasive method to detect DM and nonproliferative diabetic retinopathy (NPDR), the initial stage of DR-based on three groups of features extracted from tongue images. They include color, texture, and geometry. A noninvasive capture device with image correction first captures the tongue images. A tongue color gamut was established with 12 colors representing the tongue color features. The texture values of eight blocks strategically located on the tongue surface, with the additional mean of all eight blocks were used to characterize the nine tongue texture features. Finally, 13 features extracted from tongue images based on measurements, distances, areas, and their ratios represent the geometric features. Applying a combination of the 34 features, the proposed method can separate Healthy and DM-tongues as well as NPDR/DM-sans NPDR (DM samples without NP-DR) tongues using features from each of the three groups with average accuracies of 80.52 and 80.33%, respectively. This is based on a database consisting of 130 Healthy and 296 DM samples, where 29 of those in DM are NPDR.

17.1 Introduction

The World Health Organization (WHO) has estimated that in 2000 there were 171 million people worldwide with diabetes mellitus (DM), and the number will increase to 366 million by 2030 (Organization, 2006) making the disease among the leading causes of death, disabilities, and economic hardship in the world. Two main types of DM exist, Type 1 DM and Type 2 DM. People with Type 1 DM fail to produce insulin, and therefore require injections of it. Type 2 DM is the most common type and can be categorized by insulin resistance. Currently, there is no cure for Type 1 DM or Type 2 DM. However, Type 2 DM can be managed by eating well, exercising, and maintaining a healthy lifestyle.

D. Zhang et al., *Tongue Image Analysis*, DOI 10.1007/978-981-10-2167-1_17

A fasting plasma glucose (FPG) test is the standard method practiced by medical professionals to diagnose DM. The FPG test is performed after the patient has gone at least 12 h without food, and requires taking a sample of the patient's blood (by piercing their finger) in order to analyse its blood glucose levels. Even though this method is accurate, it is invasive, and slightly painful (the piercing process). Diabetic retinopathy (DR) is a micro vascular complication of DM that is responsible for 4.8% of the 37 million cases of blindness in the world, estimated by WHO (Organization, 2006). In its earliest stage known as nonproliferative diabetic retinopathy (NPDR), the disease if detected can be treated to prevent further progression and sight loss. Various imaging modalities such as red free (Hipwell et al., 2000; Martinez-Perez, Hughes, Bharath, & Parker, 2007), angiography (Martinez-Perez et al., 2007; Spencer, Olson, Mchardy, Sharp, & Forrester, 1996), and color (Abràmoff, Van Ginneken, & Niemeijer, 2009; Meindert, Bram, Cree, Atsushi, Gwénolé, Sanchez, Bob, Roberto, Mathieu, & Chisako, 2010; Joes, Abràmoff, Meindert, Viergever, & Bram, 2004; Zhang, Karray, Li, & Zhang, 2012a, b; Zhang, Zhang, Zhang, & Karray, 2010) fundus imaging are used to examine the human retina in order to detect DR and subsequently NPDR. These methods are based on the detection of relevant features related to DR, including but not limited to hemorrhages, micro aneurysms, various exudates, and retinal blood vessels. These imaging modalities themselves can be regarded as invasive, exposing the eye to bright flashes or having fluorescein injected into a vein in the case of angiography. Therefore, there is a need to develop a noninvasive yet accurate DM and NPDR detection method.

As a result, this chapter deals with the aforementioned problems and proposes a noninvasive automated method to detect DM and NPDR by distinguishing Healthy/DM and NPDR/DM sans NPDR (DM without NPDR) samples using an array of tongue features consisting of color, texture, and geometry. The human tongue contains numerous features that can be used to diagnose disease (Chiu, 1996; Pang, Zhang, & Wang, 2005a, b), with color, texture, and geometric features being the most prominent (Chiu, 1996; Pang et al., 2005a, b). Traditionally, medical practitioners examine these features based on years of experience (Chiu, 1996; Pang et al., 2005a, b). However, ambiguity and subjectivity are always associated with their diagnostic results. By removing these qualitative aspects, quantitative feature extraction and analysis from tongue images can be established. To the best of our knowledge, there is no other published work on detecting DM or NPDR using tongue color, texture, and geometric features.

Tongue images were captured using an especially designed in-house device taking into consideration color correction (Chiu, 1996; Pang et al., 2005a, b). Each image was segmented (Pang et al., 2005a, b) in order to locate its foreground pixels. With the relevant pixels located, three groups of features namely color, texture, and geometric were extracted from the tongue foreground. To analyse experimental results, a dataset consisting of 130 Healthy samples taken from Guangdong Provincial Hospital of Traditional Chinese Medicine, Guangdong, China, and 296 DM samples consisting of 267 DM sans NPDR, and 29 NPDR processed from the Hong Kong Foundation for Research and Development in Diabetes, Prince of

Wales Hospital, Hong Kong SAR were used. Classification was initially performed between Healthy versus DM in addition to NPDR versus DM-sans NPDR using every feature individually (from the three groups), followed by an optimal combination of all the features.

The rest of this chapter is organized as follows. Section 17.2 describes the tongue image capture device, color correction, and tongue segmentation, while Sect. 17.3 discusses tongue color feature extraction. In Sect. 17.4, tongue texture feature extraction is given in detail, with tongue geometric feature extraction presented in Sect. 17.5. Section 17.6 describes the experimental results and discussion, followed by concluding remarks in Sect. 17.7.

17.2 Capture Device and Tongue Image Preprocessing

The capture device, color correction of the tongue images, and tongue segmentation are given in this section. Figure 17.1 shows the in house designed device consisting of a three chip CCD camera with 8-bit resolution, and two D65 fluorescent tubes placed symmetrically around the camera in order to produce uniform illumination. The angle between the incident light and emergent light is 45°, as recommended by Commission International de l'Eclairage (CIE). During image capture, patients place their chin on a chinrest while showing their tongue to the camera. The images captured in JPEG format that ranged from 257 × 189 pixels to 443 × 355 pixels were color corrected (Wang & Zhang, 2010) to eliminate any variability in color images caused by changes of illumination and device dependence. This allows for consistent feature extraction and classification in the following steps. The idea of Wang and Zhang (2010) (based on the Munsell ColorChecker) is to map a matrix generated from the input RGB vector to an objective sRGB vector, thereby obtaining a transformation model. Compared with the retinal imaging modalities

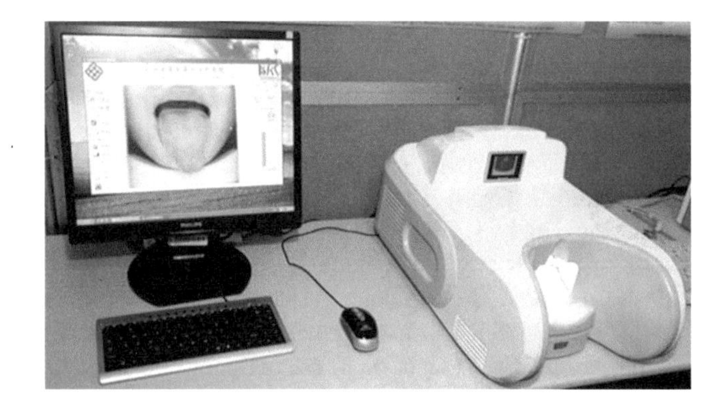

Fig. 17.1 Tongue capture device. © 2016 IEEE. Reprinted, with permission, from Zhang et al. (2013)

previously mentioned, this capture device is noninvasive, requiring neither a bright flash nor injection of dye into a patient's blood stream.

Once the tongue images are captured, automatic segmentation (Pang et al., 2005a, b) is next applied to each image in order to separate its foreground pixels from its background pixels. This is accomplished by combining a bi-elliptical deformable template (BEDT), and an active contour model known as the bi-elliptical deformable contour (BEDC). In (Pang et al., 2005a, b), the segmented tongue is obtained by first minimizing the energy function of BEDT, followed by the energy function of BEDC. BEDT captures the overall tongue shape features, while BEDC can be deformed to match the local tongue details. The result is a binary tongue image clearly defining foreground pixels (the tongue surface area and its edges) from its background pixels (the area outside the tongue edges). This allows for three groups of features, color, texture, and geometric to be extracted from a tongue foreground image in the next steps.

17.3 Tongue Color Features

The following section describes how color features are extracted from tongue images. The tongue color gamut is first summarized in Sect. 17.3.1. In Sect. 17.3.2, every foreground tongue pixel is compared to 12 colors representing the tongue color gamut and assigned its nearest color. This forms the color features.

17.3.1 Tongue Color Gamut

The tongue color gamut (Wang & Zhang, 2011) represents all possible colors that appear on the tongue surface, and exists within the red boundary shown in Fig. 17.2. It was created by plotting each tongue foreground pixel in our dataset onto the CIE 1931 chromaticity diagram (refer to Fig. 17.2), which shows all possible colors in the visible spectrum. Further investigation revealed that 98% of the tongue pixels lie inside the black boundary. To better represent the tongue color gamut, the 12 colors plotted in Fig. 17.3 were selected with the help of the RGB color space. On the RG line, a point Y (Yellow) is marked. Between RB, a point P (Purple) is marked, and C (Cyan) is marked between GB. The center of the RGB color space is calculated and designated as W (White), the first of the 12 colors (see Fig. 17.3). Then, for each R (Red), B (Blue), Y, P, and C point, a straight line is drawn to W. Each time these lines intersect the tongue color gamut, a new color is added to represent the 12 colors. This accounts for R, Y, C, B, and P.LR (Light red), LP (Light purple), and LB (Light blue) are midpoints between lines from the black boundary to W, while DR (Deep red) is selected as no previous point occupies that area. More details about the tongue color gamut can be found in

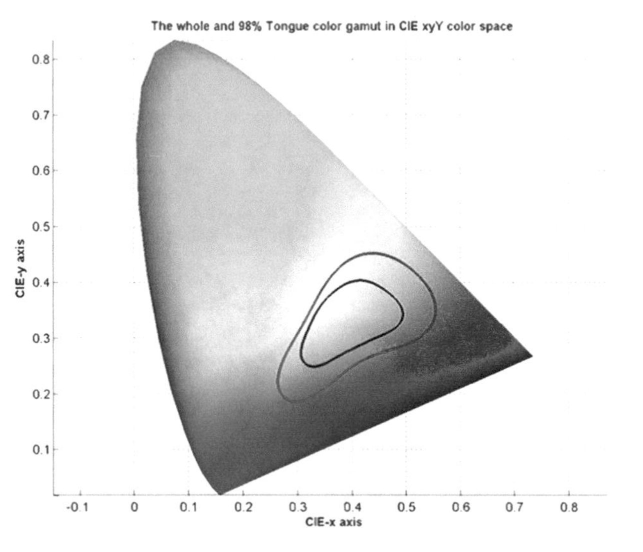

Fig. 17.2 Color gamut in the CIExyY color space depicting the tongue color gamut inside the *red* boundary. Furthermore, 98% of the tongue color gamut can be located within the *black* boundary. © 2016 IEEE. Reprinted, with permission, from Zhang et al. (2013)

(Wang & Zhang, 2011). GY (Gray) and BK (Black) are not shown in Fig. 17.3 since both belong to grayscale.

The 12 colors representing the tongue color gamut were extracted from Fig. 17.3 and shown in Fig. 17.4 as color squares with their label on top. Correspondingly, its RGB and CIELAB values are given in Table 17.1.

17.3.2 Color Feature Extraction

For the foreground pixels of a tongue image, corresponding RGB values are first extracted, and converted to CIELAB (Zhang, Wang, Jin, & Zhang, 2005) by transferring RBG to CIEXYZ using

$$\begin{bmatrix} X \\ Y \\ Z \end{bmatrix} = \begin{bmatrix} 0.4124 & 0.3576 & 0.1805 \\ 0.2126 & 0.7152 & 0.0722 \\ 0.0193 & 0.1192 & 0.9805 \end{bmatrix} \begin{bmatrix} R \\ G \\ B \end{bmatrix} \tag{17.1}$$

Followed by CIEXYZ to CIELAB via

$$\begin{aligned} L^* &= 166 \cdot f(Y/Y_0) - 16 \\ a^* &= 500 \cdot [f(X/X_0) - f(Y/Y_0)] \\ b^* &= 200 \cdot [f(Y/Y_0) - f(Z/Z_0)] \end{aligned} \tag{17.2}$$

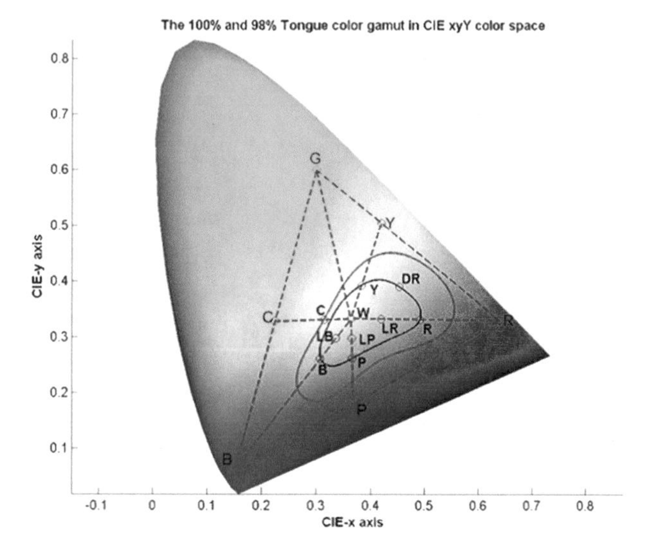

Fig. 17.3 Tongue color gamut can be represented using several points by drawing lines from the RGB color space. © 2016 IEEE. Reprinted, with permission, from Zhang et al. (2013)

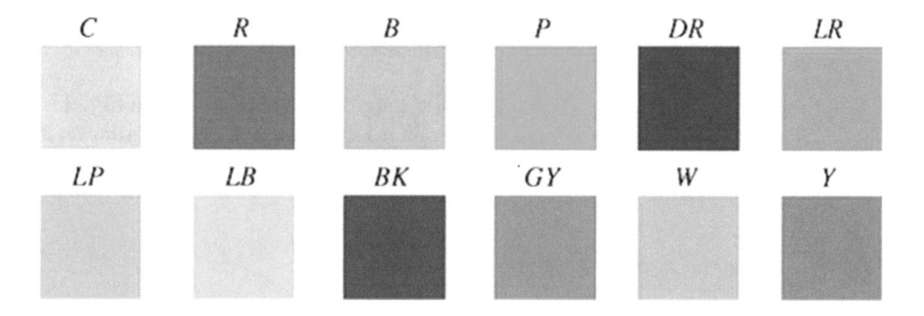

Fig. 17.4 Twelve colors representing the tongue color gamut with their label on *top*. © 2016 IEEE. Reprinted, with permission, from Zhang et al. (2013)

where $f(x) = x^{1/3}$ if $x > 0.008856$ or $f(x) = 7.787x + 16/116$ if $x \leq 0.008856$.

X_0, Y_0, and Z_0 in (17.2) are the CIEXYZ tristimulus values of the reference white point. The LAB values are then compared to 12 colors from the tongue color gamut (see Table 17.1) and assigned the color which is closest to them (measured using Euclidean distance). After evaluating all tongue foreground pixels, the total of each color is added and divided by the total number of pixels. This ratio of the 12 colors forms the tongue color feature vector$v$, where $v = [c_1, \ldots, c_{12}]$ and c_i represents the sequence of colors in Table 17.1 As an example, the color features of three tongues are shown in visual form (refer to Figs. 17.5, 17.6 and 17.7) along with their extracted color feature vector, where the original image is decomposed into one of the 12 colors. Figure 17.5 shows a Healthy sample, Fig. 17.6 shows a DM sample,

Table 17.1 RGB and CIElab values of the 12 colors

Color	[RGB]	[LAB]
C (Cyan)	[188 188 185]	[76.0693 −0.5580 1.3615]
R (Red)	[189 99 91]	[52.2540 34.8412 21.3002]
B (Blue)	[183 165 180]	[69.4695 9.5423 −5.4951]
P (Purple)	[226 142 214]	[69.4695 42.4732 −23.8880]
DR (Deep red)	[136 72 49]	[37.8424 24.5503 25.9396]
LR (Light red)	[227 150 147]	[69.4695 28.4947 13.3940]
LP (Light purple)	[225 173 207]	[76.0693 24.3246 −9.7749]
LB (Light blue)	[204 183 186]	[76.0693 7.8917 0.9885]
BK(Black)	[107 86 56]	[37.8424 3.9632 20.5874]
GF (Gray)	[163 146 143]	[61.6542 5.7160 3.7317]
W (White)	[200 167 160]	[70.9763 10.9843 8.2952]
F (Yellow)	[166 129 93]	[56.3164 9.5539 24.4546]

while an NPDR sample is given in Fig. 17.7. In these three samples, the majority of pixels are *R*.

The mean colors of Healthy, DM, and NPDR are displayed in along with their standard deviation (*std*). DM tongues have a higher ratio of DR. LR and Y are greater in Healthy samples, and GY is higher in NPDR tongues. The rest of the mean color features are similar. Only seven colors are listed out of the 12 as the remaining five have ratios less than 1% (Table 17.2).

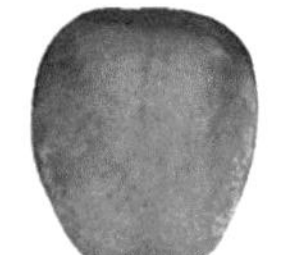

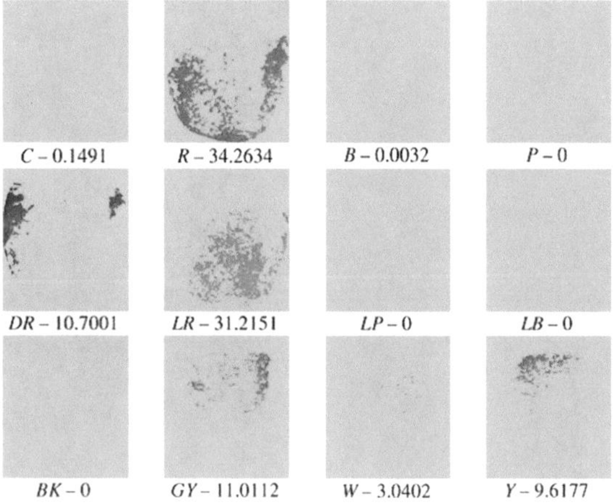

Fig. 17.5 Healthy tongue sample. Its tongue color feature vector and corresponding 12 color makeup with most of the pixels classified as *R*. © 2016 IEEE. Reprinted, with permission, from Zhang et al. (2013)

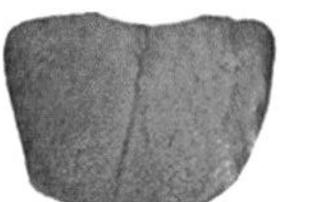

$v = [0.1256\ 31.2877\ 0.0674\ 0\ 18.4688\ 20.2692\ 0.0881\ 0.0414\ 0\ 24.2922\ 1.8107\ 3.5489]$

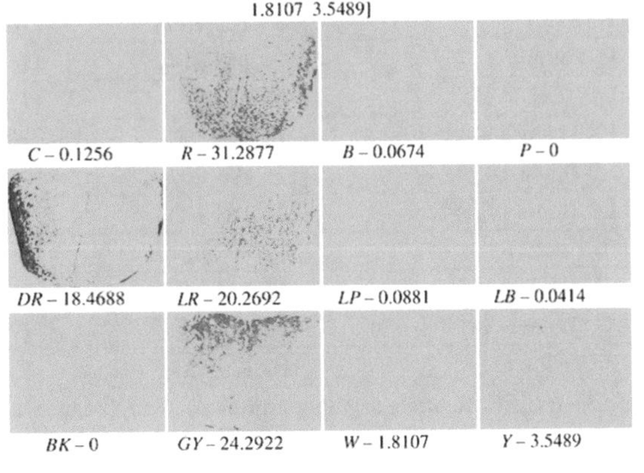

Fig. 17.6 DM tongue sample. Its tongue color feature vector and corresponding 12-color makeup with most of the pixels classified as *R*. © 2016 IEEE. Reprinted, with permission, from Zhang et al. (2013)

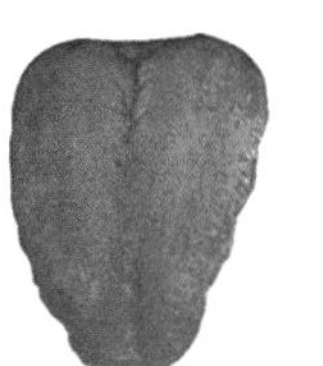

$v = [0.1484\ 40.5390\ 0.2669\ 0.0145\ 17.8854\ 13.6086\ 0.2687\ 0.0326\ 0\ 24.8616\ 0.9679\ 1.4066]$

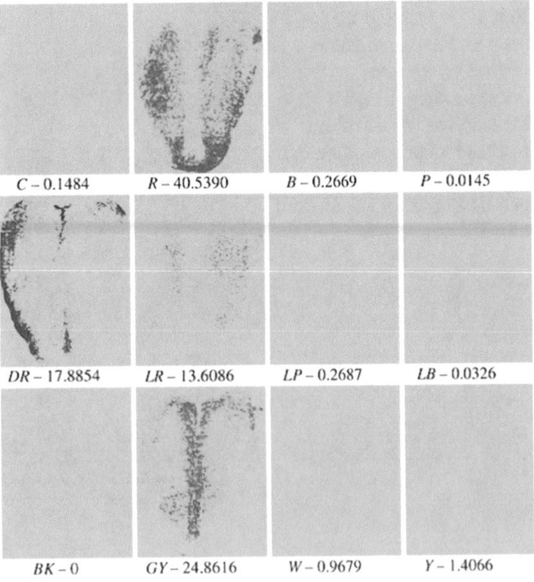

Fig. 17.7 NPDR tongue sample. Its tongue color feature vector and corresponding 12 color makeup with most of the pixels classified as *R*. © 2016 IEEE. Reprinted, with permission, from Zhang et al. (2013)

Table 17.2 Mean (*std*) of the color features for heathy ($std_{Healthy}$ = 11.71), DM (std_{DM} = 12.50), and NPDR (std_{NPDR} = 12.07)

	C	R	DR	LR	GY	W	Y
Healthy	23.77 (3.76)	30.94 (10.73)	12.71 (8.11)	14.12 (9.36)	10.54 (10.80)	1.3 (1.84)	6.53 (6.35)
DM	24.80 (4.84)	30.70 (11.47)	18.40 (12.68)	10.53 (8.73)	10.80 (12.03)	1.07 (1.79)	3.55 (5.62)
NPDR	24.14 (4.86)	28.54 (13.13)	14.31 (10.38)	11.12 (7.74)	15.50 (13.92)	1.73 (2.16)	4.48 (6.82)

17.4 Tongue Texture Features

Texture feature extraction from tongue images is presented in this section. To better represent the texture of tongue images, eight blocks (see Fig. 17.8) of size 64 × 64 strategically located on the tongue surface are used. A block size of 64 × 64 was chosen due to the fact that it covers all eight surface areas very well, while achieving minimum overlap. Larger blocks would cover areas outside the tongue boundary, and overlap more with other blocks. Smaller block sizes would prevent overlapping, but not as efficiently cover the eight areas. The blocks are calculated automatically by first locating the center of the tongue using a segmented binary tongue foreground image. Following this, the edges of the tongue are established and equal parts are measured from its center to position the eight blocks. Block 1 is located at the tip; Blocks 2 and 3, and Blocks 4 and 5 are on either side; Blocks 6 and 7 are at the root, and Block 8 is at the center.

The Gabor filter is a linear filter used in image processing, and is commonly used in texture representation. To compute the texture value of each block, the 2-D Gabor filter is applied and defined as

$$G_k(x,y) = \exp\left(\frac{x'^2 + \gamma^2 \cdot y'^2}{-2\sigma^2}\right)\cos\left(2\pi\frac{x'}{\lambda}\right) \quad (17.3)$$

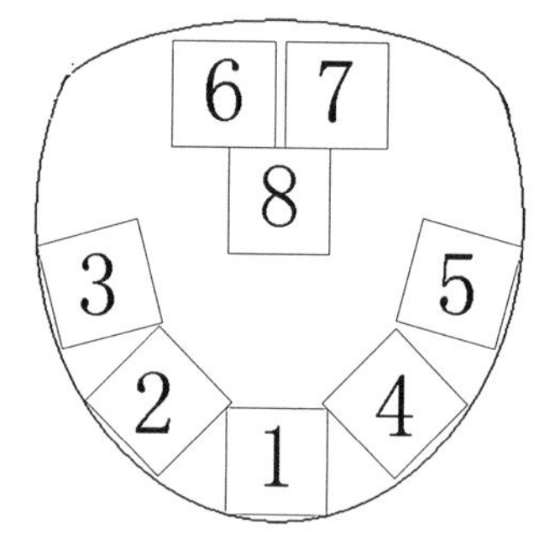

Fig. 17.8 Location of the eight texture blocks on the tongue. © 2016 IEEE. Reprinted, with permission, from Zhang et al. (2013)

where $x' = x\cos\theta + y\sin\theta$, $y' = -x\sin\theta + y{\cdot}\cos\theta$, σ is the variance, λ is the wavelength, γ is the aspect ratio of the sinusoidal function, and θ is the orientation. A total of three σ (1, 2 and 3) and four θ (0°, 45°, 90°, and 135°) choices were investigated to achieve the best result. Each filter is convolved with a texture block to produce a response R_k (x, y):

$$R_k(x, y) = G_k(x, y)^* im(x, y) \tag{17.4}$$

where im (x, y) is the texture block and * represents the 2-D convolution. Responses of a block are combined to form FR_i, and its final response evaluated as follows:

$$FR_i(x, y) = \max(R_1(x, y), R_2(x, y), \ldots, R_n(x, y)) \tag{17.5}$$

which selects the maximum pixel intensities, and represents the texture of a block by averaging the pixel values of FR_i.

Finally, σ equal to 1 and 2 with three orientations (45°, 90°, and 135°) was chosen. This is due to the fact that the sum of all texture blocks between Healthy and DM had the largest absolute difference. Figures 17.9, 17.10 and 17.11 illustrate the texture blocks for Healthy, DM, and NPDR samples, respectively. Below each block, its corresponding texture value is provided.

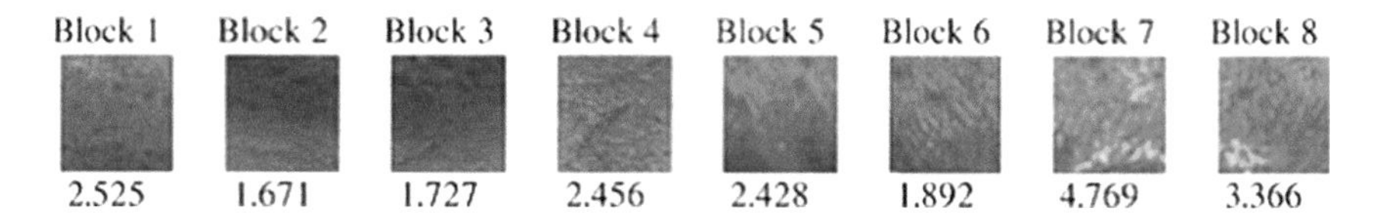

Fig. 17.9 Healthy texture blocks with their texture value *below*

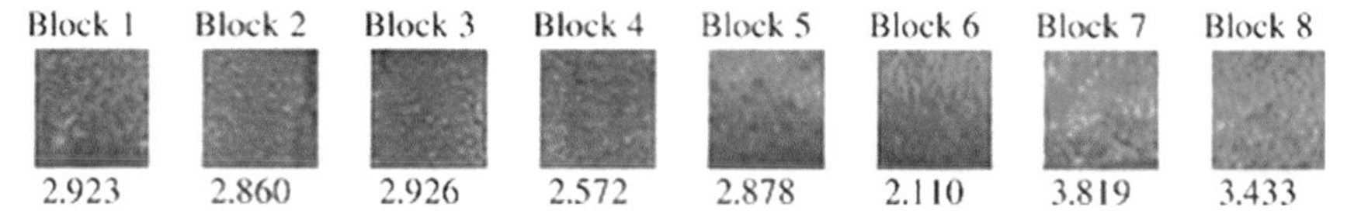

Fig. 17.10 DM texture blocks with their texture value *below*. © 2016 IEEE. Reprinted, with permission, from Zhang et al. (2013)

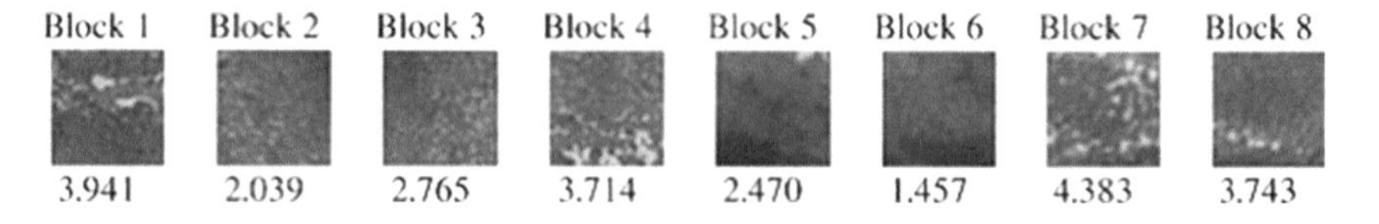

Fig. 17.11 NPDR texture blocks with their texture value *below*. © 2016 IEEE. Reprinted, with permission, from Zhang et al. (2013)

Table 17.3 Mean (*std*) of the texture features for healthy ($std_{Healthy} = 1.160$), DM ($std_{DM} = 1.238$), and NPDR ($std_{NPDR} = 1.196$)

	Block 1	Block 2	Block 3	Block 4	Block 5	Block 6	Block 7	Block 8	Mean of Blocks 1–8
Healthy	3.111 (0.978)	1.660 (0.632)	1.861 (0.677)	2.423 (0.875)	2.733 (0.989)	1.870 (0.650)	3.893 (1.167)	3.538 (1.326)	2.636 (0.486)
DM	2.952 (1.039)	2.142 (0.790)	2.359 (1.051)	2.711 (1.015)	2.522 (1.111)	1.859 (0.807)	3.710 (1.371)	3.887 (1.509)	2.768 (0.562)
NPDR	3.221 (1.118)	2.341 (0.777)	2.630 (0.892)	3.392 (1.333)	2.977 (1.130)	2.255 (1.235)	3.686 (1.343)	3.902 (1.133)	3.050 (0.521)

Table 17.3 depicts the texture value mean for Healthy, DM, and NPDR samples together with their standard deviation. Healthy samples have a higher texture value in Block 7, whereas NPDR texture values are greater for the remaining blocks. The mean of all eight blocks is also included as an additional texture value. This brings the total number of texture features extracted from tongue images to be 9.

17.5 Tongue Geometric Features

In the following section, we describe 13 geometric features extracted from tongue images. These features are based on measurements, distances, areas, and their ratios.

Width: The width w feature (see Fig. 17.12) is measured as the horizontal distance along the x-axis from a tongue's furthest right edge point (x_{max}) to its furthest left edge point (x_{min}):

$$w = x_{max} - x_{min} \tag{17.6}$$

Length: The length l feature (see Fig. 17.12) is measured as the vertical distance along the y-axis from a tongue's furthest bottom edge (y_{max}) point to its furthest top edge point (y_{min}):

$$l = y_{max} - y_{min} \tag{17.7}$$

Length–Width ratio: The length–width ratio lw is the ratio of a tongue's length to its width:

$$lw = l/w \tag{17.8}$$

Smaller half-distance: The smaller half-distance z is the half distance of l or w depending on which segment is shorter (see Fig. 17.12)

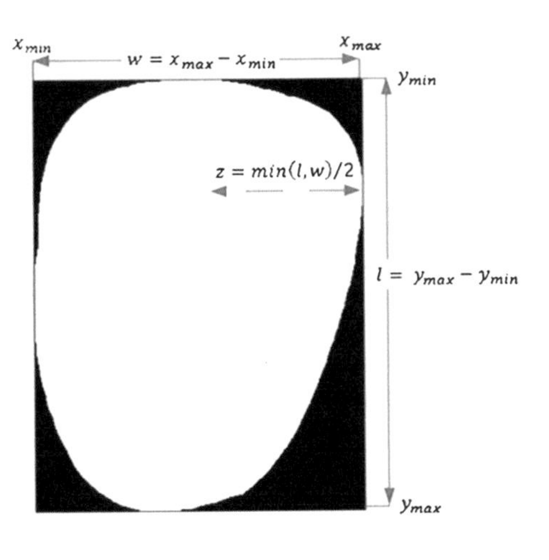

Fig. 17.12 Illustration of features 1, 2, and 4. © 2016 IEEE. Reprinted, with permission, from Zhang et al. (2013)

$$z = \min(l, w)/2 \tag{17.9}$$

Center distance: The center distance (*cd*) (refer to Fig. 17.13) is the distance from the w'^{s} *y*-axis center point to the center point of *l* (y_{cp}):

$$cd = \frac{(\max(y_{x_{\max}}) + \max(y_{x_{\min}}))}{2} - y_{cp} \tag{17.9}$$

where $y_{cp} = (y_{max} + y_{min})/2$.

Center distance ratio: The center distance ratio (*cdr*) is ratio of *cd* to *l*:

$$cdr = \frac{cd}{l} \tag{17.10}$$

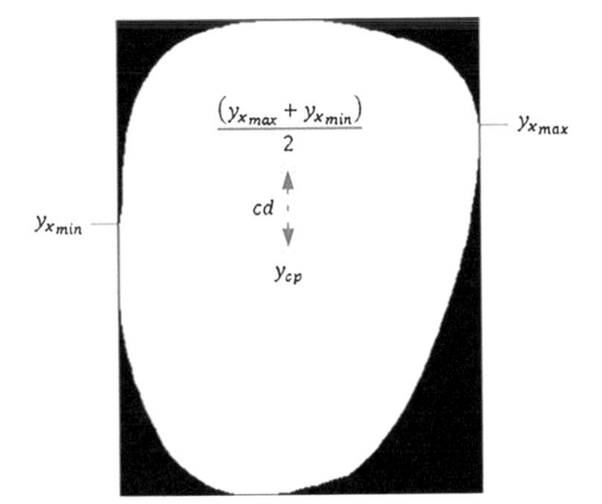

Fig. 17.13 Illustration of feature 5. © 2016 IEEE. Reprinted, with permission, from Zhang et al. (2013)

Area: The area (a) of a tongue is defined as the number of tongue foreground pixels.

Circle area: The circle area (ca) is the area of a circle within the tongue foreground using the smaller half-distance z, where $r = z$ (refer to Fig. 17.14)

$$ca = \pi r^2 \tag{17.11}$$

Circle area ratio: The circle area ratio (car) is the ratio of ca to a:

$$car = \frac{ca}{a} \tag{17.12}$$

Square area: The square area (sa) is the area of a square defined within the tongue foreground using the smaller half distance z (refer to Fig. 17.15)

$$sa = 4z^2 \tag{17.13}$$

Square area ratio: The square area ratio (sar) is the ratio of sa to a:

$$sar = \frac{sa}{a} \tag{17.14}$$

Triangle area: The triangle area (ta) is the area of a triangle defined within the tongue foreground (see Fig. 17.16) The right point of the triangle is $x_{\max}$, the left point is $x_{\min}$, and the bottom is $y_{\max}$.

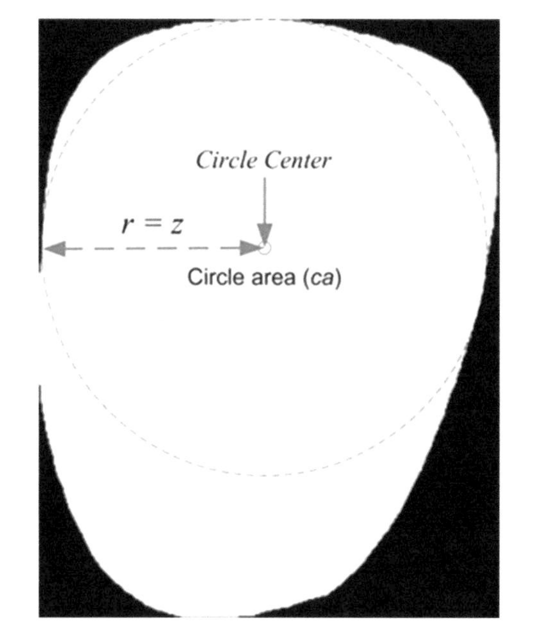

Fig. 17.14 Illustration of feature 8. © 2016 IEEE. Reprinted, with permission, from Zhang et al. (2013)

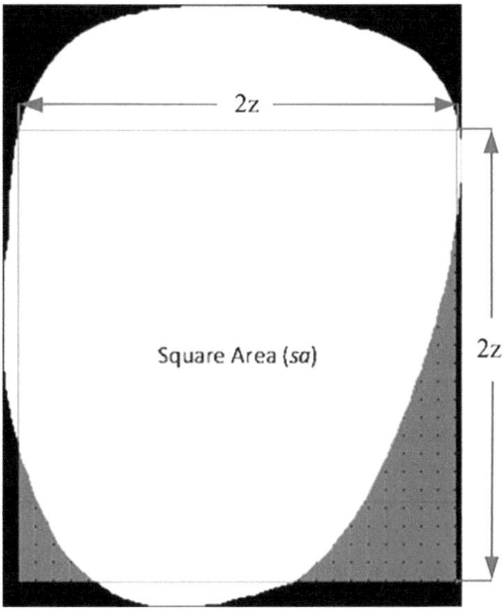

Fig. 17.15 Illustration of feature 10. © 2016 IEEE. Reprinted, with permission, from Zhang et al. (2013)

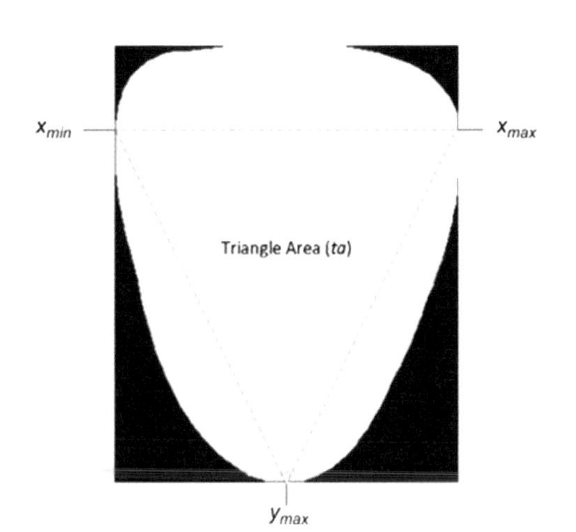

Fig. 17.16 Illustration of feature 12. © 2016 IEEE. Reprinted, with permission, from Zhang et al. (2013)

Triangle area ratio: The triangle area ratio (*tar*) is the ratio of ta to a:

$$tar = \frac{ta}{a} \tag{17.15}$$

The mean geometric features of Healthy, DM, and NPDR are shown in 2. ©2016 IEEE. Reprinted, with permission, from Zhang, Kumar, & Zhang, (2013) along with their standard deviation (Table 17.4).

Table 17.4 The mean (*std*) of the texture features for healthy (std_{Healthy} = 33,013.78), DM (std_{DM} = 33,723.85), and NPDR (std_{NPDR} = 35,673.93)

	Healthy	DM	NPDR
w	320.8077 (36.5289)	335.9189 (42.7073)	344.3103 (39.4788)
l	302.6231 (43.4015)	295.2703 (62.2306)	309.8621 (64.9713)
lw	0.9527 (0.1638)	0.8897 (0.2067)	0.9117 (0.2202)
z	144.5385 (16.6250)	141.1875 (25.1676)	146.069 (23.6574)
cd	−49.6231 (29.2308)	−66.6926 (30.9031)	−64.6552 (34.3067)
cdr	−0.1631 (0.0871)	−0.2249 (0.0900)	−0.2097 (0.1029)
a	76,709.14 (15,525.3172)	76,961.31 (21,599.4127)	83,286.67 (22,629.9217)
ca	66,493.77 (15,079.8031)	64,607.43 (21,983.2771)	68,727.14 (20,900.1437)
car	0.8635 (0.0873)	0.8232 (0.1232)	0.8155 (0.1153)
sa	84,662.52 (19,200.1304)	82,260.71 (27,989.9621)	87,506.07 (26,610.9335)
sar	0.8908 (0.0703)	0.871689 (0.0848)	0.886897 (0.0920)
ta	32,092.11 (7336.0657)	36,077.43 (10,624.3571)	37,959.16 (9973.8946)
tar	0.4212 (0.0631)	0.4722 (0.0745)	0.4624 (0.0807)

17.6 Numerical Results and Discussion

The ensuing section presents the numerical results. Healthy versus DM classification is provided in Sect. 17.6.1. This is followed by NPDR versus DM sans NPDR classification in Sect. 17.6.2.

17.6.1 Healthy Versus DM Classification

The numerical results were obtained on a tongue image database comprised of 426 images divided into 130 Healthy samples, and 296 DM samples (refer to Sect. 17.1). Healthy samples were verified through a blood test and other examinations. If indicators from these tests fell within a certain range, they were deemed healthy. In the DM class, the FPG test was used to diagnose diabetes.

Half of the images were randomly selected for training, while the other half was used for testing. This process was repeated five times. Classification was performed using the k-nearest neighbor (k-NN) (Duta, Hart, & Stork, 2000) (with $k = 1$) and a support vector machine (SVM) (Cortes & Vapnik, 1995), where the kernel function (linear) mapped the training data into kernel space. To measure the performance, average accuracy was employed

$$\text{Average Accuracy} = \frac{\text{sensitivity} + \text{specificity}}{2} \tag{17.16}$$

with the average of all five repetitions recorded as the final classification rate. In the first step, each individual feature (from the three groups) was applied to discriminate Healthy versus DM. This result can be seen in Tables 17.5, 17.6 and 17.7. It should be noted that both k-NN and SVM achieved the same average accuracy for all 34 features. The highest average accuracy of 66.26% from this step was obtained using geometric feature *ta* (refer to Table 17.7) In the next step, optimization by feature selection using sequential forward selection (SFS) was performed. SFS is a feature selection method that begins with an empty set of features. It adds additional features based on maximizing some criterion *j*, and terminates when all features have been added. In our case, *j* is the average accuracy of the classifier (k-NN and SVM). Table 17.8 (k-NN) and Table 17.9 (SVM) illustrate this result applied to each of the three main feature groups. From color features, the best combination is 3 and 12, which obtained an average accuracy of 68.76% using an SVM (see Table 17.9). In texture features, 14, 15, 16, and 17 attained an average accuracy of 67.67%, again using the SVM. With geometric features, 22, 30, 32, 33, and 34 distinguished Healthy versus DM with an average accuracy of 69.09% (in Table 17.9). Combining the features in these three groups by applying SFS, an

Table 17.5 Classification result of k-NN and SVM using each color individually to discriminate healthy versus DM

Feature number	Feature name	Average accuracy (%)
1	*C*	52.17
2	*R*	48.38
3	*B*	55.24
4	*P*	43.90
5	*DR*	60.16
6	*LR*	57.44
7	*LP*	54.30
8	*LB*	51.98
9	*BK*	50.00
10	*GY*	48.55
11	*W*	51.80
12	*Y*	64.78

Table 17.6 Classification result of *k*-NN and SVM using each texture block individually to discriminate healthy versus DM

Feature number	Feature name	Average accuracy (%)
13	Block 1	53.71
14	Block 2	62.66
15	Block 3	61.30
16	Block 4	56.63
17	Block 5	56.50
18	Block 6	48.58
19	Block 7	54.59
20	Block 8	54.17
21	Mean of Blocks 1–8	51.15

Table 17.7 Classification result of *k*-NN and SVM using each geometric feature individually to discriminate healthy versus DM

Feature number	Feature name	Average accuracy (%)
22	W	60.81
23	l	50.25
24	lw	58.44
25	Z	53.33
26	cd	60.29
27	cdr	61.61
28	A	43.76
29	ca	55.02
30	car	59.15
31	sa	55.02
32	sar	54.76
33	ta	66.26
34	tar	64.68

average accuracy of 77.39% was achieved in Table 17.9 using 3, 12, 14, 15, 17, 22, 30, 32, 33, and 34. Finally, by examining the best combination from all features (SFS), the highest average accuracy of 80.52% was accomplished (via SVM), with a sensitivity of 90.77% and a specificity of 70.27%. Receiver operating characteristic (ROC) analysis was also performed on this classification as shown by the red ROC curve in Fig. 17.17. The average accuracy of this result is higher than the optimal combination from the three feature groups (77.39%), and contains fewer features. At the same time, it significantly improves upon the use of all features without feature selection, which obtained an average accuracy of 58.06% (*k*-NN) and 44.68% (SVM). The mean of features, 3, 5, 12, 15, 22, 27, 30, 33, and 34 from the best overall grouping for Healthy and DM, is shown in Table 17.10, while Fig. 17.18 depicts three typical samples from Healthy and DM.

Table 17.8 Optimization of healthy versus DM classification using feature selection with k-NN

Grouping	Feature number	Feature name	Average accuracy (%)
Color	12	*Y*	64.78
Texture	14, 17, 16, 19	Blocks 2, 4, 5, 9	67.48
Geometry	22–30, 32–34	*w-car*, *sar-tar*	67.87
Best of color, texture, and geometry	12, 14, 16, 17, 19, 22–30, 32–34	*Y*, Blocks 2, 4, 5, 9, *w-car*, *sar-tar*	67.87
All features	1–30, 32–34	*C-car*, *sar-tar*	67.87

Table 17.9 Optimization of healthy versus DM classification using feature selection with the SVM

Grouping	Feature number	Feature name	Average accuracy (%)
Color	3,12	*B*, *Y*	68.76
Texture	14–17	Blocks 2–5	67.67
Geometry	22,30 32–34	w, car, *sar-tar*	69.09
Best of color, texture, and geometry	3, 12, 14, 15, 17, 22, 30, 32–34	*B*, *Y*, Blocks 2,3, 5, w, car, *sar-tar*	77.39
All Features	3, 5, 12, 15, 22, 27, 30, 33, 34	*B*, *DR*, *Y*, Block 3, *w*, *cdr*, *car*, *ta*, *tar*	80.52

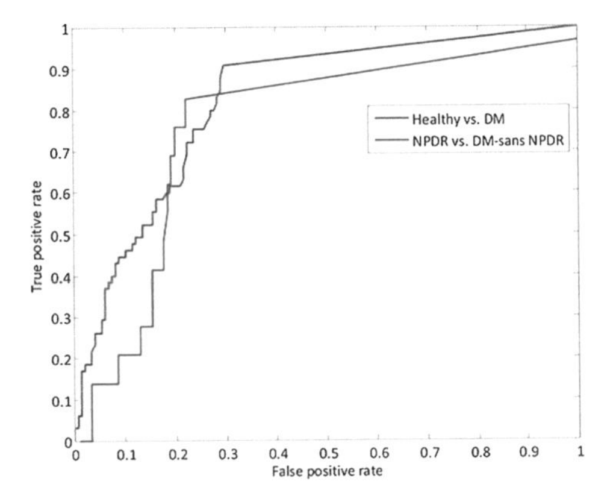

Fig. 17.17 ROC curves for Healthy versus DM (*red*), and NPDR versus DM-sans NPDR (*blue*) © 2016 IEEE. Reprinted, with permission, from Zhang et al. (2013)

Table 17.10 Mean of the optimal tongue features for healthy and DM

	3	5	12	15	22	27	30	33	34
Healthy	29.053	0.000831	1.519	1.613	2.628	−49.108	68,184.26	0.892	32,962.16
DM	29.600	0.000804	1.256	2.168	2.770	−70.392	66,629.30	0.866	37,344.22

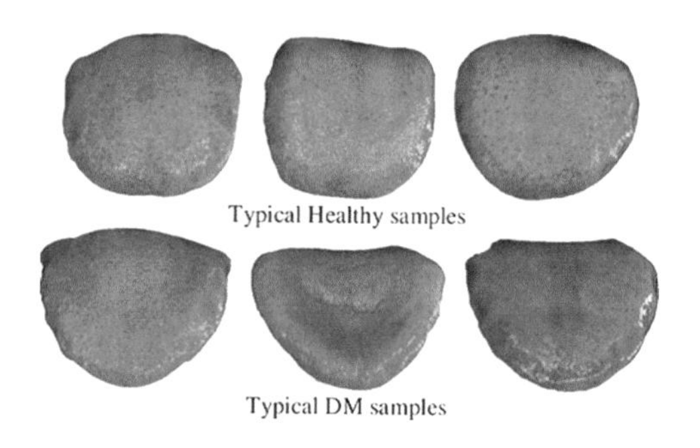

Fig. 17.18 Typical Healthy (*top*) and DM (*bottom*) tongue samples. © 2016 IEEE. Reprinted, with permission, from Zhang et al. (2013)

17.6.2 NPDR Versus DM-Sans NPDR Classification

Of the 296 DM samples, 29 were marked as NPDR (refer to Sect. 17.1). The NPDR samples were verified by medical professionals after examining the retina of patients. Using the same experimental setup as in Sect. 17.6.1, the results of NPDR versus DM-sans NPDR (267 samples) classification are illustrated in Tables 17.9, 17.10, 17.11, 17.12, 17.13 and 17.14. Since it was established in the previous section that the SVM outperforms *k*-NN, only the former classifier was used. The average accuracies of applying each feature individually from the three groups are shown in Tables 17.10, 17.11 which display the optimized result using SFS. As can be seen in the last row of Table 17.12 the best result of 80.33% was achieved with features 7, 10, 11, 14, and 25 (sensitivity of 82.76% and specificity of 77.90% based on its blue ROC curve in Fig. 17.17). This compares to 59.05 and 53.35% average accuracies for *k*-NN and SVM, respectively, using all features without

Table 17.11 Classification result of using each color individually to discriminate NPDR versus DM-SANS NPDR using the SVM

Feature number	Feature name	Average accuracy (%)
1	*C*	54.26
2	*R*	40.09
3	*B*	57.24
4	*P*	50.29
5	*DR*	61.07
6	*LR*	52.98
7	*LP*	45.19
8	*LB*	55.07
9	*BK*	49.44
10	*GY*	70.81
11	*W*	64.14
12	*Y*	53.12

Table 17.12 Classification result of using each texture block individually to discriminate NPDR versus DM-SANS NPDR using the SVM

Feature number	Feature name	Average accuracy (%)
13	Block 1	50.36
14	Block 2	58.22
15	Block 3	55.22
16	Block 4	67.07
17	Block 5	61.45
18	Block 6	52.82
19	Block 7	48.41
20	Block 8	49.15
21	Mean of Blocks 1–8	61.00

Table 17.13 Classification result of using each geometric feature individually to discriminate NPDR versus DM-SANS NPDR using the SVM

Feature number	Feature name	Average accuracy (%)
22	w	30.12
23	l	52.98
24	lw	46.08
25	z	56.43
26	cd	43.91
27	cdr	48.48
28	a	62.57
29	ca	58.30
30	car	46.45
31	sa	58.30
32	sar	58.08
33	ta	32.07
34	tar	45.49

feature selection. The mean of the five optimal features for DM sans NPDR and NPDR can be found in Table 17.13 along with three typical samples (refer to Fig. 17.19) (Table 17.15).

For completeness, the NPDR versus Healthy classification was also conducted. An average accuracy of 87.14% was accomplished using SFS with the SVM, achieving a sensitivity of 89.66% and a specificity of 84.62% via features 3, 9, 15, 16, and 33.

Table 17.14 Optimization of NPDR versus DM-SANS NPDR classification using feature selection with the SVM

Grouping	Feature number	Feature name	Average accuracy (%)
Color	1, 3, 5, 7 −11	*C, B, DR, LP-W*	75.84
Texture	13–17, 21	*Blocks* 1–5, *Mean of Blocks* 1–8	72.09
Geometry	23, 28, 32	*l, a, sar*	65.27
Best of color, texture, and geometry	3, 7, 10, 28	*B, LP, GY, a*	79.21
All features	7, 10, 11, 14, 25	*LP, GY, W, Block 2, z*	80.33

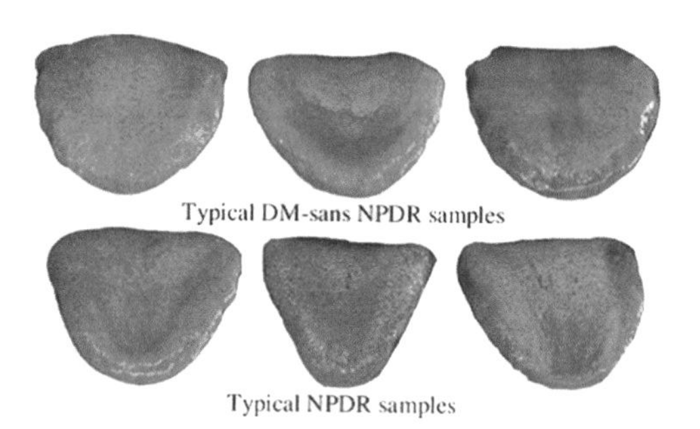

Fig. 17.19 Typical DM-sans NPDR (*top*) and NPDR (*bottom*) tongue samples.

Table 17.15 Mean of the optimal tongue features for DM-SANS NPDR and NPDR

	10	25	7	14	11
DM-sans NPDR	10.2884	140.6573	0.0647	2.1205	1.0025
NPDR	15.5041	146.0690	0.0565	2.3406	1.7322

17.7 Summary

In this chapter, a noninvasive approach to classify Healthy/DM and NPD-R/DM sans NPDR samples using three groups of features extracted from tongue images was proposed. These three groups include color, texture, and geometry. A tongue color gamut was first applied so that each tongue image can be represented by 12 colors. Afterward, eight blocks strategically located on the tongue were extracted and their texture value calculated. Finally, 13 geometric features from tongue images based on measurements, distances, areas, and their ratios were extracted. Numerical experiments were carried out using 130 Healthy and 296 DM tongue images. By individually applying each feature to separate Healthy/DM, the highest average accuracy achieved (via SVM) was only 66.26%. However, employing SFS with the SVM, nine features (with elements from all the three groups) were shown to produce the optimal result, obtaining an average accuracy of 80.52%. For the NPDR/DM-sans NPDR classification, the best result of 80.33% was attained using five features: three from color, one from texture, and one from geometry. This lays the groundwork for a potentially new way to detect DM, while providing a novel means to detect NPDR without retinal imaging or analysis.

References

Abràmoff, M. D., Van Ginneken, B., & Niemeijer, M. (2009). Automatic detection of red lesions in digital color fundus photographs (pp. 584–592). IEEE Trans Med Imaging.

Chiu, C. (1996). The development of a computerized tongue diagnosis system. *Biomedical Engineering Applications Basis Communications, 8,* 342–350.

Cortes, C., & Vapnik, V. (1995). Support-vector networks. *Machine learning, 20*(3), 273–297.

Duta, R., Hart, P., & Stork, D. (2000). *Pattern classification*. New York: Wiley.

Hipwell, J. H., Strachan, F., Olson, J. A., Mchardy, K. C., Sharp, P. F., & Forrester, J. V. (2000). Automated detection of microaneurysms in digital red-free photographs: a diabetic retinopathy screening tool. *Diabetic Medicine, 17*(8), 588–594.

Joes, S., Abràmoff, M. D., Meindert, N., Viergever, M. A., & Bram, V. G. (2004). Ridge-based vessel segmentation in color images of the retina. *IEEE Transactions on Medical Imaging, 23*(4), 501–509.

Martinez-Perez, M., Hughes, A. S., Bharath, A., & Parker, K. (2007). Segmentation of blood vessels from red-free and fluorescein retinal images. *Medical Image Analysis, 11*(1), 47–61.

Meindert, N., Bram, V. G., Cree, M. J., Atsushi, M., Gwénolé, Q., Sanchez, C. I., et al. (2010). Retinopathy online challenge: automatic detection of microaneurysms in digital color fundus photographs. *IEEE Transactions on Medical Imaging, 29*(1), 185–195.

Organization, W. H. (2006). *Prevention of blindness from diabetes mellitus*: World Health Organization.

Pang, B., Zhang, D., & Wang, K. (2005a). Tongue image analysis for appendicitis diagnosis. *Information Sciences, 175*(3), 160–176.

Pang, B., Zhang, D., & Wang, K. (2005b). The bi-elliptical deformable contour and its application to automated tongue segmentation in Chinese medicine. *IEEE Transactions on Medical Imaging, 24*(8), 946–956.

Spencer, T., Olson, J. A., Mchardy, K. C., Sharp, P. F., & Forrester, J. V. (1996). An image-processing strategy for the segmentation and quantification of microaneurysms in fluorescein angiograms of the ocular fundus. *Computers and Biomedical Research, 29*(4), 284–302.

Wang, X., & Zhang, D. (2010). An optimized tongue image color correction scheme. *IEEE Transactions on Information Technology in Biomedicine, 14*(6), 1355–1364.

Wang, X., & Zhang, D. (2011). Statistical tongue color distribution and its application. *Health, 2856,* 2566.

Zhang, H., Wang, K., Jin, X., & Zhang, D. (2005). SVR based color calibration for tongue image (pp. 5065–5070). IEEE.

Zhang, B., Zhang, L., Zhang, L., & Karray, F. (2010). Retinal vessel extraction by matched filter with first-order derivative of Gaussian. *Computers in Biology and Medicine, 40*(4), 438–445.

Zhang, B., Karray, F., Li, Q., & Zhang, L. (2012a). Sparse representation classifier for microaneurysm detection and retinal blood vessel extraction. *Information Sciences, 200*(1), 78–90.

Zhang, B., Karray, F., Li, Q., & Zhang, L. (2012b). Sparse representation classifier for microaneurysm detection and retinal blood vessel extraction. *Information Sciences, 200*(1), 78–90.

Zhang, B., Kumar, B. V., & Zhang, D. (2013). Detecting diabetes mellitus and nonproliferative diabetic retinopathy using tongue color, texture, and geometry features. *IEEE transactions on bio-medical engineering, 61*(2), 491–501.

Part V
Book Recapitulation

Chapter 18
Book Review and Future Work

Abstract In this book, four types of tongue image analysis technologies were elaborated by including the most current research findings in all aspects of tongue image acquisition, preprocessing, classification, and diagnostic support methodologies. In this chapter, we summarized these technologies from a systemic point of view and presented our thoughts on future work in the CDT research field.

18.1 Book Recapitulation

With the development of digital image processing and pattern classification technology, computer-aided tongue image analysis for medical application has been found to be an effective way to address the intrinsic problems of traditional tongue diagnosis, namely, ambiguity, subjectivity, and inconsistence, which are mainly derived from the practitioner's subjective observation and experience-based analysis. In this regard, this book introduced several essential aspects of tongue image processing and analysis technology, in a bottom-up manner, including tongue imaging hardware and system, tongue image segmentation, color correction, diagnostic classification, etc. These works are supposed to fill the blank in the research community and to promote the development of a computerized tongue diagnosis system. From the perspective of both academic research and engineering, the main contributions of this book are as follows:

A high quality and consistent tongue imaging scheme: We introduced a novel tongue imaging scheme to faithfully and precisely record tongue information for medical analysis. Based on thorough and fundamental research of the development of tongue imaging, a system was developed for medical analysis to fulfill the requirements of accurately and consistently recording each type of tongue image feature. A series of criteria were presented to guide the development of each module in the system. This is the first proposed design guideline in the research community, and it also can be regarded as a design standard in this area because most of the proposed criteria are based on international standards of color imaging technology.

D. Zhang et al., *Tongue Image Analysis*, DOI 10.1007/978-981-10-2167-1_18

A comprehensive discussion about tongue image segmentation: Due to the large diversity of the human tongue body, it is practically impossible to develop a segmentation algorithm that fits all situations. Consequently, we carried out a series of methodical, comprehensive discussions on tongue image segmentation tasks. In this book, a variety of segmentation algorithms were considered including deformable contour, gradient vector flow, and region- and edge-based methods. From an engineering point of view, popular image segmentation approaches, although partially overlapping each other, were systematically elaborated and experimentally appraised based on tongue images captured under visible and hyperspectral light. Some of the segmentation methods in this book are also beneficial to readers to upgrade their skills for future studies of the image processing field.

An optimized tongue color correction method: In this book, we elaborated the particular color correction requirement for selection of a device-independent target color space in tongue image analysis, and developed corresponding color correction algorithms which are able to reduce the color difference between images captured using different cameras or under different lighting conditions. During the research, a novel designed color checker dedicated to tongue color correction was developed to ensure a promising performance. The aforementioned method is more than an application specific one in CTD and, in a more general sense, can be smoothly extended to solve other color correction problems in the photographic field.

Computing models for tongue image classification and diagnosis: To establish the relationships between diagnostic signs in tongue appearance and the corresponding diseases, rather than syndromes, in terms of quantitative features, is the very idea mainly expressed throughout this book. This means we can take advantage of quantitative feature extraction and pattern classification techniques, and where possible prevent the validity and accuracy of tongue diagnosis from degradation caused by subjective and nonquantitative factors. For this purpose, this book elaborated how the new technologies, e.g., Bayesian networks, support vector machines, and other algorithms from biometrics help to reinforce the objective basis of tongue diagnosis. Such approaches give us hints for early diagnosis of some specific diseases, and further expedite their use in clinical applications.

18.2 Future Work

In order to solve the most essential problem in current research of a computerized tongue diagnosis system, this book mainly focused on color imaging and analyzing technology to ensure high quality color rendering and objective color feature extraction. Though some progress has been made, there are still some limitations which cannot be overcome in this book due to various reasons, but they are expected to be improved in our future studies. Instead of a detailed blueprint, here we discuss some forthcoming changes in terms of the aforementioned techniques in this book.

Tongue image acquisition: The main objective design of this tongue imaging device is to achieve high quality and consistent tongue image acquisition. Theoretically, the elements in a device that has been optimally designed and implemented, following these design criteria should produce similar high quality results. However, as far as the size is concerned, there is great room for continued improvement for all kinds of existing tongue image acquisition devices. New wearable technologies and products in recent years, e.g., Google glasses and Oculus, inspire us to develop the next generation of tongue imaging devices which should be more compact, more comfortable, more economical, and more powerful.

Algorithm performance: For tongue image segmentation, it was noted in this book that the segmentation may have an unsatisfactory performance when the tongue edge is very weak or the images include strong interference from teeth or lip features. Such difficulties need to be overcome in our future work. In the case of color correction, we evaluated the difference between two color images (before and after color correction) by calculating the color difference of their mean color. Although this evaluation method works well in this book, it still needs to be further investigated on several tasks, such as why the mean color works well? Is there a better method to calculate the color difference between images? How to design an evaluation algorithm which can fit subjective evaluation by human inspection? Can the correction perform intelligently without a color checker? All these topics are worth for our further study.

Modeling methods: To provide more accurate diagnosis, the tongue image database, from a statistical point of view, still needs to be enlarged to cover as many kinds of tongue images as possible. In the foreseeable future, computed tongue diagnosis will step on the stage of big data. The value of the application of big data techniques in analyzing and modeling such a large collection of tongue images attracts a great deal of attention from practitioners of both medical and artificial intelligence fields, which, in turn, makes computerized tongue diagnosis challenging and charming research!

Index

D. Zhang et al., *Tongue Image Analysis*, DOI 10.1007/978-981-10-2167-1

Printed in the United States
By Bookmasters